CANCER MORTALITY AND MORBIDITY STATISTICS

Gann Monograph on Cancer Research

The "Gann Monograph on Cancer Research" series is promoted by the Japanese Cancer Association. This semiannual series of monographs was initiated in 1966 by the late Dr. Tomizo Yoshida (1903–1973) and is now published jointly by Japan Scientific Societies Press, Tokyo and S. Karger AG, Basel. Each volume consists of collected contributions on current topics in cancer problems and allied research fields. The planning for each volume is done by the Monograph Committee of the Japanese Cancer Association, with the final approval of the Board of Directors. It is hoped that the series will serve as an important source of information in the field of cancer research.

The publication of these monographs owed much to the financial support given by the late Professor Kazushige Higuchi, the Jikei University School of Medicine.

Japanese Cancer Association

JAPANESE CANCER ASSOCIATION

Gann Monograph on Cancer Research No. 51

CANCER MORTALITY AND MORBIDITY STATISTICS

JAPAN AND THE WORLD-2004

Edited by
KAZUO TAJIMA, TETSUO KUROISHI and AKIRA OSHIMA

JAPAN SCIENTIFIC SOCIETIES PRESS
Tokyo

KARGER
Basel·Freiburg·Paris·London·New York·Bangalore
Bangkok·Singapore·Tokyo·Sydney

March 2004

Published jointly by
JAPAN SCIENTIFIC SOCIETIES PRESS
2-10 Hongo, 6-chome, Bunkyo-ku, Tokyo 113-0033, Japan
ISBN 4-7622-3026-X

and

S. KARGER AG
P.O. Box, CH-4009 Basel, Switzerland
ISBN 3-8055-7747-8

Sole distribution rights outside Japan granted to S. KARGER AG, Basel.

PREFACE

A recent estimate from the World Health Organization (WHO) indicated that there were more than 10 million new cancer cases in the world and more than 6 million people died of this disease. Cancer is one of the major targets of health control programs in most developed countries. In developing countries the number of cancer deaths has actually increased in compensation for successful control programs of infectious and other chronic diseases. In Japan cancer became the leading cause of death in 1981 and has continued to increase up to the present day.

Dr. Mitsuo Segi and his colleagues first published "Cancer Mortality and Morbidity Statistics: Japan and the World" (Gann Monograph on Cancer Research No. 26) in 1981. Ten years later Dr. Suketami Tominaga and his colleagues published volumes 41 and 47 of cancer statistics as of 1993 and 1999, respectively. Five years have passed since publication of the last monograph and in this volume we have updated the cancer mortality and morbidity statistics in Japan and also the cancer mortality statistics throughout the world. The 10th revision of the International Classification of Diseases (ICD) was adopted in 2000 and the trends in mortality rates of the main sites of cancer have been recalculated accordingly. We added a new chapter on "Estimation of Survival of Cancer Patients in Japan" in this volume.

Cancer statistics provide a valuable resource for persons who wish to know what is going on with respect to cancer epidemiologic research and the planning of a practical control program for cancer. Analyses of these statistics often provide etiological clues and suggest countermeasures to prevent the disease. This makes the recording of information on cancer mortality and morbidity by epidemiologists and public health workers valuable, and for clinicians and researchers it may provide clues to biological derivation and impact.

The editors hope that this latest publication of the monograph will make a substantial contribution to medical researchers and health professionals involved disease control programs in Japan and the rest of the world. The editors wish to acknowledge the support and assistance of the Statistics and Information Department of the Minister's secretariat of the Ministry of Health, Welfare and Labor of Japan, and the Dissemination Information Office of the WHO.

March 2004 Kazuo TAJIMA

CONTENTS

CANCER MORTALITY IN JAPAN (1950–2000)

Tetsuo KUROISHI,[*1,*2] Kaoru HIROSE,[*1] Toshiro TAKEZAKI,[*3]
Suketami TOMINAGA,[*4] and Kazuo TAJIMA[*1]

Division of Epidemiology and Cancer Prevention, Aichi Cancer Center Research Institute,[*1]
Nagoya Preventive Medical Institute,[*2] *School of Medicine, Kagoshima University,*[*3]
Foundation of Aichi Health Promotion[*4]

Cancer mortality statistics in Japan (1950–2000) were calculated from the "*Vital Statistics, Japan*" series published annually by the Statistics and Information Department, Minister's Secretariat, Ministry of Health, Labour and Welfare and from data edited from magnetic tape copies of "*Vital Statistics*" with the official permission of the Ministry of Management and Coordination.

This report includes the following cancer mortality statistics in Japan:

1) The number of deaths from malignant neoplasms by site, its proportion of all malignant neoplasms and the death rates in Japan (2000).

2) The number of deaths, the death rates and the average age at death from malignant neoplasms by site in Japan (1950–2000).

3) Age- and sex-specific mortality rates by site in Japan (1950, 1955, 1960, 1965, 1970, 1975, 1980, 1985, 1990, 1995, and 2000).

4) Standardized mortality ratio (SMR) of cancer by site in Japan by prefecture (2000).

This report was prepared to update data on "Cancer mortality in Japan (1950–1995)" last published in 1999 in "*Cancer Mortality and Morbidity Statistics—Japan and the World—1999,*" GANN Monograph on Cancer Research No. 47 (*2*).

Cancer mortality statistics for 1950–2000 were taken from the "*Vital Statistics, Japan*" series (*3*) which is published annually by the Statistics and Information Department, Minister's Secretariat, Ministry of Health, Labour and Welfare. Mortality statistics for 2000 by prefecture were based on fundamental data edited from magnetic tape copies of "*Vital Statistics*" provided by the Ministry of Health, Labour and Welfare after obtaining official permission from the Ministry of Management and Coordination.

The Statistics and Information Department, Minister's Secretariat, Ministry of Health, Labour and Welfare of Japan recommended use of the 'model' population for the year 1985 in Japan (Table A) as a standard population for calculation of age-adjusted death rates (*1*), and this 1985 'model' population was employed for the age-adjusted death rates by site for 1950–2000.

[*1] 1-1 Kanokoden, Chikusa-ku, Nagoya 464-8681, Japan
[*2] 4-23 Nagaosa-cho, Nakamura-ku, Nagoya 453-8521, Japan
[*3] 8-35-1 Sakuragaoka, Kagoshima 890-8521, Japan
[*4] 1-1 Gengoyama, Morioka, Higashiura-cho, Aichi, 470-2101, Japan

TABLE A. Standard Population

Age group in years	'Model' population for 1985 in Japan in thousands
0–4	8,180
5–9	8,338
10–14	8,497
15–19	8,655
20–24	8,814
25–29	8,972
30–34	9,130
35–39	9,289
40–44	9,400
45–49	8,651
50–54	7,616
55–59	6,581
60–64	5,546
65–69	4,511
70–74	3,476
75–79	2,441
80–84	1,406
85 and over	784
Total	120,287

Number of Deaths from Malignant Neoplasms by Site, Its Proportion of All Malignant Neoplasms and the Death Rates in Japan (2000)

The number of deaths from malignant neoplasms by sex and site and the proportion of all malignant neoplasms in Japan for 2000 are shown in Table I-1. The 10th revision of the International Classification of Diseases (ICD) was adopted in since 1995. There were 179,140 male cancer deaths and 116,344 female cancer deaths in Japan for 2000, accounting for 34.1% and 26.7% of all deaths, respectively. Major cancers which rank top to tenth in proportion among all malignant neoplasms for both sexes are shown in Fig. 1.

The crude and age-adjusted death rates per 100,000 populations from malignant neoplasms by sex and site in Japan for 2000 are shown in Table I-2. The age-adjusted death rates in Table I-2 are standardized on the age distribution of the 'model' population for the year 1985 in Japan.

Number of Deaths, Death Rates and Average Age at Death from Malignant Neoplasms by Site in Japan (1950–2000)

The number of deaths, the crude and age-adjusted death rates and the average age at death from malignant neoplasms by site in Japan for 1950–2000 are given in Tables II-1 to II-21. The age-adjusted death rates are standardized on the age distribution of the 'model' population for the year 1985 in Japan. Trends in this rate and the average age at death for cancer of major sites are illustrated in Figs. 2-1 and 2-2, respectively.

The contents of Tables II-1 to II-21 are as follows:

	Site of cancer	ICD			
		7th revision	8th revision	9th revision	10th revision
TABLE II-1	All sites	140–205	140–209	140–208	C00–C97
TABLE II-2	Buccal cavity and pharynx	140–148	140–149	140–149	C00–C14
TABLE II-3	Esophagus	150	150	150	C15
TABLE II-4	Stomach	151	151	151	C16
TABLE II-5	Colon	153	153	153	C18
TABLE II-6	Rectum	154	154	154	C19–C21
TABLE II-7	Liver	155.0, 156	155, 197.7, 197.8	155	C22
TABLE II-8	Biliary passages	155.1	156	156	C23, C24
TABLE II-9	Pancreas	157	157	157	C25
TABLE II-10	Larynx	161	161	161	C32
TABLE II-11	Trachea, bronchus, and lung	162, 163	162	162	C33, C34
TABLE II-12	Bone	196	170	170	C40, C41
TABLE II-13	Skin	190, 191	172,173	172,173	C43, C44
TABLE II-14	Breast	170	174	174	C50
TABLE II-15	Uterus	171–174	180–182	179–182	C53–C55, C58
TABLE II-16	Ovary	175a	183.0	183.0	C56
TABLE II-17	Prostate	177	185	185	C61
TABLE II-18	Urinary Bladder	181a	188	188	C67
TABLE II-19	Kidney	180	189.0, 189.1	189.0, 189.1	C64, C65
TABLE II-20	Lymphatic tissue	200–205	200–203, 208, 209	200–203	C81–C90, C96
TABLE II-21	Leukemia	204	204–207	204–208	C91–C95

ICD: International Classification of Diseases.

Age- and Sex-specific Mortality Rates by Site in Japan (Each 5 Years from 1950–2000)

The age- and sex-specific mortality rates by site in Japan for 1950, 1955, 1960, 1965, 1970, 1975, 1980, 1985, 1990, 1995, and 2000 are given in Tables III-1 to III-21, and illustrated by age group (1950–2000) (A) and by year (1950, 1960, 1970, 1980, 1990, and 2000) (B) in Figs. 3-1 to 3-21. The contents of these tables and figures are as follows:

		Site of cancer	ICD (10th revision)
TABLE III-1	FIG. 3-1	All sites	C00–C97
TABLE III-2	FIG. 3-2	Buccal cavity and pharynx	C00–C14
TABLE III-3	FIG. 3-3	Esophagus	C15
TABLE III-4	FIG. 3-4	Stomach	C16
TABLE III-5	FIG. 3-5	Colon	C18
TABLE III-6	FIG. 3-6	Rectum	C19–C21
TABLE III-7	FIG. 3-7	Liver	C22
TABLE III-8	FIG. 3-8	Biliary passages	C23, C24
TABLE III-9	FIG. 3-9	Pancreas	C25
TABLE III-10	FIG. 3-10	Larynx	C32
TABLE III-11	FIG. 3-11	Trachea, bronchus, and lung	C33, C34
TABLE III-12	FIG. 3-12	Bone	C40, C41
TABLE III-13	FIG. 3-13	Skin	C43, C44
TABLE III-14	FIG. 3-14	Breast	C50
TABLE III-15	FIG. 3-15	Uterus	C53–C55, C58
TABLE III-16	FIG. 3-16	Ovary	C56
TABLE III-17	FIG. 3-17	Prostate	C61
TABLE III-18	FIG. 3-18	Urinary Bladder	C67
TABLE III-19	FIG. 3-19	Kidney	C64, C65
TABLE III-20	FIG. 3-20	Lymphatic tissue	C81–C90, C96
TABLE III-21	FIG. 3-21	Leukemia	C91–C95

Standardized Mortality Ratio (SMR) of Cancer by Site by Prefecture (2000)

The SMR of cancer by site in Japan for 2000 was calculated for each prefecture. Locations of each prefecture are shown in Fig. A. Maps of distribution of SMR are shown in Figs. 4-1 to 4-11. SMRs of cancer by prefecture are omitted. The contents of figures are as follows:

		Site of cancer	ICD (10th revision)
TABLE IV-1	FIG. 4-1	A All sites B Buccal cavity and pharynx	C00–C97 C00–C14
TABLE IV-2	FIG. 4-2	A Esophagus B Stomach	C15 C16
TABLE IV-3	FIG. 4-3	A Colon B Rectum	C18 C19–C21
TABLE IV-4	FIG. 4-4	A Liver B Biliary passages	C22 C23, C24
TABLE IV-5	FIG. 4-5	A Pancreas B Larynx	C25 C32
TABLE IV-6	FIG. 4-6	A Trachea, bronchus, and lung B Bone	C33, C34 C40, C41
TABLE IV-7	FIG. 4-7	A Skin B Breast	C43, C44 C50
TABLE IV-8	FIG. 4-8	A Uterus B Ovary	C53–C55, C58 C56
TABLE IV-9	FIG. 4-9	A Prostate B Urinary Bladder	C61 C67
TABLE IV-10	FIG. 4-10	A Kidney B Lymphatic tissue	C64, C65 C81–C90, C96
TABLE IV-11	FIG. 4-11	A Leukemia	C91–C95

Acknowledgments

We would like to thank the Statistics and Information Department, Ministry of Health, Labour and Welfare of Japan for providing us magnetic tape copies of "*Vital Statistics*" with the official permission of the Ministry of Management and Coordination.

REFERENCES

1. Abe, Y., Onodera, M., Kamiya, K., Saito, F., and Matsue, T. On the revision of the age-adjusted death rate. *Kousei no Shihyo*, **38**(5), 12–16 (1991) (in Japanese).
2. Kuroishi, T., Hirose, K., Tajima, K., and Tominaga, S. (1950–1995). GANN Monograph on Cancer Research No.47, Japan Scientific Societies Press, Tokyo, 1999.
3. Statistics and Information Department, Minister's Secretariat, Ministry of Health, Labour and Welfare. *In* "Vital Statistics 1950–2000 Japan" (1952–2002). Kousei Tokei Kyokai, Tokyo (in Japanese).

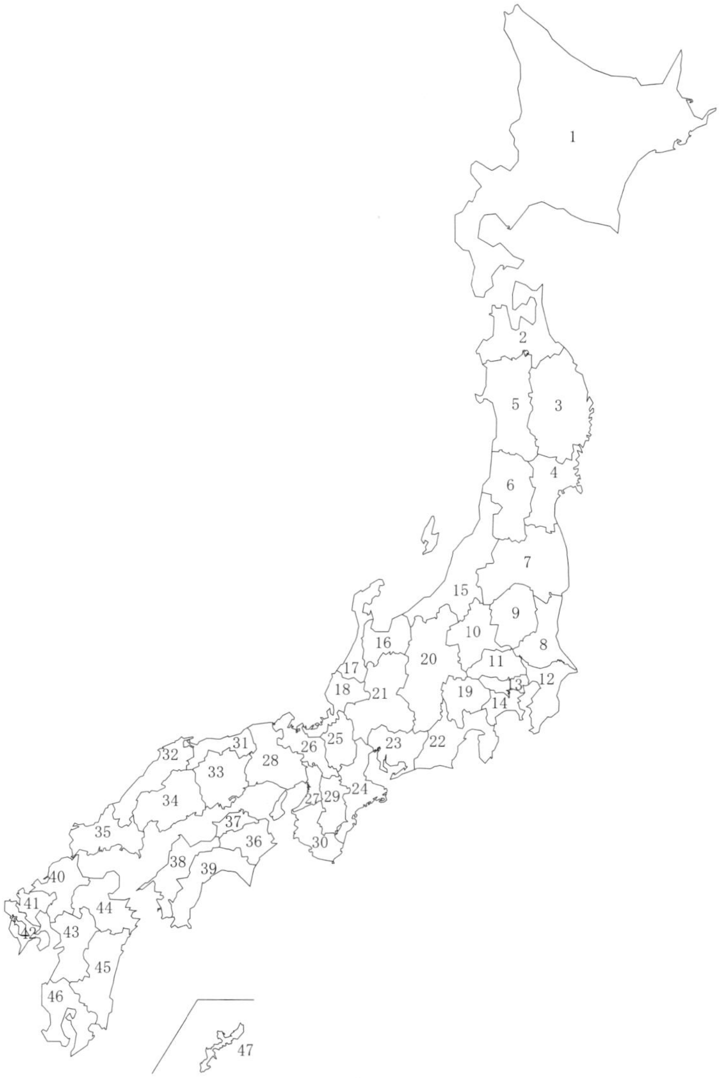

1 Hokkaido
2 Aomori
3 Iwate
4 Miyagi
5 Akita
6 Yamagata
7 Fukushima
8 Ibaraki
9 Tochigi
10 Gunma
11 Saitama
12 Chiba
13 Tokyo
14 Kanagawa
15 Niigata
16 Toyama
17 Ishikawa
18 Fukui
19 Yamanashi
20 Nagano
21 Gifu
22 Shizuoka
23 Aichi
24 Mie
25 Shiga
26 Kyoto
27 Osaka
28 Hyogo
29 Nara
30 Wakayama
31 Tottori
32 Shimane
33 Okayama
34 Hiroshima
35 Yamaguchi
36 Tokushima
37 Kagawa
38 Ehime
39 Kochi
40 Fukuoka
41 Saga
42 Nagasaki
43 Kumamoto
44 Oita
45 Miyazaki
46 Kagoshima
47 Okinawa

FIG. A. Map of 47 prefectures in Japan.

TABLE I-1. Number of Deaths from Malignant Neoplasms by Site and

ICD (10th revision)	Site of malignant neoplasm	Male		Female	
		No.	%	No.	%
C00–C97	All sites	179,140	100.0	116,344	100.0
C00–C14	Lip, oral cavity and pharynx	3,610	2.0	1,456	1.3
C00	Lip	14	0.0	14	0.0
C01	Base of tongue	20	0.0	3	0.0
C02	Other and unspecified parts of tongue	681	0.4	444	0.4
C03	Gum	472	0.3	366	0.3
C04	Floor of mouth	164	0.1	49	0.0
C05	Palate	31	0.0	28	0.0
C06	Other and unspecified parts of mouth	144	0.1	124	0.1
C07	Parotid gland	186	0.1	83	0.1
C08	Other and unspecified major salivary glands	71	0.0	45	0.0
C09	Tonsil	22	0.0	5	0.0
C10	Oropharynx	442	0.2	64	0.1
C11	Nasopharynx	259	0.1	73	0.1
C12	Pyriform sinus	0	0.0	0	0.0
C13	Hypopharynx	830	0.5	110	0.1
C14	Other and ill-defined sites in the lip, oral cavity and pharynx	274	0.2	48	0.0
C15–C26	Digestive organs	103,502	57.8	63,622	54.7
C15	Esophagus	8,706	4.9	1,550	1.3
C16	Stomach	32,798	18.3	17,852	15.3
C17	Small intestine	528	0.3	363	0.3
C18–C21	Large intestine	20,002	11.2	16,201	13.9
C18	Colon	12,139	6.8	11,498	9.9
C19–C21	Rectum, rectosigmoid junction, and anus	7,863	4.4	4,703	4.0
C19	Rectosigmoid junction	197	0.1	88	0.1
C20	Rectum	7,532	4.2	4,494	3.9
C21	Anus and anal canal	134	0.1	121	0.1
C22	Liver and intrahepatic bile ducts	23,602	13.2	10,379	8.9
C23, C24	Gallbladder and extrahepatic bile ducts	6,913	3.9	8,240	7.1
C23	Gallbladder	2,295	1.3	4,155	3.6
C24	Other and unspecified parts of biliary tract	4,618	2.6	4,085	3.5
C25	Pancreas	10,380	5.8	8,714	7.5
C26	Other and ill-defined digestive organs	573	0.3	323	0.3
C30–C39	Respiratory and intrathoracic organs	40,568	22.6	15,049	12.9
C30	Nasal cavity and middle ear	72	0.0	56	0.0
C31	Accessory sinuses	178	0.1	101	0.1
C32	Larynx	958	0.5	88	0.1
C33–C34	Trachea, bronchus, and lung	39,053	21.8	14,671	12.6
C33	Trachea	13	0.0	9	0.0
C34	Bronchus and lung	39,040	21.8	14,662	12.6
C37	Thymus	173	0.1	81	0.1
C38	Heart, mediastinum and pleura	129	0.1	49	0.0
C39	Other and ill-defined sites in the respiratory system and intrathoracic organs	5	0.0	3	0.0
C40, C41	Bone and articular cartilage	218	0.1	159	0.1
C40	Bone and articular cartilage of limbs	56	0.0	46	0.0
C41	Bone and articular cartilage of other and unspecified sites	162	0.1	113	0.1
C43, C44	Skin	502	0.3	484	0.4
C43	Malignant melanoma of skin	244	0.1	204	0.2
C44	Other malignant neoplasms of skin	258	0.1	280	0.2
C45–C49	Mesothelial and soft tissue	1,209	0.7	728	0.6
C45	Mesothelioma	537	0.3	173	0.1
C46	Kaposi's sarcoma	0	0.0	0	0.0
C47	Peripheral nerves and autonomic nervous system	41	0.0	33	0.0
C48	Retroperitoneum and peritoneum	145	0.1	199	0.2
C49	Other connective and soft tissue	486	0.3	323	0.3
C50	Breast	77	0.0	9,171	7.9

ICD: International Classification of Diseases.

Its Proportion of All Malignant Neoplasms in Japan (2000)

ICD (10th revision)	Site of malignant neoplasm	Male		Female	
		No.	%	No.	%
C51–C58	Female genital organs			9,608	8.3
C51	Vulva			175	0.2
C52	Vagina			105	0.1
C53–C55, C58	Uterus			5,216	4.5
C53	Cervix uteri			2,393	2.1
C54	Corpus uteri			1,139	1.0
C55	Uterus, part unspecified			1,670	1.4
C56	Ovary			3,993	3.4
C57	Other and unspecified female genital organs			119	0.1
C58	Placenta			14	0.0
C60–C63	Male genital organs	7,743	4.3		
C60	Penis	103	0.1		
C61	Prostate	7,514	4.2		
C62	Testis	113	0.1		
C63	Other and unspecified male genital organs	13	0.0		
C64–C68	Urinary tract	6,266	3.5	3,142	2.7
C64, C65	Kidney	2,583	1.4	1,280	1.1
C64	Kidney, except renal pelvis	2,134	1.2	1,028	0.9
C65	Renal pelvis	449	0.3	252	0.2
C66	Ureter	397	0.2	298	0.3
C67	Bladder	3,184	1.8	1,496	1.3
C68	Other and unspecified urinary organs	102	0.1	68	0.1
C69–C72	Eye, brain and other parts of central nervous system	883	0.5	713	0.6
C69	Eye and adnexa	26	0.0	14	0.0
C70	Meninges	20	0.0	26	0.0
C71	Brain	823	0.5	659	0.6
C72	Spinal cord, cranial nerves and other parts of central nervous system	14	0.0	14	0.0
C73–C75	Thyroid and other endocrine glands	562	0.3	977	0.8
C73	Thyroid gland	411	0.2	887	0.8
C74	Adrenal gland	133	0.1	83	0.1
C75	Other endocrine glands and related structures	18	0.0	7	0.0
C76–C80	Ill-defined, secondary and unspecified sites	3,295	1.8	3,245	2.8
C76	Other and ill-defined sites	202	0.1	224	0.2
C77	Lymph nodes specified as secondary and unspecified	40	0.0	22	0.0
C78	Respiratory and digestive systems specified as secondary	1,274	0.7	1,451	1.2
C79	Other sites, secondary as specified	381	0.2	262	0.2
C80	Without specification of site	1,398	0.8	1,286	1.1
C81–C96	Lymphoid, hematopoietic and related tissue	10,322	5.8	7,787	6.7
C81–C90, C96	Lymphatic and hematopoietic systems	6,352	3.5	4,991	4.3
C81	Hodgkin's disease	76	0.0	51	0.0
C82	Follicular [nodular] non-Hodgkin's lymphoma	3	0.0	8	0.0
C83	Diffuse non-Hodgkin's lymphoma	71	0.0	47	0.0
C84	Peripheral and cutaneous T-cell lymphomas	54	0.0	37	0.0
C85	Other and unspecified types of non-Hodgkin's lymphoma	4,374	2.4	3,197	2.7
C88	Malignant immunoproliferative diseases	63	0.0	20	0.0
C90	Multiple myeloma and malignant plasma cell neoplasms	1,673	0.9	1,605	1.4
C91–C95	Leukemia	3,970	2.2	2,796	2.4
C91	Lymphoid leukemia	1,030	0.6	908	0.8
C92	Myeloid leukemia	2,485	1.4	1,552	1.3
C93	Monocytic leukemia	32	0.0	21	0.0
C94	Other leukemias of specified cell type	25	0.0	7	0.0
C95	Leukemia of unspecified cell type	398	0.2	308	0.3
C96	Other and unspecified malignant neoplasms of lymphoid, hematopoietic and related tissue	38	0.0	26	0.0
C97	Independent (primary) multiple sites	383	0.2	203	0.2

TABLE I-2. Death Rates from Malignant Neoplasms

ICD (10th revision)	Site of malignant neoplasm	Male		Female	
		CDR	ADR	CDR	ADR
C00–C97	All sites	291.3	214.0	181.4	103.5
C00–C14	Lip, oral cavity and pharynx	5.9	4.4	2.3	1.3
C00	Lip	0.0	0.0	0.0	0.0
C01	Base of tongue	0.0	0.0	0.0	0.0
C02	Other and unspecified parts of tongue	1.1	0.9	0.7	0.4
C03	Gum	0.8	0.6	0.6	0.3
C04	Floor of mouth	0.3	0.2	0.1	0.0
C05	Palate	0.1	0.0	0.0	0.0
C06	Other and unspecified parts of mouth	0.2	0.2	0.2	0.1
C07	Parotid gland	0.3	0.2	0.1	0.1
C08	Other and unspecified major salivary glands	0.1	0.1	0.1	0.0
C09	Tonsil	0.0	0.0	0.0	0.0
C10	Oropharynx	0.7	0.5	0.1	0.1
C11	Nasopharynx	0.4	0.3	0.1	0.1
C12	Pyriform sinus	0.0	0.0	0.0	0.0
C13	Hypopharynx	1.3	1.0	0.2	0.1
C14	Other and ill-defined sites in the lip, oral cavity and pharynx	0.4	0.3	0.1	0.0
C15–C26	Digestive organs	168.3	123.4	99.2	53.8
C15	Esophagus	14.2	10.4	2.4	1.3
C16	Stomach	53.3	39.1	27.8	15.3
C17	Small intestine	0.9	0.6	0.6	0.3
C18–C21	Large intestine	32.5	23.9	25.3	13.7
C18	Colon	19.7	14.4	17.9	9.5
C19–C21	Rectum, rectosigmoid junction, and anus	12.8	9.5	7.3	4.2
C19	Rectosigmoid junction	0.3	0.2	0.1	0.1
C20	Rectum	12.2	9.1	7.0	4.0
C21	Anus and anal canal	0.2	0.2	0.2	0.1
C22	Liver and intrahepatic bile ducts	38.4	28.2	16.2	8.8
C23, C24	Gallbladder and extrahepatic bile ducts	11.2	8.2	12.8	6.8
C23	Gallbladder	3.7	2.7	6.5	3.8
C24	Other and unspecified parts of biliary tract	7.5	5.5	6.4	3.1
C25	Pancreas	16.9	12.4	13.6	7.2
C26	Other and ill-defined digestive organs	0.9	0.7	0.5	0.2
C30–C39	Respiratory and intrathoracic organs	66.0	48.2	23.5	12.7
C30	Nasal cavity and middle ear	0.1	0.1	0.1	0.1
C31	Accessory sinuses	0.3	0.2	0.2	0.1
C32	Larynx	1.6	1.1	0.1	0.1
C33, C34	Trachea, bronchus, and lung	63.5	46.3	22.9	12.3
C33	Trachea	0.0	0.0	0.0	0.0
C34	Bronchus and lung	63.5	46.3	22.9	12.3
C37	Thymus	0.3	0.2	0.1	0.1
C38	Heart, mediastinum and pleura	0.2	0.2	0.1	0.1
C39	Other and ill-defined sites in the respiratory system and intrathoracic organs	0.0	0.0	0.0	0.0
C40, C41	Bone and articular cartilage	0.4	0.3	0.2	0.2
C40	Bone and articular cartilage of limbs	0.1	0.1	0.1	0.1
C41	Bone and articular cartilage of other and unspecified sites	0.3	0.2	0.2	0.1
C43, C44	Skin	0.8	0.6	0.8	0.4
C43	Malignant melanoma of skin	0.4	0.3	0.3	0.2
C44	Other malignant neoplasms of skin	0.4	0.3	0.4	0.2
C45–C49	Mesothelial and soft tissue	2.0	1.5	1.1	0.8
C45	Mesothelioma	0.9	0.6	0.3	0.2
C46	Kaposi's sarcoma	0.0	0.0	0.0	0.0
C47	Peripheral nerves and autonomic nervous system	0.1	0.1	0.1	0.0
C48	Retroperitoneum and peritoneum	0.2	0.2	0.3	0.2
C49	Other connective and soft tissue	0.8	0.6	0.5	0.3
C50	Breast	0.1	0.1	14.3	10.7

CDR: crude death rate per 100,000 population.
ADR: age-adjusted death rate per 100,000 population standardized on the age distribution of the 'model' population for the year 1985 in Japan.

by Site in Japan (2000)

ICD (10th revision)	Site of malignant neoplasm	Male		Female	
		CDR	ADR	CDR	ADR
C51–C58	Female genital organs			15.0	10.0
C51	Vulva			0.3	0.1
C52	Vagina			0.2	0.1
C53–C55, C58	Uterus			8.1	5.3
C53	Cervix uteri			3.7	2.7
C54	Corpus uteri			1.8	1.2
C55	Uterus, part unspecified			2.6	1.4
C56	Ovary			6.2	4.3
C57	Other and unspecified female genital organs			0.2	0.1
C58	Placenta			0.0	0.0
C60–C63	Male genital organs	12.6	8.9		
C60	Penis	0.2	0.1		
C61	Prostate	12.2	8.6		
C62	Testis	0.2	0.2		
C63	Other and unspecified male genital organs	0.0	0.0		
C64–C68	Urinary tract	10.2	7.4	4.9	2.4
C64, C65	Kidney	4.2	3.1	2.0	1.1
C64	Kidney, except renal pelvis	3.5	2.6	1.6	0.9
C65	Renal pelvis	0.7	0.5	0.4	0.2
C66	Ureter	0.6	0.5	0.5	0.2
C67	Bladder	5.2	3.7	2.3	1.0
C68	Other and unspecified urinary organs	0.2	0.1	0.1	0.1
C69–C72	Eye, brain and other parts of central nervous system	1.4	1.2	1.1	0.9
C69	Eye and adnexa	0.0	0.0	0.0	0.0
C70	Meninges	0.0	0.0	0.0	0.0
C71	Brain	1.3	1.1	1.0	0.8
C72	Spinal cord, cranial nerves and other parts of central nervous system	0.0	0.0	0.0	0.0
C73–C75	Thyroid and other endocrine glands	0.9	0.7	1.5	0.8
C73	Thyroid gland	0.7	0.5	1.4	0.7
C74	Adrenal gland	0.2	0.2	0.1	0.1
C75	Other endocrine glands and related structures	0.0	0.0	0.0	0.0
C76–C80	Ill-defined, secondary and unspecified sites	5.4	3.9	5.1	2.5
C76	Other and ill-defined sites	0.3	0.2	0.3	0.2
C77	Lymph nodes specified as secondary and unspecified	0.1	0.1	0.0	0.0
C78	Respiratory and digestive systems specified as secondary	2.1	1.5	2.3	1.1
C79	Other sites, secondary as specified	0.6	0.5	0.4	0.2
C80	Without specification of site	2.3	1.7	2.0	1.1
C81–C96	Lymphoid, hematopoietic and related tissue	16.8	12.9	12.1	7.4
C81–90, C96	Lympatic, and hematopoietic systems	10.3	7.7	7.8	4.4
C81	Hodgkin's disease	0.1	0.1	0.1	0.1
C82	Follicular [nodular] non-Hodgkin's lymphoma	0.0	0.0	0.0	0.0
C83	Diffuse non-Hodgkin's lymphoma	0.1	0.1	0.1	0.0
C84	Peripheral and cutaneous T-cell lymphomas	0.1	0.1	0.1	0.0
C85	Other and unspecified types of non-Hodgkin's lymphoma	7.1	5.3	5.0	2.9
C88	Malignant immunoproliferative diseases	0.1	0.1	0.0	0.0
C90	Multiple myeloma and malignant plasma cell neoplasms	2.7	2.0	2.5	1.4
C91–C95	Leukemia	6.5	5.2	4.4	3.0
C91	Lymphoid leukemia	1.7	1.4	1.4	1.0
C92	Myeloid leukemia	4.0	3.2	2.4	1.6
C93	Monocytic leukemia	0.1	0.0	0.0	0.0
C94	Other leukemias of specified cell type	0.0	0.0	0.0	0.0
C95	Leukemia of unspecified cell type	0.6	0.5	0.5	0.3
C96	Other and unspecified malignant neoplasms of lymphoid, hematopoietic and related tissue	0.1	0.0	0.0	0.0
C97	Independent (primary) multiple sites	0.6	0.5	0.3	0.2

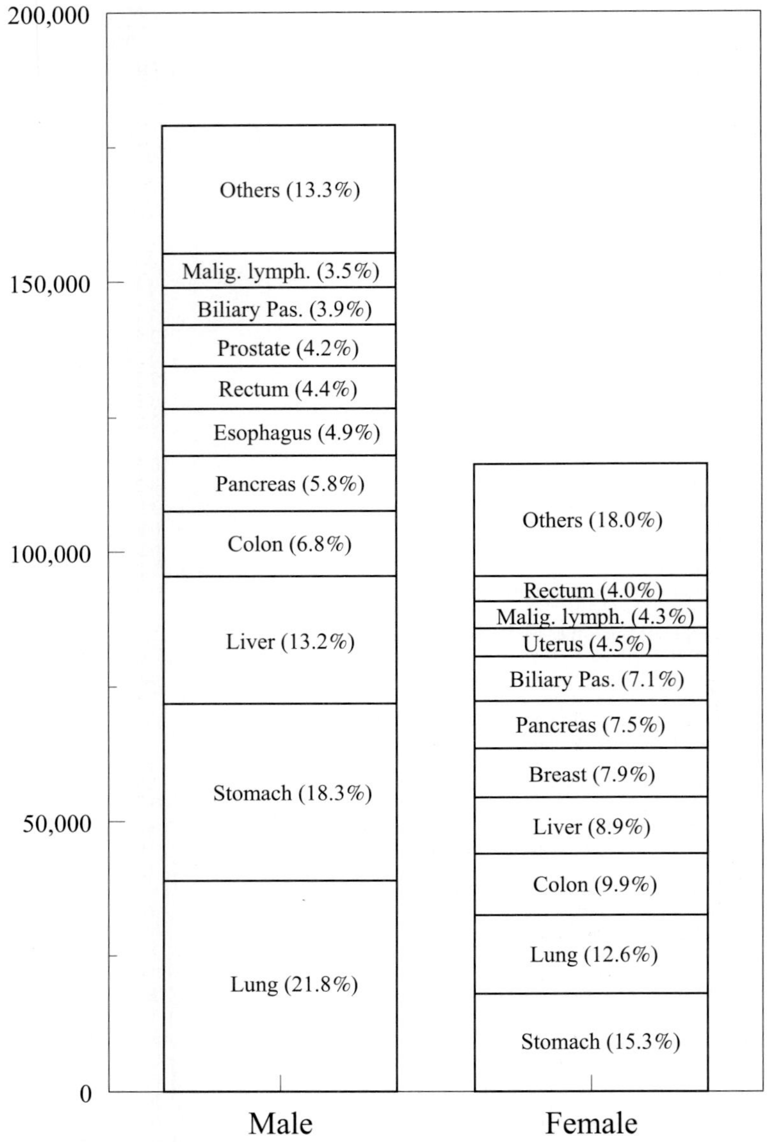

FIG. 1. Number of deaths from malignant neoplasms and its proportion of all malignant neoplasms for major sites by sex in Japan (2000)

TABLE II-1. Cancer Mortality Statistics in Japan (1950–2000)
Cancer of all sites (ICD, 10th revision: C00–C97)

Year	No. of deaths		Crude death rate per 100,000		Age-adjusted death rate per 100,000[a]		Average age at death in years	
	Male	Female	Male	Female	Male	Female	Male	Female
1950	32,670	31,758	80.1	74.9	148.2	121.4	59.6	57.7
1951	33,872	32,482	81.6	75.4	150.3	122.4	59.8	58.1
1952	35,845	33,643	85.1	77.0	155.7	123.9	59.9	58.4
1953	37,386	34,192	87.5	77.2	160.1	122.7	60.1	58.4
1954	39,703	35,606	91.6	79.3	166.1	124.7	60.2	58.6
1955	41,223	36,498	94.0	80.4	167.9	125.4	60.4	59.2
1956	43,628	38,251	98.4	83.3	174.7	128.5	60.6	59.3
1957	44,777	38,378	100.0	82.9	175.7	126.0	60.9	59.2
1958	47,237	40,658	104.4	86.9	182.7	130.7	61.1	59.6
1959	49,215	42,071	107.7	89.0	186.0	132.3	61.3	59.8
1960	50,898	42,875	110.9	90.2	188.3	132.0	61.5	60.1
1961	52,254	44,188	112.9	92.1	188.8	132.3	61.7	60.2
1962	53,499	44,725	114.4	92.3	188.0	130.6	61.7	60.2
1963	55,567	45,859	117.7	93.7	192.6	131.2	61.8	60.3
1964	57,705	46,619	120.9	94.3	195.9	130.0	62.1	60.5
1965	58,899	47,637	122.1	95.2	195.6	130.3	62.2	60.7
1966	60,803	49,002	125.0	97.2	197.3	130.5	62.5	60.8
1967	62,308	50,285	127.4	99.1	197.9	130.8	62.6	61.2
1968	64,244	51,218	129.8	99.8	200.0	129.7	62.9	61.4
1969	66,270	52,289	132.3	100.7	202.1	129.1	63.2	61.7
1970	67,074	52,903	132.6	100.7	199.2	126.9	63.2	61.8
1971	68,399	54,451	133.5	102.5	198.2	126.5	63.5	62.1
1972	71,298	56,001	137.5	103.9	202.3	126.4	63.7	62.3
1973	73,401	57,563	138.5	104.5	201.9	125.2	64.1	62.7
1974	75,456	58,295	139.7	104.0	202.0	123.0	64.3	63.0
1975	76,922	59,461	140.6	105.2	198.9	121.1	64.3	63.1
1976	79,995	60,898	144.6	106.7	202.0	120.7	64.5	63.5
1977	83,088	62,684	148.7	108.8	203.4	120.0	64.8	64.0
1978	85,630	64,706	151.9	111.3	203.8	120.0	65.1	64.3
1979	90,136	66,525	158.6	113.5	208.6	119.6	65.4	64.8
1980	93,501	68,263	163.5	115.5	210.9	118.8	65.6	65.2
1981	96,524	69,875	167.4	117.3	211.6	117.8	65.9	65.5
1982	99,114	71,016	170.7	118.5	210.7	115.7	66.2	66.0
1983	103,330	72,876	176.8	120.8	213.3	114.9	66.4	66.3
1984	107,175	75,105	182.3	123.7	215.0	114.6	66.7	66.7
1985	110,660	77,054	187.2	125.9	214.8	113.1	67.0	67.2
1986	113,589	78,065	191.1	126.9	213.8	110.9	67.1	67.6
1987	119,161	80,402	199.5	130.1	216.9	110.1	67.4	68.0
1988	122,015	83,455	203.5	134.5	215.5	110.5	67.8	68.4
1989	127,211	85,414	211.4	137.1	217.8	109.4	67.9	68.7
1990	130,395	87,018	216.4	139.3	215.6	107.7	68.1	69.2
1991	134,475	89,252	222.6	142.4	215.6	107.1	68.4	69.3
1992	139,674	92,243	230.5	146.7	216.8	107.0	68.6	69.7
1993	142,222	93,485	234.2	148.3	214.1	105.0	68.8	70.0
1994	146,896	96,774	241.5	153.1	214.7	105.1	69.1	70.5
1995	159,623	103,399	262.0	163.1	226.2	108.3	69.5	71.0
1996	164,824	106,359	269.7	167.2	225.7	107.8	69.7	71.3
1997	167,076	108,337	273.0	169.9	221.3	106.4	70.1	71.5
1998	172,306	111,615	281.0	174.6	221.0	105.9	70.4	72.0
1999	175,817	114,739	286.5	179.1	219.0	105.2	70.7	72.4
2000	179,140	116,344	291.3	181.4	214.0	103.5	71.0	72.6

[a] Standardized on the age distribution of the model population for the year 1985 in Japan.

TABLE II-2. Cancer Mortality Statistics in Japan (1950–2000)
Cancer of the buccal cavity and pharynx (ICD, 10th revision: C00–C14)

Year	No. of deaths		Crude death rate per 100,000		Age-adjusted death rate per 100,000[a]		Average age at death in years	
	Male	Female	Male	Female	Male	Female	Male	Female
1950	432	267	1.1	0.6	2.1	1.1	59.0	60.9
1951	409	235	1.0	0.6	2.0	0.9	60.8	59.7
1952	427	217	1.0	0.5	1.9	0.9	61.1	61.9
1953	468	237	1.1	0.5	2.0	0.9	59.1	59.6
1954	410	246	1.0	0.6	1.8	0.9	60.2	60.1
1955	414	236	0.9	0.5	1.7	0.9	60.4	61.7
1956	413	238	0.9	0.5	1.7	0.8	60.4	59.6
1957	430	285	1.0	0.6	1.8	1.0	60.8	61.0
1958	443	252	1.0	0.5	1.7	0.8	60.9	63.4
1959	509	280	1.1	0.6	2.0	0.9	60.7	61.5
1960	484	277	1.1	0.6	1.8	0.9	60.9	61.4
1961	522	263	1.1	0.6	1.9	0.8	61.8	61.1
1962	498	287	1.1	0.6	1.7	0.9	60.5	61.9
1963	592	296	1.3	0.6	2.0	0.9	59.7	62.4
1964	580	331	1.2	0.7	2.0	0.9	61.7	61.8
1965	561	333	1.2	0.7	1.9	0.9	61.9	62.5
1966	579	321	1.2	0.6	1.9	0.9	60.7	62.3
1967	640	337	1.3	0.7	2.0	0.9	61.4	62.4
1968	675	362	1.4	0.7	2.1	0.9	61.3	62.7
1969	695	384	1.4	0.7	2.1	1.0	62.2	62.3
1970	738	374	1.5	0.7	2.2	0.9	61.7	62.3
1971	813	374	1.6	0.7	2.3	0.9	61.6	63.1
1972	786	371	1.5	0.7	2.2	0.8	62.1	62.8
1973	784	429	1.5	0.8	2.1	0.9	62.1	63.7
1974	874	424	1.6	0.8	2.3	0.9	62.4	64.1
1975	943	505	1.7	0.9	2.4	1.0	62.5	63.9
1976	1,012	466	1.8	0.8	2.5	0.9	61.9	65.2
1977	1,007	478	1.8	0.8	2.4	0.9	62.3	63.6
1978	1,052	499	1.9	0.9	2.4	0.9	62.2	64.8
1979	1,218	588	2.1	1.0	2.8	1.1	62.6	65.4
1980	1,233	592	2.2	1.0	2.7	1.0	62.8	66.4
1981	1,320	528	2.3	0.9	2.8	0.9	63.6	66.2
1982	1,283	593	2.2	1.0	2.7	1.0	63.4	66.2
1983	1,408	584	2.4	1.0	2.8	0.9	63.4	66.8
1984	1,450	598	2.5	1.0	2.9	0.9	64.0	67.3
1985	1,462	627	2.5	1.0	2.8	0.9	63.9	68.1
1986	1,611	633	2.7	1.0	3.0	0.9	63.6	68.3
1987	1,643	650	2.8	1.1	2.9	0.9	64.3	68.0
1988	1,787	659	3.0	1.1	3.1	0.9	64.3	68.3
1989	1,755	691	2.9	1.1	2.9	0.9	64.4	68.2
1990	1,866	741	3.1	1.2	3.0	0.9	64.4	69.5
1991	2,119	750	3.5	1.2	3.3	0.9	64.5	69.8
1992	2,170	824	3.6	1.3	3.3	0.9	65.2	70.4
1993	2,258	897	3.7	1.4	3.4	1.0	65.3	70.8
1994	2,408	859	4.0	1.4	3.5	0.9	65.0	70.4
1995	2,980	1,119	4.9	1.8	4.2	1.1	65.9	72.0
1996	3,178	1,169	5.2	1.8	4.4	1.2	66.0	72.0
1997	3,295	1,268	5.4	2.0	4.4	1.2	66.1	73.3
1998	3,409	1,361	5.6	2.1	4.4	1.3	66.4	73.0
1999	3,485	1,361	5.7	2.1	4.4	1.2	66.9	73.4
2000	3,610	1,456	5.9	2.3	4.4	1.3	67.2	73.6

[a] Standardized on the age distribution of the model population for the year 1985 in Japan.

TABLE II-3. Cancer Mortality Statistics in Japan (1950–2000)
Cancer of the esophagus (ICD, 10th revision: C15)

Year	No. of deaths		Crude death rate per 100,000		Age-adjusted death rate per 100,000[a]		Average age at death in years	
	Male	Female	Male	Female	Male	Female	Male	Female
1950	1,961	802	4.8	1.9	9.5	3.2	63.9	63.3
1951	1,899	785	4.6	1.8	9.1	3.2	64.2	63.8
1952	2,070	845	4.9	1.9	9.6	3.3	64.3	64.0
1953	2,101	875	4.9	2.0	9.7	3.3	64.4	64.1
1954	2,155	849	5.0	1.9	9.8	3.1	65.1	64.6
1955	2,102	871	4.8	1.9	9.3	3.2	65.4	65.8
1956	2,272	962	5.1	2.1	9.9	3.4	65.6	65.6
1957	2,297	931	5.1	2.0	9.6	3.2	65.1	65.7
1958	2,329	965	5.1	2.1	9.7	3.3	65.6	66.2
1959	2,412	950	5.3	2.0	9.8	3.1	65.9	65.6
1960	2,472	995	5.4	2.1	9.6	3.3	65.5	67.3
1961	2,675	1,041	5.8	2.2	10.2	3.3	66.0	66.5
1962	2,683	994	5.7	2.1	9.9	3.1	66.0	66.7
1963	2,797	1,018	5.9	2.1	10.2	3.1	65.9	66.8
1964	2,931	1,102	6.1	2.2	10.5	3.3	66.4	67.3
1965	2,870	1,088	5.9	2.2	10.1	3.2	66.5	67.8
1966	3,076	1,090	6.3	2.2	10.5	3.1	66.7	68.3
1967	3,180	1,164	6.5	2.3	10.6	3.2	66.8	68.4
1968	3,447	1,183	7.0	2.3	11.2	3.2	66.7	69.1
1969	3,526	1,225	7.0	2.4	11.2	3.2	67.0	69.2
1970	3,673	1,150	7.3	2.2	11.4	2.9	67.2	68.7
1971	3,737	1,263	7.3	2.4	11.3	3.1	67.4	68.9
1972	3,739	1,182	7.2	2.2	11.0	2.8	67.3	69.7
1973	3,903	1,207	7.4	2.2	11.1	2.7	67.7	69.7
1974	3,946	1,262	7.3	2.3	10.9	2.8	67.6	70.4
1975	3,862	1,135	7.1	2.0	10.3	2.4	67.4	70.2
1976	3,924	1,166	7.1	2.0	10.1	2.4	67.2	70.9
1977	4,057	1,184	7.3	2.1	10.2	2.3	67.9	71.7
1978	4,130	1,195	7.3	2.1	10.0	2.2	67.8	71.8
1979	4,347	1,132	7.6	1.9	10.3	2.0	68.0	71.8
1980	4,490	1,243	7.8	2.1	10.3	2.2	68.1	71.7
1981	4,454	1,184	7.7	2.0	9.9	2.0	67.8	72.1
1982	4,646	1,208	8.0	2.0	10.0	1.9	67.7	71.8
1983	4,776	1,220	8.2	2.0	9.9	1.9	67.8	73.0
1984	4,791	1,167	8.1	1.9	9.6	1.7	67.7	73.4
1985	5,046	1,151	8.5	1.9	9.8	1.6	67.4	73.4
1986	5,202	1,183	8.8	1.9	9.7	1.6	67.3	73.4
1987	5,573	1,127	9.3	1.8	10.1	1.5	67.7	72.9
1988	5,625	1,199	9.4	1.9	9.8	1.5	67.7	73.9
1989	5,798	1,243	9.6	2.0	9.8	1.5	67.4	74.4
1990	6,004	1,270	10.0	2.0	9.8	1.5	67.4	73.4
1991	6,263	1,294	10.4	2.1	9.9	1.5	67.3	73.5
1992	6,557	1,297	10.8	2.1	10.0	1.4	67.3	73.9
1993	6,734	1,306	11.1	2.1	10.0	1.4	67.4	74.0
1994	6,778	1,365	11.1	2.2	9.8	1.4	67.6	73.7
1995	7,253	1,385	11.9	2.2	10.1	1.3	67.8	74.8
1996	7,671	1,467	12.6	2.3	10.4	1.4	67.9	74.2
1997	8,113	1,486	13.3	2.3	10.6	1.4	68.0	74.0
1998	8,241	1,464	13.4	2.3	10.5	1.3	68.3	74.2
1999	8,449	1,542	13.8	2.4	10.5	1.3	68.3	74.5
2000	8,706	1,550	14.2	2.4	10.4	1.3	68.5	74.5

[a] Standardized on the age distribution of the model population for the year 1985 in Japan.

TABLE II-4. Cancer Mortality Statistics in Japan (1950–2000)
Cancer of the stomach (ICD, 10th revision: C16)

Year	No. of deaths		Crude death rate per 100,000		Age-adjusted death rate per 100,000[a]		Average age at death in years	
	Male	Female	Male	Female	Male	Female	Male	Female
1950	19,023	12,188	46.6	28.8	87.3	48.0	61.1	60.9
1951	19,865	12,491	47.9	29.0	89.1	48.4	61.2	61.3
1952	20,814	13,101	49.4	30.0	91.8	49.7	61.4	61.7
1953	21,347	13,418	49.9	30.3	92.8	49.4	61.7	61.3
1954	22,116	13,875	51.0	30.9	93.8	50.0	61.9	61.6
1955	22,899	14,407	52.2	31.7	94.4	50.8	62.0	62.0
1956	23,642	15,081	53.3	32.9	95.9	51.8	62.2	61.9
1957	24,380	15,104	54.5	32.6	96.9	50.7	62.4	61.7
1958	25,151	15,598	55.6	33.3	98.3	51.3	62.6	62.1
1959	25,757	16,127	56.4	34.1	98.4	51.9	62.8	62.4
1960	26,283	16,467	57.3	34.6	98.5	51.8	62.9	62.5
1961	26,469	16,772	57.2	35.0	96.7	51.2	63.2	62.4
1962	26,585	16,918	56.9	34.9	94.5	50.4	63.2	62.5
1963	27,284	17,252	57.8	35.3	95.9	50.3	63.3	62.4
1964	28,219	17,474	59.1	35.3	96.8	49.5	63.4	62.4
1965	28,636	17,749	59.4	35.5	96.0	49.4	63.6	62.6
1966	28,923	17,849	59.5	35.4	94.7	48.3	63.9	62.7
1967	29,160	18,505	59.6	36.5	93.5	48.8	63.9	62.9
1968	30,043	19,257	60.7	37.5	94.5	49.4	64.2	63.1
1969	30,322	19,216	60.5	37.0	93.4	47.9	64.5	63.2
1970	29,653	19,170	58.6	36.5	88.9	46.5	64.5	63.4
1971	29,882	19,563	58.3	36.8	87.4	45.8	64.8	63.5
1972	30,380	19,563	58.6	36.3	87.1	44.5	65.0	63.8
1973	30,603	20,075	57.7	36.4	85.0	44.0	65.2	64.2
1974	30,599	19,791	56.7	35.3	82.7	42.0	65.4	64.4
1975	30,403	19,454	55.6	34.4	79.4	39.8	65.5	64.3
1976	30,537	19,555	55.2	34.3	77.6	38.9	65.6	64.6
1977	30,326	19,806	54.3	34.4	74.9	38.0	65.9	65.0
1978	30,136	19,428	53.5	33.4	72.3	36.1	66.0	65.2
1979	30,777	19,843	54.1	33.8	71.8	35.7	66.3	65.7
1980	30,845	19,598	53.9	33.2	69.9	34.1	66.5	66.0
1981	30,876	19,258	53.6	32.3	68.0	32.4	66.7	66.2
1982	30,036	18,977	51.7	31.7	64.1	30.9	66.8	66.5
1983	30,591	18,775	52.4	31.1	63.3	29.5	66.9	66.7
1984	30,876	18,909	52.5	31.1	62.2	28.8	67.3	67.2
1985	30,146	18,756	51.0	30.7	58.7	27.4	67.6	67.8
1986	30,127	18,139	50.7	29.5	56.9	25.7	67.7	68.0
1987	30,237	18,103	50.6	29.3	55.2	24.7	68.1	68.4
1988	30,009	17,995	50.0	29.0	53.1	23.7	68.2	68.9
1989	30,271	17,954	50.3	28.8	51.9	22.9	68.5	69.1
1990	29,909	17,562	49.6	28.1	49.5	21.6	68.6	69.7
1991	30,296	17,600	50.1	28.1	48.7	20.9	68.8	69.9
1992	30,507	17,534	50.3	27.9	47.4	20.1	69.2	70.3
1993	29,998	17,313	49.4	27.5	45.2	19.2	69.4	70.8
1994	30,564	17,227	50.2	27.2	44.7	18.4	69.6	71.5
1995	32,015	18,061	52.6	28.5	45.4	18.5	70.1	71.9
1996	32,384	17,781	53.0	28.0	44.3	17.6	70.2	72.3
1997	32,218	17,521	52.6	27.5	42.6	16.8	70.6	72.6
1998	32,858	17,822	53.6	27.9	42.1	16.4	70.7	73.1
1999	32,788	17,888	53.4	27.9	40.8	15.9	71.1	73.5
2000	32,798	17,852	53.3	27.8	39.1	15.3	71.4	73.9

[a] Standardized on the age distribution of the model population for the year 1985 in Japan.

TABLE II-5. Cancer Mortality Statistics in Japan (1950–2000)
Cancer of the colon (ICD, 10th revision: C18)

Year	No. of deaths		Crude death rate per 100,000		Age-adjusted death rate per 100,000[a]		Average age at death in years	
	Male	Female	Male	Female	Male	Female	Male	Female
1950	620	837	1.5	2.0	2.9	3.3	60.4	62.0
1951	663	797	1.6	1.9	3.0	3.1	60.4	61.7
1952	606	828	1.4	1.9	2.7	3.1	60.5	62.0
1953	608	808	1.4	1.8	2.6	3.0	60.4	62.9
1954	644	862	1.5	1.9	2.8	3.1	60.6	62.3
1955	723	905	1.6	2.0	3.1	3.2	61.3	62.9
1956	772	946	1.7	2.1	3.2	3.3	62.5	63.6
1957	783	967	1.7	2.1	3.1	3.3	61.5	63.7
1958	815	1,090	1.8	2.3	3.3	3.6	61.6	64.0
1959	867	1,131	1.9	2.4	3.5	3.7	62.4	64.2
1960	910	1,129	2.0	2.4	3.6	3.6	62.6	64.2
1961	968	1,246	2.1	2.6	3.7	3.9	62.3	64.8
1962	1,047	1,296	2.2	2.7	3.8	3.9	62.6	64.1
1963	1,057	1,325	2.2	2.7	3.8	3.9	62.1	64.5
1964	1,250	1,420	2.6	2.9	4.3	4.1	61.4	64.3
1965	1,272	1,532	2.6	3.1	4.3	4.3	61.8	64.5
1966	1,349	1,654	2.8	3.3	4.5	4.6	62.1	64.8
1967	1,445	1,729	3.0	3.4	4.6	4.7	61.9	65.2
1968	1,580	1,819	3.2	3.5	5.0	4.7	62.5	64.8
1969	1,666	2,036	3.3	3.9	5.1	5.2	62.1	65.5
1970	1,766	2,052	3.5	3.9	5.2	5.0	62.3	65.2
1971	1,931	2,230	3.8	4.2	5.7	5.3	63.3	65.9
1972	2,089	2,360	4.0	4.4	6.0	5.4	63.6	65.5
1973	2,322	2,669	4.4	4.8	6.4	5.9	63.9	65.5
1974	2,508	2,761	4.6	4.9	6.7	5.9	64.3	65.9
1975	2,662	2,911	4.9	5.1	7.0	6.0	64.4	65.7
1976	2,901	3,214	5.2	5.6	7.4	6.4	64.9	66.4
1977	3,105	3,355	5.6	5.8	7.7	6.5	65.0	66.8
1978	3,353	3,763	5.9	6.5	8.0	7.0	65.3	67.0
1979	3,553	3,772	6.3	6.4	8.2	6.8	65.7	67.4
1980	3,842	4,090	6.7	6.9	8.7	7.1	66.2	67.5
1981	4,168	4,462	7.2	7.5	9.2	7.5	66.6	68.2
1982	4,494	4,729	7.7	7.9	9.6	7.7	66.6	68.1
1983	4,763	4,983	8.2	8.3	9.9	7.8	67.1	68.6
1984	5,196	5,350	8.8	8.8	10.5	8.1	67.3	69.0
1985	5,522	5,703	9.3	9.3	10.8	8.3	67.7	69.0
1986	5,895	5,983	9.9	9.7	11.2	8.4	68.0	69.5
1987	6,453	6,255	10.8	10.1	11.8	8.4	68.2	69.9
1988	6,747	6,893	11.3	11.1	12.0	9.0	68.2	70.4
1989	7,274	7,371	12.1	11.8	12.5	9.3	68.5	70.5
1990	7,791	7,718	12.9	12.4	12.9	9.3	68.8	71.0
1991	8,236	8,031	13.6	12.8	13.2	9.4	69.1	71.1
1992	8,804	8,578	14.5	13.6	13.7	9.7	69.2	71.6
1993	9,197	8,901	15.1	14.1	13.8	9.7	69.3	71.8
1994	9,646	9,417	15.9	14.9	14.1	9.8	69.6	72.6
1995	10,420	9,866	17.1	15.6	14.8	9.9	70.5	73.2
1996	11,055	10,327	18.1	16.2	15.1	9.9	70.6	73.5
1997	11,162	10,538	18.2	16.5	14.7	9.8	70.7	73.6
1998	11,581	10,820	18.9	16.9	14.8	9.6	71.1	74.3
1999	11,862	11,383	19.3	17.8	14.7	9.8	71.5	74.8
2000	12,139	11,498	19.7	17.9	14.4	9.5	71.8	75.1

[a] Standardized on the age distribution of the model population for the year 1985 in Japan.

TABLE II-6. Cancer Mortality Statistics in Japan (1950–2000)
Cancer of the rectum (ICD, 10th revision: C19–C21)

Year	No. of deaths		Crude death rate per 100,000		Age-adjusted death rate per 100,000[a]		Average age at death in years	
	Male	Female	Male	Female	Male	Female	Male	Female
1950	1,199	1,072	2.9	2.5	5.6	4.2	61.2	59.6
1951	1,251	1,101	3.0	2.6	5.9	4.3	61.8	60.9
1952	1,236	1,163	2.9	2.7	5.6	4.4	61.8	61.6
1953	1,239	1,144	2.9	2.6	5.6	4.3	62.1	61.8
1954	1,351	1,207	3.1	2.7	6.1	4.4	62.5	62.0
1955	1,356	1,255	3.1	2.8	6.0	4.5	63.3	62.2
1956	1,439	1,297	3.2	2.8	6.1	4.5	63.3	63.0
1957	1,456	1,360	3.3	2.9	6.1	4.6	63.2	62.6
1958	1,500	1,417	3.3	3.0	6.2	4.7	63.7	62.9
1959	1,615	1,467	3.5	3.1	6.4	4.7	63.1	62.9
1960	1,480	1,518	3.2	3.2	5.9	4.8	64.6	63.9
1961	1,677	1,589	3.6	3.3	6.4	4.9	63.9	63.7
1962	1,679	1,579	3.6	3.3	6.2	4.8	63.3	63.9
1963	1,839	1,628	3.9	3.3	6.7	4.8	63.7	63.5
1964	1,868	1,653	3.9	3.3	6.7	4.8	63.9	64.1
1965	1,993	1,803	4.1	3.6	7.0	5.1	64.1	63.8
1966	1,961	1,879	4.0	3.7	6.7	5.1	64.2	63.1
1967	2,146	1,978	4.4	3.9	7.1	5.3	63.8	63.8
1968	2,266	2,128	4.6	4.1	7.4	5.5	64.4	64.8
1969	2,417	2,165	4.8	4.2	7.6	5.4	64.2	64.1
1970	2,555	2,162	5.0	4.1	7.8	5.3	63.7	64.3
1971	2,611	2,355	5.1	4.4	7.7	5.5	63.8	64.0
1972	2,692	2,374	5.2	4.4	7.8	5.4	64.1	64.7
1973	2,964	2,542	5.6	4.6	8.4	5.6	65.2	65.2
1974	3,178	2,739	5.9	4.9	8.7	5.9	65.1	65.4
1975	3,148	2,756	5.8	4.9	8.3	5.7	65.0	65.5
1976	3,324	2,694	6.0	4.7	8.6	5.4	65.8	66.2
1977	3,493	2,780	6.3	4.8	8.6	5.4	65.3	65.9
1978	3,504	2,898	6.2	5.0	8.5	5.4	65.5	66.3
1979	3,838	3,070	6.8	5.2	9.0	5.5	65.9	66.8
1980	3,933	2,984	6.9	5.0	9.0	5.2	66.2	67.1
1981	4,123	3,156	7.2	5.3	9.1	5.3	66.4	67.7
1982	4,131	3,153	7.1	5.3	8.9	5.1	67.0	68.0
1983	4,299	3,319	7.4	5.5	8.9	5.2	66.6	68.1
1984	4,477	3,343	7.6	5.5	9.0	5.1	66.7	67.7
1985	4,643	3,291	7.9	5.4	9.0	4.8	66.8	68.6
1986	4,732	3,420	8.0	5.6	8.9	4.8	66.7	68.5
1987	4,884	3,484	8.2	5.6	8.8	4.7	66.9	69.2
1988	5,070	3,589	8.5	5.8	8.9	4.7	67.1	68.8
1989	5,352	3,666	8.9	5.9	9.1	4.7	67.2	69.3
1990	5,569	3,701	9.2	5.9	9.2	4.6	67.4	69.6
1991	5,693	3,823	9.4	6.1	9.0	4.6	67.3	69.4
1992	6,157	3,933	10.2	6.3	9.5	4.6	67.6	69.8
1993	6,122	3,841	10.1	6.1	9.1	4.3	67.6	70.0
1994	6,189	3,836	10.2	6.1	9.0	4.1	67.5	70.7
1995	6,984	4,232	11.5	6.7	9.8	4.4	68.1	71.1
1996	7,147	4,290	11.7	6.7	9.7	4.3	68.3	71.3
1997	7,302	4,411	11.9	6.9	9.6	4.3	68.4	71.5
1998	7,588	4,647	12.4	7.3	9.7	4.4	68.7	72.1
1999	7,678	4,690	12.5	7.3	9.6	4.3	68.8	72.6
2000	7,863	4,703	12.8	7.3	9.5	4.2	69.0	72.3

[a] Standardized on the age distribution of the model population for the year 1985 in Japan.

TABLE II-7. Cancer Mortality Statistics in Japan (1950–2000)
Cancer of the liver (ICD, 10th revision: C22)

Year	No. of deaths		Crude death rate per 100,000		Age-adjusted death rate per 100,000[a]		Average age at death in years	
	Male	Female	Male	Female	Male	Female	Male	Female
1950								
1951								
1952								
1953								
1954								
1955								
1956								
1957								
1958	4,806	3,485	10.6	7.4	19.0	11.7	62.6	64.2
1959	4,878	3,534	10.7	7.5	18.7	11.6	62.7	64.5
1960	5,204	3,613	11.3	7.6	19.4	11.6	62.7	64.7
1961	5,064	3,530	10.9	7.4	18.6	11.0	62.8	64.9
1962	5,175	3,454	11.1	7.1	18.4	10.5	62.9	65.1
1963	5,190	3,516	11.0	7.2	18.3	10.5	63.0	64.9
1964	5,194	3,497	10.9	7.1	17.9	10.1	62.9	65.2
1965	5,006	3,497	10.4	7.0	17.0	9.9	63.3	65.0
1966	5,341	3,566	11.0	7.1	17.6	9.9	63.3	65.4
1967	5,320	3,449	10.9	6.8	16.9	9.3	62.9	65.9
1968	5,468	3,544	11.1	6.9	17.1	9.3	63.4	65.6
1969	5,838	3,635	11.7	7.0	18.0	9.3	63.5	66.1
1970	5,908	3,608	11.7	6.9	17.7	8.9	63.5	66.0
1971	6,038	3,723	11.8	7.0	17.5	8.9	63.5	66.2
1972	6,100	3,688	11.8	6.8	17.3	8.5	63.4	66.5
1973	6,333	3,699	11.9	6.7	17.3	8.2	63.4	66.2
1974	6,443	3,673	11.9	6.6	17.1	7.9	63.5	67.0
1975	6,795	3,793	12.4	6.7	17.4	7.8	63.4	66.8
1976	7,520	3,972	13.6	7.0	18.7	8.0	63.3	67.4
1977	7,937	4,062	14.2	7.0	19.0	7.9	63.2	67.7
1978	8,743	4,308	15.5	7.4	20.3	8.0	63.1	67.9
1979	9,198	4,225	16.2	7.2	20.8	7.6	63.3	68.2
1980	9,741	4,227	17.0	7.1	21.3	7.4	63.1	68.8
1981	10,332	4,515	17.9	7.6	21.9	7.6	63.1	68.8
1982	11,278	4,582	19.4	7.6	23.1	7.4	63.1	69.2
1983	12,160	4,726	20.8	7.8	24.2	7.4	63.7	69.2
1984	12,906	4,915	22.0	8.1	25.0	7.4	63.5	70.0
1985	13,780	5,192	23.3	8.5	25.7	7.5	63.4	69.7
1986	14,574	5,288	24.5	8.6	26.4	7.4	63.7	70.1
1987	15,624	5,560	26.2	9.0	27.4	7.5	63.8	70.6
1988	16,238	5,830	27.1	9.4	27.7	7.6	64.2	70.7
1989	17,040	6,045	28.3	9.7	28.2	7.6	64.4	70.9
1990	17,786	6,447	29.5	10.3	28.4	7.8	64.7	71.4
1991	18,172	6,482	30.1	10.3	28.2	7.6	65.0	71.4
1992	18,907	6,864	31.2	10.9	28.5	7.8	65.3	71.8
1993	19,410	7,181	32.0	11.4	28.4	7.8	65.7	72.0
1994	20,105	7,367	33.0	11.7	28.7	7.8	66.0	72.2
1995	22,773	8,934	37.4	14.1	31.6	9.1	66.4	72.4
1996	22,904	9,271	37.5	14.6	30.8	9.1	66.7	72.8
1997	22,937	9,422	37.5	14.8	29.9	9.0	67.2	72.8
1998	23,553	9,880	38.4	15.5	29.9	9.0	67.6	73.5
1999	23,492	10,324	38.3	16.1	29.0	9.1	67.8	73.8
2000	23,602	10,379	38.4	16.2	28.2	8.8	68.4	74.3

[a] Standardized on the age distribution of the model population for the year 1985 in Japan.

TABLE II-8. Cancer Mortality Statistics in Japan (1950–2000)
Cancer of the biliary passages (ICD, 10th revision: C23, C24)

Year	No. of deaths		Crude death rate per 100,000		Age-adjusted death rate per 100,000[a]		Average age at death in years	
	Male	Female	Male	Female	Male	Female	Male	Female
1950								
1951								
1952								
1953								
1954								
1955								
1956								
1957								
1958	427	493	0.9	1.1	1.7	1.6	64.0	63.6
1959	483	543	1.1	1.1	1.8	1.8	62.3	64.5
1960	556	588	1.2	1.2	2.1	1.9	63.7	63.9
1961	609	747	1.3	1.6	2.3	2.3	64.5	65.1
1962	677	831	1.4	1.7	2.5	2.5	64.3	65.0
1963	742	932	1.6	1.9	2.6	2.8	64.2	64.8
1964	870	1,049	1.8	2.1	3.0	3.0	64.5	65.2
1965	991	1,050	2.1	2.1	3.4	3.0	64.7	65.4
1966	993	1,271	2.0	2.5	3.3	3.5	65.1	65.0
1967	1,083	1,411	2.2	2.8	3.6	3.8	65.5	65.7
1968	1,139	1,436	2.3	2.8	3.7	3.7	65.8	65.4
1969	1,252	1,519	2.5	2.9	3.9	3.8	65.2	66.0
1970	1,340	1,764	2.6	3.4	4.1	4.3	65.6	65.6
1971	1,420	1,912	2.8	3.6	4.2	4.5	66.2	66.7
1972	1,626	2,124	3.1	3.9	4.8	4.9	66.7	66.5
1973	1,674	2,254	3.2	4.1	4.8	5.0	67.1	66.8
1974	1,750	2,326	3.2	4.2	4.7	5.0	66.8	67.0
1975	1,905	2,579	3.5	4.6	5.1	5.3	67.1	67.5
1976	2,101	2,806	3.8	4.9	5.4	5.6	67.2	67.7
1977	2,267	3,087	4.1	5.4	5.7	6.0	67.5	67.7
1978	2,350	3,261	4.2	5.6	5.8	6.1	68.0	68.2
1979	2,488	3,505	4.4	6.0	5.9	6.3	68.4	69.0
1980	2,791	3,808	4.9	6.4	6.5	6.6	68.6	69.1
1981	2,961	4,095	5.1	6.9	6.6	6.9	68.6	69.2
1982	3,148	4,370	5.4	7.3	6.8	7.1	69.0	70.1
1983	3,405	4,763	5.8	7.9	7.2	7.4	69.4	70.4
1984	3,634	5,168	6.2	8.5	7.5	7.8	69.9	70.6
1985	3,949	5,521	6.7	9.0	7.9	7.9	70.4	71.4
1986	4,201	5,680	7.1	9.2	8.1	7.9	70.4	71.7
1987	4,502	6,185	7.5	10.0	8.4	8.2	70.6	72.3
1988	4,655	6,445	7.8	10.4	8.4	8.2	71.1	72.5
1989	5,034	6,571	8.4	10.5	8.8	8.1	71.2	73.0
1990	5,069	6,802	8.4	10.9	8.5	8.0	71.1	73.7
1991	5,426	7,147	9.0	11.4	8.8	8.1	71.5	73.6
1992	5,609	7,307	9.3	11.6	8.8	8.0	71.7	73.8
1993	5,779	7,489	9.5	11.9	8.8	7.8	71.6	74.2
1994	5,924	7,601	9.7	12.0	8.7	7.6	72.4	74.9
1995	6,189	7,557	10.2	11.9	8.8	7.2	72.6	75.6
1996	6,286	7,781	10.3	12.2	8.6	7.1	72.9	75.8
1997	6,522	7,823	10.7	12.3	8.6	6.8	73.0	76.4
1998	6,670	8,178	10.9	12.8	8.5	6.9	73.3	76.6
1999	6,748	8,149	11.0	12.7	8.3	6.6	73.7	76.9
2000	6,913	8,240	11.2	12.9	8.2	6.8	73.7	75.1

[a] Standardized on the age distribution of the model population for the year 1985 in Japan.

TABLE II-9. Cancer Mortality Statistics in Japan (1950–2000)
Cancer of the pancreas (ICD, 10th revision: C25)

Year	No. of deaths		Crude death rate per 100,000		Age-adjusted death rate per 100,000[a]		Average age at death in years	
	Male	Female	Male	Female	Male	Female	Male	Female
1950	328	198	0.8	0.5	1.4	0.8	56.0	56.4
1951	318	265	0.8	0.6	1.3	1.0	56.6	57.0
1952	364	286	0.9	0.7	1.5	1.0	57.8	56.8
1953	509	359	1.2	0.8	2.0	1.3	57.6	57.5
1954	570	448	1.3	1.0	2.2	1.6	58.1	58.8
1955	625	477	1.4	1.1	2.4	1.6	58.8	59.0
1956	719	576	1.6	1.3	2.7	1.9	59.3	59.2
1957	851	626	1.9	1.4	3.1	2.1	58.7	59.5
1958	909	711	2.0	1.5	3.4	2.3	60.1	60.3
1959	975	800	2.1	1.7	3.5	2.5	60.3	60.0
1960	1,150	825	2.5	1.7	4.1	2.5	60.4	60.8
1961	1,220	859	2.6	1.8	4.2	2.6	61.0	61.9
1962	1,353	977	2.9	2.0	4.5	2.9	60.8	61.6
1963	1,376	1,058	2.9	2.2	4.6	3.1	61.1	62.5
1964	1,613	1,173	3.4	2.4	5.3	3.3	61.9	62.3
1965	1,748	1,318	3.6	2.6	5.6	3.6	61.9	62.1
1966	1,845	1,410	3.8	2.8	5.7	3.8	61.5	62.8
1967	2,087	1,498	4.3	3.0	6.4	3.9	62.3	63.3
1968	2,257	1,543	4.6	3.0	6.8	3.9	62.1	63.4
1969	2,385	1,698	4.8	3.3	7.1	4.3	63.0	64.3
1970	2,549	1,850	5.0	3.5	7.4	4.5	63.0	63.9
1971	2,670	1,870	5.2	3.5	7.6	4.4	63.4	64.5
1972	2,857	2,073	5.5	3.8	8.0	4.7	63.7	64.3
1973	2,948	2,140	5.6	3.9	8.0	4.7	64.0	64.8
1974	3,139	2,263	5.8	4.0	8.3	4.8	64.1	65.8
1975	3,155	2,480	5.8	4.4	8.0	5.1	64.4	65.7
1976	3,430	2,499	6.2	4.4	8.6	5.0	64.8	66.1
1977	3,688	2,657	6.6	4.6	8.9	5.1	64.8	66.3
1978	3,894	2,913	6.9	5.0	9.2	5.4	65.0	67.0
1979	4,147	3,063	7.3	5.2	9.5	5.5	65.3	67.3
1980	4,483	3,352	7.8	5.7	10.0	5.8	65.4	67.9
1981	4,764	3,488	8.3	5.9	10.3	5.9	66.0	68.4
1982	5,033	3,743	8.7	6.2	10.7	6.1	66.7	68.8
1983	5,229	4,032	8.9	6.7	10.7	6.3	66.6	69.3
1984	5,389	4,096	9.2	6.7	10.8	6.2	67.1	69.8
1985	5,953	4,488	10.1	7.3	11.5	6.5	67.3	70.2
1986	6,273	4,893	10.6	8.0	11.8	6.8	67.8	71.3
1987	6,829	5,196	11.4	8.4	12.5	6.9	68.1	71.5
1988	6,906	5,649	11.5	9.1	12.2	7.2	68.6	72.2
1989	7,251	5,737	12.1	9.2	12.4	7.1	68.5	72.4
1990	7,317	6,001	12.1	9.6	12.1	7.1	68.6	72.6
1991	7,581	6,024	12.5	9.6	12.2	6.9	68.9	72.8
1992	7,810	6,337	12.9	10.1	12.1	7.0	69.2	72.9
1993	8,139	6,574	13.4	10.4	12.3	7.0	69.0	73.2
1994	8,294	6,696	13.6	10.6	12.1	6.9	69.0	73.4
1995	8,965	7,054	14.7	11.1	12.7	7.0	69.3	74.0
1996	9,059	7,554	14.8	11.9	12.4	7.2	69.5	74.0
1997	9,268	7,738	15.1	12.1	12.3	7.1	69.6	74.4
1998	9,760	7,883	15.9	12.3	12.5	7.0	69.8	74.4
1999	10,204	8,450	16.6	13.2	12.7	7.3	70.1	74.7
2000	10,380	8,714	16.9	13.6	12.4	7.2	70.2	75.0

[a] Standardized on the age distribution of the model population for the year 1985 in Japan.

TABLE II-10. Cancer Mortality Statistics in Japan (1950–2000)
Cancer of the larynx (ICD, 10th revision: C32)

Year	No. of deaths		Crude death rate per 100,000		Age-adjusted death rate per 100,000[a]		Average age at death in years	
	Male	Female	Male	Female	Male	Female	Male	Female
1950	575	225	1.4	0.5	2.7	0.9	62.0	60.7
1951	487	155	1.2	0.4	2.3	0.6	63.3	61.3
1952	556	194	1.3	0.4	2.5	0.7	62.7	62.0
1953	583	179	1.4	0.4	2.6	0.7	63.8	62.4
1954	539	188	1.2	0.4	2.4	0.7	64.3	64.9
1955	536	181	1.2	0.4	2.3	0.6	64.1	64.3
1956	556	199	1.3	0.4	2.4	0.7	65.2	62.6
1957	564	187	1.3	0.4	2.4	0.6	64.9	64.0
1958	537	175	1.2	0.4	2.2	0.6	65.3	66.4
1959	546	182	1.2	0.4	2.2	0.6	64.8	66.7
1960	557	181	1.2	0.4	2.2	0.6	65.4	65.9
1961	615	160	1.3	0.3	2.3	0.5	66.0	65.6
1962	569	164	1.2	0.3	2.1	0.5	65.7	65.1
1963	561	168	1.2	0.3	2.0	0.5	66.0	65.6
1964	608	146	1.3	0.3	2.2	0.4	66.8	65.3
1965	624	168	1.3	0.3	2.2	0.5	67.1	66.9
1966	665	168	1.4	0.3	2.3	0.5	66.9	68.5
1967	643	178	1.3	0.4	2.2	0.5	67.6	67.6
1968	643	148	1.3	0.3	2.1	0.4	67.5	68.0
1969	673	149	1.3	0.3	2.2	0.4	68.2	67.7
1970	773	170	1.5	0.3	2.4	0.4	68.2	66.1
1971	718	140	1.4	0.3	2.1	0.3	67.6	68.8
1972	763	144	1.5	0.3	2.3	0.3	68.4	70.0
1973	746	134	1.4	0.2	2.1	0.3	68.2	67.5
1974	818	148	1.5	0.3	2.3	0.3	68.0	68.3
1975	738	124	1.3	0.2	2.0	0.3	69.2	70.8
1976	751	146	1.4	0.3	2.0	0.3	69.0	71.3
1977	742	127	1.3	0.2	1.9	0.2	68.8	69.7
1978	766	107	1.4	0.2	1.9	0.2	69.6	72.8
1979	748	111	1.3	0.2	1.8	0.2	69.1	72.4
1980	736	130	1.3	0.2	1.7	0.2	70.2	70.9
1981	729	120	1.3	0.2	1.6	0.2	69.7	73.0
1982	736	106	1.3	0.2	1.6	0.2	70.8	72.8
1983	716	91	1.2	0.2	1.5	0.1	70.7	73.1
1984	785	87	1.3	0.1	1.6	0.1	70.3	72.3
1985	747	88	1.3	0.1	1.5	0.1	70.2	71.7
1986	740	66	1.2	0.1	1.4	0.1	70.4	72.0
1987	729	87	1.2	0.1	1.3	0.1	70.4	74.2
1988	760	96	1.3	0.2	1.4	0.1	70.6	73.8
1989	752	90	1.2	0.1	1.3	0.1	70.8	75.2
1990	770	77	1.3	0.1	1.3	0.1	70.3	75.0
1991	770	76	1.3	0.1	1.2	0.1	70.4	74.7
1992	801	79	1.3	0.1	1.2	0.1	71.3	76.0
1993	800	56	1.3	0.1	1.2	0.1	70.8	73.7
1994	842	83	1.4	0.1	1.2	0.1	71.8	74.4
1995	872	87	1.4	0.1	1.2	0.1	72.4	76.8
1996	938	92	1.5	0.1	1.3	0.1	71.9	77.2
1997	976	88	1.6	0.1	1.3	0.1	71.3	75.1
1998	951	98	1.6	0.2	1.2	0.1	72.4	76.2
1999	909	86	1.5	0.1	1.1	0.1	72.9	75.8
2000	958	88	1.6	0.1	1.1	0.1	72.9	75.2

[a] Standardized on the age distribution of the model population for the year 1985 in Japan.

TABLE II-11. Cancer Mortality Statistics in Japan (1950–2000)
Cancer of the trachea, bronchus, and lung (ICD, 10th revision: C33, C34)

Year	No. of deaths		Crude death rate per 100,000		Age-adjusted death rate per 100,000[a]		Average age at death in years	
	Male	Female	Male	Female	Male	Female	Male	Female
1950	789	330	1.9	0.8	3.6	1.3	61.7	58.9
1951	809	387	1.9	0.9	3.6	1.5	60.8	60.1
1952	1,084	496	2.6	1.1	4.6	1.8	59.9	58.7
1953	1,234	518	2.9	1.2	5.2	1.9	60.3	59.1
1954	1,599	685	3.7	1.5	6.5	2.4	61.0	58.9
1955	1,893	818	4.3	1.8	7.8	2.8	62.4	59.3
1956	2,318	999	5.2	2.2	9.3	3.4	62.5	60.4
1957	2,568	1,085	5.7	2.3	10.0	3.6	62.4	61.0
1958	2,919	1,352	6.5	2.9	11.3	4.4	63.1	61.0
1959	3,329	1,410	7.3	3.0	12.6	4.5	63.3	61.6
1960	3,638	1,533	7.9	3.2	13.6	4.8	63.6	62.0
1961	3,932	1,766	8.5	3.7	14.3	5.3	63.7	61.6
1962	4,336	1,891	9.3	3.9	15.3	5.6	63.7	62.3
1963	4,768	1,968	10.1	4.0	16.5	5.8	64.1	63.0
1964	5,067	2,105	10.6	4.3	17.3	6.0	64.3	62.9
1965	5,404	2,321	11.2	4.6	18.1	6.5	64.7	63.2
1966	5,857	2,508	12.0	5.0	19.1	6.8	64.8	63.5
1967	6,296	2,566	12.9	5.1	20.2	6.8	65.2	63.0
1968	6,666	2,699	13.5	5.3	20.9	6.9	65.4	63.7
1969	7,209	2,924	14.4	5.6	22.2	7.3	65.7	64.2
1970	7,502	2,987	14.8	5.7	22.5	7.3	65.9	64.6
1971	8,042	3,087	15.7	5.8	23.6	7.3	66.2	64.7
1972	8,837	3,453	17.0	6.4	25.3	7.9	66.5	65.2
1973	9,256	3,600	17.5	6.5	25.8	7.9	66.9	65.7
1974	9,986	3,730	18.5	6.7	27.1	8.0	67.1	66.0
1975	10,711	4,048	19.6	7.2	28.1	8.3	67.2	66.0
1976	11,440	4,429	20.7	7.8	29.6	8.9	67.6	66.8
1977	12,542	4,693	22.5	8.1	31.3	9.0	67.8	67.0
1978	13,417	5,113	23.8	8.8	32.5	9.5	68.2	67.5
1979	14,600	5,323	25.7	9.1	34.5	9.6	68.5	67.8
1980	15,438	5,856	27.0	9.9	35.5	10.2	68.6	68.3
1981	16,638	6,161	28.9	10.3	37.2	10.4	68.9	68.5
1982	17,555	6,661	30.2	11.1	38.0	10.8	69.1	69.0
1983	18,644	7,007	31.9	11.6	39.3	11.0	69.4	69.5
1984	19,877	7,479	33.8	12.3	40.7	11.3	69.5	69.6
1985	20,837	7,753	35.3	12.7	41.2	11.2	69.9	70.3
1986	21,447	8,088	36.1	13.1	41.1	11.3	70.0	70.3
1987	23,132	8,597	38.7	13.9	42.8	11.5	70.2	70.7
1988	24,333	9,055	40.6	14.6	43.7	11.8	70.5	70.9
1989	25,870	9,607	43.0	15.4	45.0	12.0	70.5	71.6
1990	26,872	9,614	44.6	15.4	45.0	11.6	70.6	71.8
1991	27,968	10,231	46.3	16.3	45.3	11.9	70.7	71.9
1992	29,223	10,940	48.2	17.4	45.8	12.3	70.9	72.1
1993	30,398	11,129	50.1	17.6	46.1	12.1	70.9	72.3
1994	31,724	11,752	52.1	18.6	46.7	12.3	71.3	72.7
1995	33,389	12,356	54.8	19.5	47.5	12.5	71.6	73.0
1996	35,023	13,018	57.3	20.5	48.1	12.6	71.6	73.4
1997	35,700	13,294	58.3	20.9	47.3	12.5	71.8	73.6
1998	36,880	13,991	60.2	21.9	47.3	12.6	72.1	74.0
1999	37,934	14,243	61.8	22.2	47.0	12.5	72.5	74.2
2000	39,053	14,671	63.5	22.9	46.3	12.3	72.6	74.6

[a] Standardized on the age distribution of the model population for the year 1985 in Japan.

TABLE II-12. Cancer Mortality Statistics in Japan (1950–2000)
Cancer of the bone (ICD, 10th revision: C40, C41)

Year	No. of deaths		Crude death rate per 100,000		Age-adjusted death rate per 100,000[a]		Average age at death in years	
	Male	Female	Male	Female	Male	Female	Male	Female
1950	226	186	0.6	0.4	0.9	0.7	51.5	52.3
1951	249	215	0.6	0.5	1.0	0.8	53.9	52.8
1952	386	284	0.9	0.6	1.5	1.0	53.3	52.3
1953	472	396	1.1	0.9	1.9	1.4	55.0	54.7
1954	503	396	1.2	0.9	1.9	1.3	53.3	53.5
1955	470	341	1.1	0.8	1.8	1.1	54.7	53.3
1956	536	369	1.2	0.8	2.0	1.2	53.1	55.0
1957	561	411	1.3	0.9	2.0	1.3	53.5	53.8
1958	554	405	1.2	0.9	1.9	1.2	52.9	54.4
1959	580	426	1.3	0.9	1.9	1.2	53.6	53.7
1960	586	428	1.3	0.9	1.9	1.2	52.5	54.5
1961	617	440	1.3	0.9	2.0	1.2	54.4	53.5
1962	586	489	1.3	1.0	1.8	1.3	52.7	54.1
1963	639	460	1.4	0.9	2.0	1.2	54.4	54.8
1964	583	456	1.2	0.9	1.8	1.2	54.2	55.4
1965	610	434	1.3	0.9	1.8	1.1	54.1	54.1
1966	565	412	1.2	0.8	1.6	1.0	52.9	54.4
1967	538	420	1.1	0.8	1.6	1.0	54.3	53.1
1968	506	414	1.0	0.8	1.4	1.0	52.6	54.0
1969	475	339	0.9	0.7	1.2	0.8	49.5	53.8
1970	537	365	1.1	0.7	1.4	0.8	50.8	53.6
1971	492	338	1.0	0.6	1.3	0.8	51.8	56.1
1972	476	349	0.9	0.6	1.2	0.7	54.9	53.1
1973	479	324	0.9	0.6	1.2	0.7	51.2	53.9
1974	447	344	0.8	0.6	1.1	0.7	54.1	54.1
1975	424	280	0.8	0.5	1.0	0.6	52.6	54.1
1976	398	281	0.7	0.5	0.9	0.5	53.6	54.3
1977	404	280	0.7	0.5	0.9	0.5	52.9	54.5
1978	370	300	0.7	0.5	0.8	0.5	53.9	51.8
1979	334	238	0.6	0.4	0.7	0.4	51.1	52.3
1980	288	221	0.5	0.4	0.6	0.4	51.2	46.4
1981	291	214	0.5	0.4	0.6	0.4	48.4	50.7
1982	275	183	0.5	0.3	0.5	0.3	49.1	54.5
1983	279	203	0.5	0.3	0.5	0.3	49.6	49.9
1984	248	185	0.4	0.3	0.5	0.3	49.4	51.7
1985	278	209	0.5	0.3	0.5	0.3	48.5	52.3
1986	239	201	0.4	0.3	0.4	0.3	46.7	51.4
1987	282	195	0.5	0.3	0.5	0.3	48.7	52.0
1988	262	172	0.4	0.3	0.4	0.2	48.5	51.7
1989	261	197	0.4	0.3	0.4	0.3	44.8	52.0
1990	265	190	0.4	0.3	0.4	0.3	47.8	52.2
1991	247	189	0.4	0.3	0.4	0.3	49.1	53.5
1992	264	175	0.4	0.3	0.4	0.2	50.3	56.2
1993	220	167	0.4	0.3	0.3	0.2	47.2	55.9
1994	272	175	0.4	0.3	0.4	0.2	49.5	52.8
1995	225	143	0.4	0.2	0.4	0.2	47.4	53.5
1996	239	148	0.4	0.2	0.4	0.2	50.0	48.0
1997	215	183	0.4	0.3	0.3	0.2	48.8	53.8
1998	204	170	0.3	0.3	0.3	0.2	49.2	54.9
1999	227	173	0.4	0.3	0.3	0.2	51.0	57.2
2000	218	159	0.4	0.3	0.3	0.2	52.4	53.6

[a] Standardized on the age distribution of the model population for the year 1985 in Japan.

TABLE II-13. Cancer Mortality Statistics in Japan (1950–2000)
Cancer of the skin (ICD, 10th revision: C43, C44)

Year	No. of deaths		Crude death rate per 100,000		Age-adjusted death rate per 100,000[a]		Average age at death in years	
	Male	Female	Male	Female	Male	Female	Male	Female
1950	292	225	0.7	0.5	1.5	0.9	59.4	59.4
1951	226	239	0.5	0.6	1.1	1.0	60.7	63.0
1952	286	277	0.7	0.6	1.4	1.1	61.1	61.4
1953	279	236	0.7	0.5	1.4	0.9	60.1	63.2
1954	288	272	0.7	0.6	1.4	1.0	61.9	60.7
1955	300	263	0.7	0.6	1.3	1.0	60.5	63.0
1956	308	279	0.7	0.6	1.5	1.0	63.3	63.9
1957	303	310	0.7	0.7	1.4	1.1	62.7	63.7
1958	320	311	0.7	0.7	1.5	1.1	64.8	63.9
1959	344	297	0.8	0.6	1.5	1.0	63.3	64.2
1960	300	310	0.7	0.7	1.3	1.0	64.3	65.6
1961	297	287	0.6	0.6	1.3	0.9	63.2	64.8
1962	328	322	0.7	0.7	1.4	1.0	63.6	65.6
1963	331	319	0.7	0.7	1.3	1.0	62.4	67.9
1964	335	269	0.7	0.5	1.3	0.8	65.2	67.1
1965	325	301	0.7	0.6	1.2	0.9	64.0	68.7
1966	320	306	0.7	0.6	1.2	0.9	64.3	66.7
1967	333	354	0.7	0.7	1.2	1.0	64.7	68.8
1968	352	304	0.7	0.6	1.2	0.8	64.5	67.4
1969	374	301	0.7	0.6	1.3	0.8	65.5	68.2
1970	381	326	0.8	0.6	1.3	0.8	65.1	69.1
1971	362	345	0.7	0.6	1.2	0.9	66.0	69.9
1972	383	324	0.7	0.6	1.2	0.8	64.7	68.2
1973	401	349	0.8	0.6	1.2	0.8	65.6	68.6
1974	378	326	0.7	0.6	1.1	0.7	66.7	68.5
1975	371	333	0.7	0.6	1.0	0.7	66.1	69.0
1976	425	319	0.8	0.6	1.1	0.7	66.0	69.4
1977	409	376	0.7	0.7	1.1	0.7	66.1	68.5
1978	395	353	0.7	0.6	1.0	0.7	67.2	70.8
1979	333	286	0.6	0.5	0.8	0.5	66.0	70.7
1980	327	292	0.6	0.5	0.8	0.5	66.5	71.8
1981	348	293	0.6	0.5	0.8	0.5	67.1	70.6
1982	343	278	0.6	0.5	0.8	0.4	68.2	70.2
1983	324	267	0.6	0.4	0.7	0.4	67.3	70.8
1984	357	289	0.6	0.5	0.7	0.4	67.1	70.8
1985	367	312	0.6	0.5	0.7	0.4	66.5	72.5
1986	335	255	0.6	0.4	0.6	0.3	67.6	72.1
1987	345	338	0.6	0.5	0.6	0.4	67.7	71.5
1988	359	277	0.6	0.4	0.6	0.4	67.4	70.3
1989	343	297	0.6	0.5	0.6	0.4	68.3	71.0
1990	381	304	0.6	0.5	0.6	0.4	69.2	73.6
1991	328	330	0.5	0.5	0.5	0.4	68.4	71.7
1992	379	342	0.6	0.5	0.6	0.4	68.5	72.4
1993	372	345	0.6	0.5	0.6	0.4	69.1	72.6
1994	345	307	0.6	0.5	0.5	0.3	69.7	75.6
1995	451	418	0.7	0.7	0.6	0.4	69.4	73.5
1996	469	461	0.8	0.7	0.7	0.4	69.6	74.3
1997	473	427	0.8	0.7	0.6	0.4	69.3	75.3
1998	459	472	0.7	0.7	0.6	0.4	71.0	75.3
1999	482	440	0.8	0.7	0.6	0.4	70.2	76.3
2000	502	484	0.8	0.8	0.6	0.4	70.6	76.6

[a] Standardized on the age distribution of the model population for the year 1985 in Japan.

TABLE II-14. Cancer Mortality Statistics in Japan (1950–2000)
Cancer of the breast (ICD, 10th revision: C50)

Year	No. of deaths		Crude death rate per 100,000		Age-adjusted death rate per 100,000[a]		Average age at death in years	
	Male	Female	Male	Female	Male	Female	Male	Female
1950	29	1,419	0.1	3.3	0.1	5.4	59.9	55.8
1951	20	1,402	0.0	3.3	0.1	5.2	58.3	55.6
1952	35	1,446	0.1	3.3	0.2	5.3	61.6	55.5
1953	17	1,452	0.0	3.3	0.1	5.2	57.5	55.7
1954	26	1,526	0.1	3.4	0.1	5.2	61.0	55.1
1955	17	1,572	0.0	3.5	0.1	5.3	69.0	56.2
1956	17	1,544	0.0	3.4	0.1	5.1	62.5	56.7
1957	21	1,458	0.0	3.1	0.1	4.7	64.2	56.4
1958	14	1,692	0.0	3.6	0.1	5.3	65.0	55.8
1959	21	1,652	0.0	3.5	0.1	5.1	62.0	55.8
1960	20	1,683	0.0	3.5	0.1	5.1	61.5	56.4
1961	23	1,741	0.0	3.6	0.1	5.1	67.7	56.3
1962	18	1,740	0.0	3.6	0.1	4.9	65.8	55.8
1963	22	1,857	0.0	3.8	0.1	5.1	66.6	55.5
1964	18	1,853	0.0	3.7	0.1	5.0	68.1	55.9
1965	29	1,966	0.1	3.9	0.1	5.2	64.4	55.4
1966	29	2,100	0.1	4.2	0.1	5.4	64.9	55.6
1967	24	2,107	0.0	4.2	0.1	5.3	66.0	55.9
1968	36	2,248	0.1	4.4	0.1	5.5	66.1	55.9
1969	29	2,208	0.1	4.3	0.1	5.3	62.0	56.1
1970	23	2,486	0.0	4.7	0.1	5.8	64.9	56.3
1971	29	2,689	0.1	5.1	0.1	6.0	65.4	55.6
1972	31	2,762	0.1	5.1	0.1	6.1	65.9	56.0
1973	31	2,995	0.1	5.4	0.1	6.3	67.5	56.1
1974	22	3,059	0.0	5.5	0.1	6.3	67.5	55.8
1975	27	3,262	0.0	5.8	0.1	6.5	65.8	55.9
1976	22	3,347	0.0	5.9	0.1	6.5	71.1	56.2
1977	39	3,570	0.1	6.2	0.1	6.8	68.3	56.6
1978	33	3,755	0.1	6.5	0.1	6.9	71.0	56.8
1979	44	3,878	0.1	6.6	0.1	7.0	67.6	56.6
1980	44	4,141	0.1	7.0	0.1	7.2	66.0	56.9
1981	44	4,364	0.1	7.3	0.1	7.5	70.0	57.1
1982	31	4,311	0.1	7.2	0.1	7.2	68.0	57.5
1983	35	4,417	0.1	7.3	0.1	7.2	68.9	57.5
1984	38	4,825	0.1	7.9	0.1	7.7	68.2	57.5
1985	36	4,922	0.1	8.0	0.1	7.6	70.3	57.8
1986	37	5,127	0.1	8.3	0.1	7.8	69.4	57.9
1987	44	5,231	0.1	8.5	0.1	7.8	68.4	58.3
1988	43	5,602	0.1	9.0	0.1	8.1	68.8	58.2
1989	54	5,746	0.1	9.2	0.1	8.2	72.4	58.3
1990	34	5,848	0.1	9.4	0.1	8.2	70.7	58.5
1991	43	6,309	0.1	10.1	0.1	8.7	74.0	58.9
1992	56	6,451	0.1	10.3	0.1	8.7	70.2	59.2
1993	56	6,758	0.1	10.7	0.1	8.9	66.0	59.6
1994	64	7,131	0.1	11.3	0.1	9.3	72.0	59.7
1995	56	7,763	0.1	12.2	0.1	9.9	70.9	60.1
1996	63	7,900	0.1	12.4	0.1	9.9	69.7	60.7
1997	73	8,393	0.1	13.2	0.1	10.4	71.6	60.7
1998	76	8,589	0.1	13.4	0.1	10.4	73.8	60.9
1999	67	8,882	0.1	13.9	0.1	10.5	70.8	61.7
2000	77	9,171	0.1	14.3	0.1	10.7	74.2	61.8

[a] Standardized on the age distribution of the model population for the year 1985 in Japan.

TABLE II-15. Cancer Mortality Statistics in Japan (1950–2000)
Cancer of the uterus (ICD, 10th revision: C53–C55, C58)

Year	No. of deaths	Crude death rate per 100,000	Age-adjusted death rate per 100,000[a]	Average age at death in years
1950	8,356	19.7	31.0	54.1
1951	8,197	19.0	29.9	54.3
1952	8,061	18.4	28.8	54.8
1953	7,638	17.2	26.8	55.4
1954	7,703	17.2	26.4	55.6
1955	7,289	16.0	24.6	56.4
1956	7,343	16.0	24.1	56.3
1957	7,144	15.4	23.0	56.4
1958	7,105	15.2	22.4	57.0
1959	6,999	14.8	21.5	57.1
1960	7,068	14.9	21.3	57.4
1961	6,964	14.5	20.4	57.7
1962	6,940	14.3	19.9	57.8
1963	6,940	14.2	19.4	58.0
1964	6,736	13.6	18.4	58.2
1965	6,689	13.4	18.0	58.9
1966	6,667	13.2	17.5	58.8
1967	6,668	13.1	17.1	59.1
1968	6,610	12.9	16.5	59.4
1969	6,534	12.6	15.9	59.8
1970	6,373	12.1	15.1	60.1
1971	6,194	11.7	14.3	60.5
1972	6,332	11.7	14.2	61.0
1973	6,056	11.0	13.1	61.2
1974	6,149	11.0	12.9	61.7
1975	6,075	10.7	12.4	62.3
1976	5,879	10.3	11.6	62.6
1977	5,694	9.9	10.9	63.2
1978	5,710	9.8	10.6	63.5
1979	5,644	9.6	10.2	64.0
1980	5,465	9.2	9.5	64.5
1981	5,354	9.0	9.1	64.7
1982	5,179	8.6	8.5	65.1
1983	5,133	8.5	8.1	65.4
1984	4,975	8.2	7.6	65.9
1985	4,912	8.0	7.3	65.8
1986	4,744	7.7	6.8	66.0
1987	4,614	7.5	6.4	66.1
1988	4,724	7.6	6.4	66.8
1989	4,632	7.4	6.1	66.9
1990	4,600	7.4	5.8	67.2
1991	4,610	7.4	5.7	67.1
1992	4,665	7.4	5.6	67.1
1993	4,445	7.0	5.2	67.5
1994	4,575	7.2	5.2	67.4
1995	4,877	7.7	5.4	67.8
1996	4,984	7.8	5.5	67.6
1997	5,008	7.9	5.3	68.2
1998	5,015	7.8	5.3	67.9
1999	5,159	8.1	5.3	68.1
2000	5,216	8.1	5.3	67.5

[a] Standardized on the age distribution of the model population for the year 1985 in Japan.

TABLE II-16. Cancer Mortality Statistics in Japan (1950–2000)
Cancer of the ovary (ICD, 10th revision: C56)

Year	No. of deaths	Crude death rate per 100,000	Age-adjusted death rate per 100,000[a]	Average age at death in years
1950	346	0.8	1.2	47.7
1951	326	0.8	1.1	48.7
1952	329	0.8	1.0	46.0
1953	400	0.9	1.3	47.1
1954	449	1.0	1.4	48.0
1955	473	1.0	1.4	48.3
1956	533	1.2	1.6	47.8
1957	553	1.2	1.6	47.8
1958	557	1.2	1.6	48.5
1959	641	1.4	1.8	48.5
1960	647	1.4	1.7	48.3
1961	731	1.5	2.0	49.6
1962	743	1.5	1.9	49.0
1963	829	1.7	2.1	48.6
1964	842	1.7	2.1	49.6
1965	840	1.7	2.1	50.1
1966	935	1.9	2.3	50.3
1967	964	1.9	2.3	51.2
1968	1,052	2.1	2.4	50.8
1969	1,090	2.1	2.5	50.6
1970	1,129	2.1	2.5	51.7
1971	1,244	2.3	2.7	52.3
1972	1,299	2.4	2.8	53.1
1973	1,392	2.5	2.9	53.5
1974	1,428	2.5	2.9	53.7
1975	1,516	2.7	3.0	54.0
1976	1,730	3.0	3.3	53.9
1977	1,788	3.1	3.4	55.4
1978	1,963	3.4	3.6	56.0
1979	2,070	3.5	3.7	56.4
1980	2,098	3.5	3.7	57.1
1981	2,305	3.9	3.9	57.2
1982	2,349	3.9	3.9	57.5
1983	2,434	4.0	3.9	58.4
1984	2,561	4.2	4.1	58.7
1985	2,675	4.4	4.1	59.1
1986	2,686	4.4	4.0	60.5
1987	3,052	4.9	4.4	61.1
1988	3,118	5.0	4.4	61.3
1989	3,251	5.2	4.5	61.9
1990	3,279	5.2	4.4	61.7
1991	3,379	5.4	4.5	62.3
1992	3,514	5.6	4.5	62.4
1993	3,518	5.6	4.4	62.4
1994	3,871	6.1	4.7	63.2
1995	3,892	6.1	4.6	63.6
1996	4,006	6.3	4.7	63.9
1997	4,194	6.6	4.8	64.2
1998	4,173	6.5	4.6	65.0
1999	4,076	6.4	4.5	65.0
2000	3,993	6.2	4.3	65.2

[a] Standardized on the age distribution of the model population for the year 1985 in Japan.

TABLE II-17. Cancer Mortality Statistics in Japan (1950–2000)
Cancer of the prostate (ICD, 10th revision: C61)

Year	No. of deaths	Crude death rate per 100,000	Age-adjusted death rate per 100,000[a]	Average age at death in years
1950	83	0.2	0.5	66.5
1951	128	0.3	0.6	64.5
1952	147	0.3	0.8	67.5
1953	196	0.5	1.0	67.6
1954	235	0.5	1.1	65.8
1955	273	0.6	1.3	68.1
1956	305	0.7	1.5	69.3
1957	358	0.8	1.8	69.6
1958	431	1.0	2.1	70.6
1959	453	1.0	2.2	70.9
1960	480	1.0	2.2	71.0
1961	487	1.1	2.3	71.8
1962	578	1.2	2.5	70.5
1963	599	1.3	2.6	71.1
1964	703	1.5	3.0	72.4
1965	683	1.4	2.8	71.1
1966	717	1.5	2.9	72.2
1967	730	1.5	2.9	72.0
1968	825	1.7	3.1	72.2
1969	937	1.9	3.4	72.3
1970	883	1.7	3.2	72.6
1971	886	1.7	3.0	72.6
1972	975	1.9	3.3	72.8
1973	1,107	2.1	3.6	73.5
1974	1,179	2.2	3.7	73.3
1975	1,267	2.3	3.8	73.7
1976	1,296	2.3	3.8	73.6
1977	1,448	2.6	4.1	74.5
1978	1,499	2.7	4.0	74.5
1979	1,666	2.9	4.4	74.9
1980	1,736	3.0	4.4	75.0
1981	1,866	3.2	4.6	75.4
1982	2,053	3.5	4.8	75.7
1983	2,168	3.7	4.9	76.1
1984	2,315	3.9	5.1	76.3
1985	2,640	4.5	5.5	76.8
1986	2,756	4.6	5.6	76.4
1987	2,969	5.0	5.8	76.9
1988	3,035	5.1	5.7	77.0
1989	3,420	5.7	6.1	76.6
1990	3,460	5.7	6.0	77.2
1991	3,836	6.3	6.4	77.3
1992	4,073	6.7	6.5	77.0
1993	4,262	7.0	6.6	77.4
1994	4,730	7.8	7.0	77.6
1995	5,399	8.9	7.7	77.9
1996	6,009	9.8	8.2	78.1
1997	6,251	10.2	8.2	78.4
1998	6,819	11.1	8.6	78.5
1999	7,005	11.4	8.5	78.8
2000	7,514	12.2	8.6	78.6

[a] Standardized on the age distribution of the model population for the year 1985 in Japan.

TABLE II-18. Cancer Mortality Statistics in Japan (1950–2000)
Cancer of the urinary bladder (ICD, 10th revision: C67)

Year	No. of deaths		Crude death rate per 100,000		Age-adjusted death rate per 100,000[a]		Average age at death in years	
	Male	Female	Male	Female	Male	Female	Male	Female
1950	311	203	0.8	0.5	1.7	0.8	64.8	62.5
1951	357	218	0.9	0.5	1.8	0.8	65.1	62.6
1952	348	263	0.8	0.6	1.7	1.0	65.5	64.0
1953	401	267	0.9	0.6	2.0	1.0	66.5	63.4
1954	509	292	1.2	0.7	2.5	1.1	65.9	63.5
1955	528	309	1.2	0.7	2.6	1.1	66.9	65.2
1956	554	352	1.2	0.8	2.6	1.2	67.2	64.7
1957	538	384	1.2	0.8	2.5	1.3	68.0	65.5
1958	612	331	1.4	0.7	2.7	1.1	67.1	66.7
1959	646	379	1.4	0.8	2.9	1.3	68.0	65.8
1960	673	435	1.5	0.9	2.9	1.4	68.7	67.4
1961	736	407	1.6	0.8	3.1	1.3	67.8	67.5
1962	794	466	1.7	1.0	3.3	1.4	68.7	67.3
1963	770	448	1.6	0.9	3.1	1.4	68.6	68.0
1964	810	440	1.7	0.9	3.2	1.3	68.3	68.8
1965	837	454	1.7	0.9	3.2	1.3	68.3	67.2
1966	929	506	1.9	1.0	3.4	1.4	68.4	69.0
1967	951	534	1.9	1.1	3.5	1.5	69.4	68.9
1968	1,005	524	2.0	1.0	3.5	1.4	69.0	68.2
1969	1,019	577	2.0	1.1	3.6	1.5	69.5	69.4
1970	1,030	540	2.0	1.0	3.4	1.4	68.8	69.8
1971	1,000	595	2.0	1.1	3.3	1.5	69.6	70.3
1972	1,177	621	2.3	1.2	3.8	1.5	69.6	70.7
1973	1,198	621	2.3	1.1	3.7	1.4	70.5	70.8
1974	1,267	603	2.3	1.1	3.8	1.3	70.6	71.2
1975	1,174	656	2.1	1.2	3.4	1.4	70.6	72.2
1976	1,304	662	2.4	1.2	3.7	1.4	70.8	72.4
1977	1,373	640	2.5	1.1	3.7	1.3	70.9	72.3
1978	1,440	638	2.6	1.1	3.7	1.2	70.9	73.0
1979	1,515	676	2.7	1.2	3.8	1.2	71.8	73.4
1980	1,606	755	2.8	1.3	3.9	1.3	72.1	73.9
1981	1,615	732	2.8	1.2	3.8	1.2	72.5	74.4
1982	1,671	750	2.9	1.3	3.8	1.2	72.1	74.8
1983	1,670	826	2.9	1.4	3.7	1.3	72.6	75.4
1984	1,669	772	2.8	1.3	3.5	1.1	72.9	74.8
1985	1,705	872	2.9	1.4	3.5	1.2	73.2	75.1
1986	1,807	795	3.0	1.3	3.6	1.1	73.4	76.0
1987	1,815	806	3.0	1.3	3.4	1.0	73.6	76.9
1988	1,851	874	3.1	1.4	3.4	1.1	73.9	76.9
1989	1,999	939	3.3	1.5	3.5	1.1	74.5	77.8
1990	2,110	938	3.5	1.5	3.6	1.0	74.6	77.8
1991	2,165	1,008	3.6	1.6	3.6	1.1	74.6	77.7
1992	2,179	1,017	3.6	1.6	3.5	1.0	74.7	78.4
1993	2,217	1,062	3.7	1.7	3.4	1.0	75.0	78.4
1994	2,415	1,116	4.0	1.8	3.6	1.0	75.2	78.4
1995	2,700	1,231	4.4	1.9	3.9	1.1	75.8	79.5
1996	2,785	1,194	4.6	1.9	3.8	1.0	75.5	79.1
1997	2,856	1,277	4.7	2.0	3.8	1.0	76.3	80.0
1998	2,952	1,344	4.8	2.1	3.7	1.0	76.2	79.7
1999	3,296	1,485	5.4	2.3	4.0	1.1	76.3	80.5
2000	3,184	1,496	5.2	2.3	3.7	1.1	76.3	80.2

[a] Standardized on the age distribution of the model population for the year 1985 in Japan.

TABLE II-19. Cancer Mortality Statistics in Japan (1950–2000)
Cancer of the kidney (ICD, 10th revision: C64, C65)

Year	No. of deaths		Crude death rate per 100,000		Age-adjusted death rate per 100,000[a]		Average age at death in years	
	Male	Female	Male	Female	Male	Female	Male	Female
1950	114	91	0.3	0.2	0.4	0.3	44.3	49.4
1951	110	73	0.3	0.2	0.4	0.3	48.9	53.3
1952	116	86	0.3	0.2	0.4	0.3	47.9	50.2
1953	134	94	0.3	0.2	0.5	0.3	53.9	42.2
1954	165	114	0.4	0.3	0.6	0.4	50.8	48.3
1955	150	112	0.3	0.2	0.5	0.4	52.1	51.7
1956	179	145	0.4	0.3	0.6	0.4	51.0	50.9
1957	205	147	0.5	0.3	0.7	0.4	50.2	50.7
1958	220	162	0.5	0.3	0.8	0.5	53.6	49.4
1959	236	157	0.5	0.3	0.8	0.4	52.8	51.1
1960	277	175	0.6	0.4	0.9	0.5	54.7	50.8
1961	251	204	0.5	0.4	0.8	0.6	54.1	51.9
1962	306	202	0.7	0.4	1.0	0.6	55.8	53.2
1963	307	217	0.7	0.4	1.0	0.6	56.3	54.4
1964	333	191	0.7	0.4	1.0	0.5	56.6	53.5
1965	342	210	0.7	0.4	1.0	0.5	55.4	53.5
1966	361	221	0.7	0.4	1.1	0.6	57.9	54.6
1967	392	227	0.8	0.4	1.1	0.6	57.0	54.6
1968	404	229	0.8	0.4	1.2	0.6	56.0	57.2
1969	417	233	0.8	0.4	1.2	0.6	58.5	57.7
1970	436	248	0.9	0.5	1.2	0.6	59.4	56.9
1971	472	251	0.9	0.5	1.3	0.6	59.9	58.6
1972	509	280	1.0	0.5	1.4	0.6	58.7	55.6
1973	556	311	1.0	0.6	1.5	0.7	61.1	57.0
1974	556	307	1.0	0.5	1.4	0.6	60.4	58.5
1975	618	322	1.1	0.6	1.5	0.7	62.1	64.0
1976	643	307	1.2	0.5	1.6	0.6	60.9	62.1
1977	674	309	1.2	0.5	1.6	0.6	61.9	61.9
1978	754	401	1.3	0.7	1.7	0.7	62.2	62.7
1979	812	414	1.4	0.7	1.8	0.7	63.2	64.0
1980	944	422	1.7	0.7	2.1	0.7	63.9	63.6
1981	932	460	1.6	0.8	2.0	0.8	64.5	64.2
1982	1,079	491	1.9	0.8	2.3	0.8	64.3	63.8
1983	1,151	530	2.0	0.9	2.3	0.8	65.4	66.5
1984	1,275	566	2.2	0.9	2.5	0.9	65.5	67.2
1985	1,338	629	2.3	1.0	2.6	0.9	65.1	67.2
1986	1,384	682	2.3	1.1	2.6	1.0	66.0	69.0
1987	1,477	713	2.5	1.2	2.7	1.0	66.1	68.9
1988	1,580	731	2.6	1.2	2.8	1.0	67.2	70.0
1989	1,608	755	2.7	1.2	2.7	1.0	67.5	70.6
1990	1,763	850	2.9	1.4	2.9	1.0	67.4	70.2
1991	1,876	811	3.1	1.3	3.0	1.0	67.8	70.3
1992	1,907	895	3.1	1.4	3.0	1.0	67.6	70.9
1993	2,045	952	3.4	1.5	3.1	1.0	68.2	72.3
1994	2,097	1,005	3.4	1.6	3.1	1.1	68.5	72.3
1995	2,240	1,062	3.7	1.7	3.2	1.1	69.0	72.4
1996	2,367	1,128	3.9	1.8	3.2	1.1	69.1	72.5
1997	2,436	1,084	4.0	1.7	3.2	1.0	69.2	74.0
1998	2,554	1,192	4.2	1.9	3.3	1.1	69.8	72.8
1999	2,601	1,280	4.2	2.0	3.2	1.1	70.1	74.5
2000	2,583	1,280	4.2	2.0	3.1	1.1	70.2	74.3

[a] Standardized on the age distribution of the model population for the year 1985 in Japan.

TABLE II-20. Cancer Mortality Statistics in Japan (1950–2000)
Cancer of the lymphatic and hematopoietic systems other than leukemia (ICD, 10th revision: C81-C90, C96)

Year	No. of deaths		Crude death rate per 100,000		Age-adjusted death rate per 100,000[a]		Average age at death in years	
	Male	Female	Male	Female	Male	Female	Male	Female
1950	472	307	1.2	0.7	1.7	1.0	46.0	47.5
1951	512	316	1.2	0.7	1.8	1.1	46.0	48.1
1952	591	346	1.4	0.8	2.0	1.1	45.2	47.2
1953	633	366	1.5	0.8	2.2	1.1	46.9	46.6
1954	619	436	1.4	1.0	2.1	1.4	47.5	48.4
1955	718	430	1.6	0.9	2.4	1.3	48.1	47.4
1956	723	446	1.6	1.0	2.3	1.3	46.6	49.5
1957	756	447	1.7	1.0	2.4	1.3	48.3	48.3
1958	816	495	1.8	1.1	2.6	1.4	47.6	49.4
1959	919	563	2.0	1.2	2.9	1.6	48.9	51.4
1960	961	560	2.1	1.2	3.0	1.6	49.5	53.1
1961	1,009	619	2.2	1.3	3.2	1.7	50.6	52.6
1962	1,025	632	2.2	1.3	3.1	1.7	50.5	51.8
1963	1,158	697	2.5	1.4	3.3	1.9	49.3	53.5
1964	1,245	726	2.6	1.5	3.6	1.9	51.0	53.3
1965	1,283	763	2.7	1.5	3.7	1.9	51.7	52.0
1966	1,398	822	2.9	1.6	4.0	2.1	53.3	53.8
1967	1,518	848	3.1	1.7	4.2	2.1	52.4	53.3
1968	1,601	1,027	3.2	2.0	4.5	2.5	54.8	54.9
1969	1,652	1,075	3.3	2.1	4.4	2.5	53.3	56.1
1970	1,649	1,034	3.3	2.0	4.4	2.4	55.1	56.9
1971	1,711	1,057	3.3	2.0	4.5	2.4	55.8	57.5
1972	1,974	1,196	3.8	2.2	5.1	2.6	55.5	57.6
1973	1,933	1,279	3.6	2.3	4.9	2.7	56.0	57.8
1974	2,112	1,323	3.9	2.4	5.2	2.7	57.4	59.5
1975	2,272	1,450	4.2	2.6	5.4	2.9	57.2	59.6
1976	2,364	1,513	4.3	2.7	5.6	2.9	57.6	59.6
1977	2,528	1,599	4.5	2.8	5.8	3.0	58.4	61.4
1978	2,605	1,674	4.6	2.9	5.9	3.1	59.3	61.3
1979	2,731	1,844	4.8	3.1	6.0	3.3	59.7	61.7
1980	2,939	1,953	5.1	3.3	6.3	3.4	60.0	62.8
1981	3,001	2,133	5.2	3.6	6.3	3.6	60.7	64.0
1982	3,096	2,183	5.3	3.6	6.4	3.6	61.6	64.1
1983	3,387	2,264	5.8	3.8	6.8	3.6	61.6	63.9
1984	3,337	2,432	5.7	4.0	6.5	3.7	62.1	65.2
1985	3,552	2,450	6.0	4.0	6.8	3.6	63.7	66.5
1986	3,683	2,682	6.2	4.4	6.8	3.8	63.7	66.8
1987	3,816	2,792	6.4	4.5	6.9	3.8	64.2	67.5
1988	3,823	2,854	6.4	4.6	6.7	3.8	64.9	68.0
1989	3,936	2,932	6.5	4.7	6.7	3.8	65.7	68.5
1990	4,259	3,100	7.1	5.0	7.0	3.9	65.7	68.6
1991	4,348	3,270	7.2	5.2	7.0	3.9	66.4	69.1
1992	4,523	3,332	7.5	5.3	7.1	3.9	66.7	69.9
1993	4,505	3,495	7.4	5.5	6.9	3.9	67.1	70.0
1994	4,725	3,796	7.8	6.0	7.0	4.1	67.7	70.5
1995	5,300	4,050	8.7	6.4	7.6	4.2	67.9	71.6
1996	5,532	4,228	9.1	6.6	7.7	4.2	68.7	71.9
1997	5,527	4,455	9.0	7.0	7.4	4.3	68.9	72.4
1998	5,892	4,553	9.6	7.1	7.7	4.3	69.4	72.4
1999	6,178	4,788	10.1	7.5	7.8	4.3	69.8	72.8
2000	6,352	4,991	10.3	7.8	7.7	4.4	70.0	72.9

[a] Standardized on the age distribution of the model population for the year 1985 in Japan.

TABLE II-21. Cancer Mortality Statistics in Japan (1950–2000)
Leukemia (ICD, 10th revision: C91–C95)

Year	No. of deaths		Crude death rate per 100,000		Age-adjusted death rate per 100,000[a]		Average age at death in years	
	Male	Female	Male	Female	Male	Female	Male	Female
1950	718	508	1.8	1.2	1.8	1.1	26.2	25.2
1951	787	548	1.9	1.3	1.9	1.2	26.3	25.6
1952	796	634	1.9	1.5	1.8	1.4	24.6	26.7
1953	936	723	2.2	1.6	2.2	1.6	27.4	27.4
1954	1,122	747	2.6	1.7	2.6	1.7	26.5	28.0
1955	1,214	824	2.8	1.8	2.7	1.8	26.4	26.7
1956	1,273	900	2.9	2.0	2.9	2.0	28.0	28.5
1957	1,251	971	2.8	2.1	2.9	2.1	29.7	28.6
1958	1,363	1,075	3.0	2.3	3.1	2.4	28.8	30.1
1959	1,380	1,106	3.0	2.3	3.1	2.5	29.6	31.3
1960	1,473	1,155	3.2	2.4	3.4	2.5	30.7	29.9
1961	1,504	1,218	3.2	2.5	3.4	2.7	30.7	32.7
1962	1,606	1,306	3.4	2.7	3.5	2.8	30.5	31.6
1963	1,640	1,316	3.5	2.7	3.7	2.8	31.4	32.2
1964	1,696	1,404	3.6	2.8	3.8	3.0	33.1	33.8
1965	1,765	1,394	3.7	2.8	3.9	2.9	32.8	33.1
1966	1,801	1,465	3.7	2.9	4.0	3.0	33.9	33.8
1967	1,804	1,498	3.7	3.0	4.0	3.1	34.7	35.4
1968	1,848	1,486	3.7	2.9	4.0	3.0	35.4	35.1
1969	1,865	1,561	3.7	3.0	4.1	3.1	36.7	36.3
1970	2,005	1,554	4.0	3.0	4.3	3.1	36.7	36.6
1971	1,957	1,592	3.8	3.0	4.2	3.1	37.7	37.2
1972	2,073	1,735	4.0	3.2	4.4	3.4	38.2	38.3
1973	2,185	1,694	4.1	3.1	4.5	3.2	38.6	39.9
1974	2,223	1,739	4.1	3.1	4.6	3.2	40.2	39.5
1975	2,321	1,843	4.2	3.3	4.7	3.4	40.2	40.9
1976	2,458	1,844	4.4	3.2	5.0	3.3	41.6	42.0
1977	2,527	1,884	4.5	3.3	5.0	3.3	42.5	42.5
1978	2,505	1,849	4.4	3.2	5.0	3.3	44.5	44.1
1979	2,568	1,976	4.5	3.4	5.0	3.4	44.9	46.2
1980	2,624	1,943	4.6	3.3	5.1	3.3	46.0	46.0
1981	2,713	1,978	4.7	3.3	5.2	3.3	47.1	48.0
1982	2,789	2,074	4.8	3.5	5.3	3.4	49.5	49.9
1983	2,783	2,110	4.8	3.5	5.2	3.4	49.6	50.7
1984	2,943	2,269	5.0	3.7	5.4	3.6	51.3	52.0
1985	2,983	2,196	5.0	3.6	5.4	3.4	51.6	52.4
1986	3,116	2,290	5.2	3.7	5.5	3.5	53.1	54.3
1987	3,334	2,308	5.6	3.7	5.8	3.4	53.6	55.4
1988	3,223	2,358	5.4	3.8	5.5	3.4	55.3	54.9
1989	3,397	2,379	5.6	3.8	5.7	3.4	54.8	56.0
1990	3,225	2,408	5.4	3.9	5.3	3.4	55.5	56.9
1991	3,190	2,395	5.3	3.8	5.1	3.2	57.0	58.9
1992	3,360	2,356	5.5	3.7	5.3	3.1	56.9	58.8
1993	3,350	2,469	5.5	3.9	5.2	3.2	57.9	58.4
1994	3,348	2,562	5.5	4.1	5.1	3.2	59.0	60.4
1995	3,645	2,484	6.0	3.9	5.4	3.0	59.6	61.3
1996	3,617	2,658	5.9	4.2	5.2	3.1	60.5	63.2
1997	3,649	2,707	6.0	4.2	5.1	3.1	62.2	63.2
1998	3,781	2,765	6.2	4.3	5.2	3.1	62.0	64.4
1999	3,885	2,815	6.3	4.4	5.2	3.1	62.3	64.8
2000	3,970	2,796	6.5	4.4	5.2	3.0	63.3	65.4

[a] Standardized on the age distribution of the model population for the year 1985 in Japan.

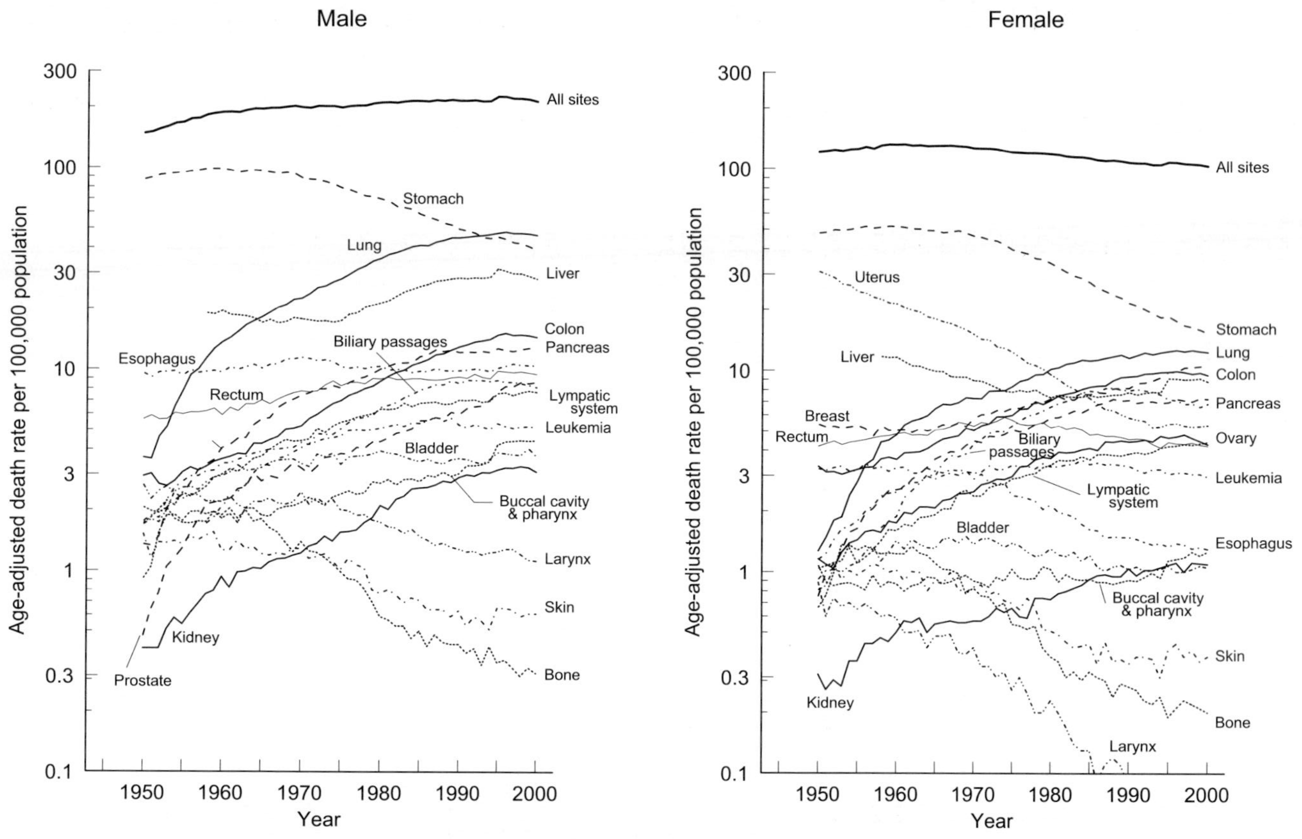

FIG. 2-1. Trends in the age-adjusted death rates* from cancer for selected sites in Japan (1950–2000)
*standardized on the age distribution of the 'model' population for the year 1985 in Japan

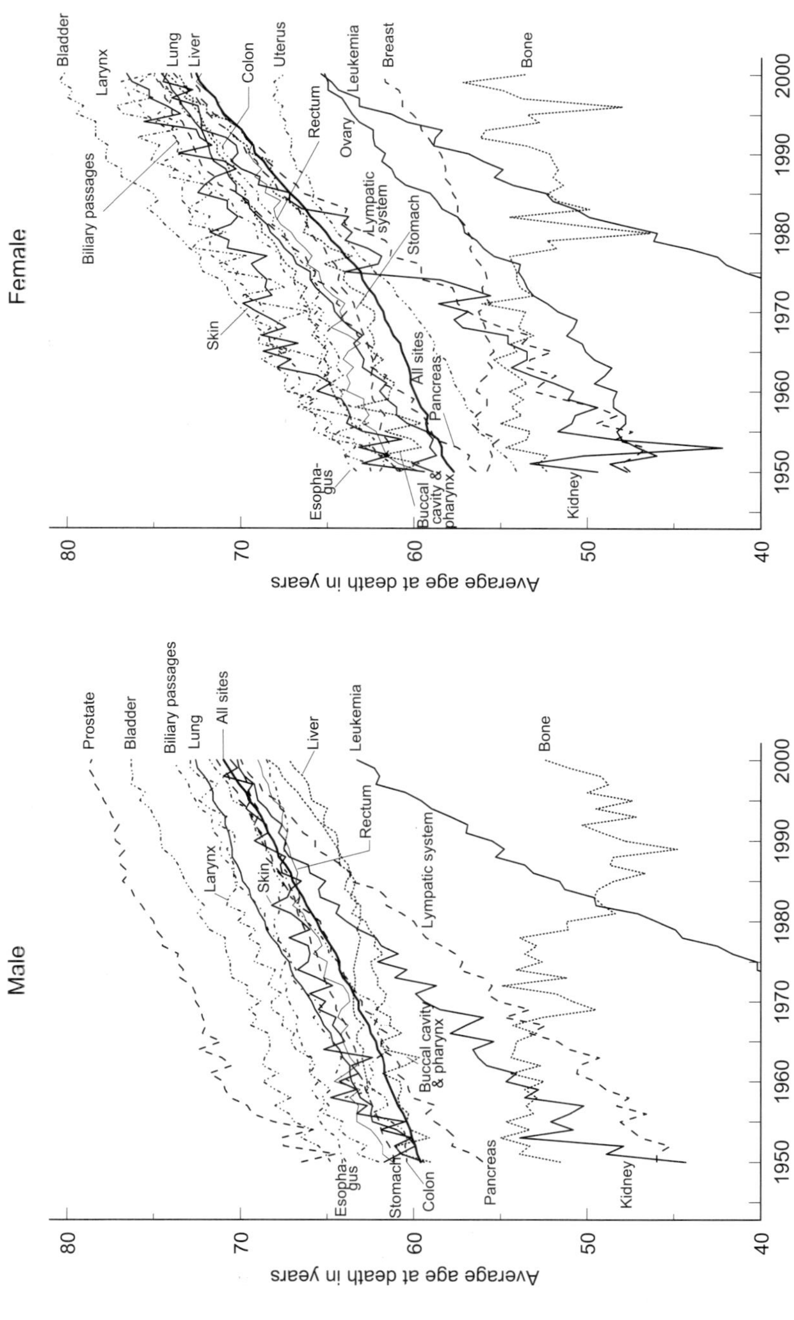

FIG. 2-2. Trends in the average age at death in years for selected sites in Japan (1950–2000)

TABLE III-1. Age- and Sex-specific Cancer Mortality Rates in Japan (1950–2000)
Cancer of all sites (ICD, 10th revision: C00–C97)

	1950	1955	1960	1965	1970	1975	1980	1985	1990	1995	2000
Male											
0–4	5.7	6.9	8.7	8.5	8.5	7.8	6.0	4.2	3.8	2.9	2.6
5–9	2.7	4.4	4.8	6.1	5.6	5.5	5.7	4.7	3.3	3.7	2.7
10–14	2.9	4.0	4.8	5.3	4.7	4.7	4.8	4.2	3.8	3.3	2.2
15–19	4.1	5.3	6.2	7.2	7.3	6.5	6.4	6.2	5.4	5.1	3.7
20–24	4.6	5.7	6.9	8.7	8.8	8.5	6.5	5.9	6.1	5.2	4.6
25–29	7.7	9.0	10.0	12.5	12.7	11.3	10.9	9.0	8.1	8.1	6.1
30–34	15.0	17.3	18.7	19.8	20.7	19.3	17.3	15.1	12.4	11.8	11.1
35–39	29.1	33.5	33.4	35.4	36.0	33.4	32.7	29.1	26.4	22.9	19.1
40–44	63.4	65.2	65.0	60.3	63.0	60.7	55.9	53.8	49.2	47.2	41.9
45–49	116.4	126.5	124.2	119.7	114.2	112.6	118.4	102.7	98.3	94.1	87.0
50–54	211.8	218.7	230.4	219.6	205.2	187.6	214.3	212.8	181.9	183.4	168.8
55–59	354.0	351.7	386.9	366.3	357.3	345.8	333.7	363.4	372.6	327.0	310.3
60–64	523.1	570.2	592.2	606.8	579.5	541.2	558.8	543.0	596.8	601.3	508.9
65–69	713.1	787.8	858.2	884.8	902.0	853.9	850.5	837.3	828.6	921.6	869.5
70–74	775.1	974.1	1,106.7	1,128.7	1,176.9	1,207.6	1,247.3	1,216.1	1,200.1	1,271.1	1,255.6
75–79	713.5	910.7	1,166.7	1,317.0	1,393.5	1,468.8	1,634.1	1,701.8	1,640.4	1,766.3	1,685.3
80–84	519.9	721.5	996.2	1,234.1	1,359.4	1,535.6	1,850.9	2,070.3	2,149.1	2,359.8	2,312.4
85–	445.1	501.5	726.3	869.3	1,078.6	1,285.0	1,677.2	2,104.8	2,443.5	2,922.0	2,971.9
Female											
0–4	4.2	5.4	6.7	6.6	6.7	6.1	5.0	3.8	3.1	2.9	2.0
5–9	1.9	3.0	3.5	4.3	4.2	4.1	3.8	3.3	2.8	2.3	1.9
10–14	2.0	3.3	4.0	4.0	4.0	3.8	4.0	3.6	2.8	2.5	1.8
15–19	3.3	3.5	5.0	5.2	5.5	4.7	4.7	3.8	3.0	2.9	2.7
20–24	4.9	5.3	7.4	7.8	7.3	6.8	6.0	4.5	4.5	3.1	3.8
25–29	11.6	11.8	12.7	13.6	13.9	12.6	11.8	9.8	7.2	6.4	6.6
30–34	26.4	23.6	26.3	27.0	24.5	24.8	20.8	18.9	16.4	14.5	13.3
35–39	56.0	49.9	49.6	45.5	41.9	38.8	36.7	31.6	32.0	28.4	27.1
40–44	104.8	91.6	84.2	74.0	71.0	63.4	57.3	55.3	49.7	50.2	46.9
45–49	152.4	138.1	138.3	120.6	111.9	101.7	89.8	83.8	80.4	83.3	80.0
50–54	215.5	201.8	189.5	188.6	163.2	156.4	141.5	128.2	118.5	125.7	124.2
55–59	283.7	273.3	270.6	262.3	243.1	221.2	204.2	185.6	175.7	171.2	170.1
60–64	375.4	367.1	369.4	358.1	347.7	308.6	296.4	275.4	248.5	248.9	229.6
65–69	470.6	485.3	495.0	488.7	471.1	446.1	421.8	388.2	362.9	358.5	340.2
70–74	484.3	578.6	636.5	642.7	639.7	615.4	612.1	563.5	527.2	513.4	482.9
75–79	463.4	600.0	714.2	756.0	788.3	773.8	814.4	788.6	741.2	736.9	691.7
80–84	379.6	524.1	667.7	739.2	793.5	850.4	961.8	1,004.7	1,018.8	1,054.4	992.9
85–	295.6	375.9	567.9	557.2	624.2	738.2	893.3	1,117.7	1,268.4	1,421.6	1,458.1

Mortality rates per 100,000 population.

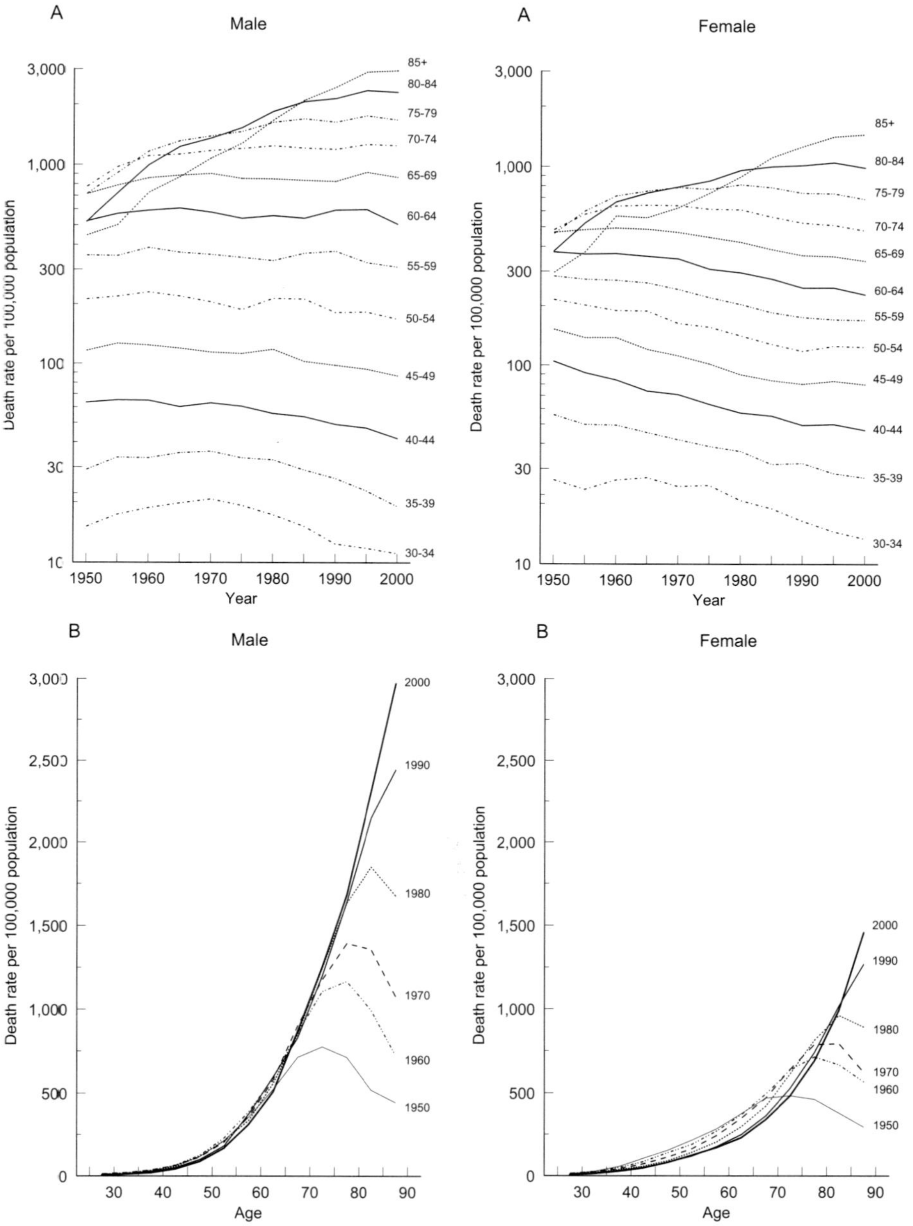

FIG. 3-1. Trends in the age- and sex-specific cancer mortality rate by age group (1950–2000) (A) and by year (1950, 1960, 1970, 1980, 1990, and 2000) (B) in Japan
Cancer of all sites (ICD, 10th revision: C00–C97)

TABLE III-2. Age- and Sex-specific Cancer Mortality Rates in Japan (1950–2000)
Cancer of the buccal cavity and pharynx (ICD, 10th revision: C00–C14)

	1950	1955	1960	1965	1970	1975	1980	1985	1990	1995	2000
Male											
0–4	0.1	0.0	0.0	0.0	0.0	0.0	0.0	0.0	0.0	0.0	0.0
5–9	0.0	0.1	0.0	0.0	0.0	0.0	0.0	0.0	0.0	0.0	0.0
10–14	0.0	0.1	0.0	0.1	0.0	0.1	0.0	0.0	0.0	0.0	0.1
15–19	0.1	0.1	0.0	0.1	0.1	0.0	0.0	0.0	0.1	0.0	0.0
20–24	0.1	0.1	0.0	0.0	0.1	0.1	0.2	0.1	0.1	0.2	0.1
25–29	0.1	0.1	0.1	0.1	0.1	0.1	0.2	0.1	0.2	0.3	0.3
30–34	0.3	0.3	0.3	0.2	0.4	0.3	0.4	0.3	0.3	0.4	0.5
35–39	0.4	0.5	0.4	0.4	0.5	0.7	0.7	0.6	0.5	0.6	0.7
40–44	0.8	0.7	0.7	0.7	1.2	1.0	1.1	1.1	1.2	1.8	1.5
45–49	1.8	0.9	1.9	1.5	1.7	1.9	2.5	2.5	2.7	3.0	3.7
50–54	3.2	2.4	2.5	2.4	2.9	3.2	4.2	4.0	4.1	5.5	5.4
55–59	4.7	3.4	3.8	3.3	4.8	4.9	5.3	5.8	6.9	8.5	9.7
60–64	6.2	4.9	5.4	5.5	6.4	7.1	7.7	7.8	9.5	12.2	12.7
65–69	7.9	7.7	5.4	8.7	9.1	8.9	11.2	11.4	12.5	18.8	18.6
70–74	8.5	8.1	8.9	8.6	9.9	12.2	11.3	13.0	15.4	21.2	21.0
75–79	10.5	12.9	13.8	12.2	12.1	16.5	16.4	16.7	15.0	22.6	27.3
80–84	10.5	9.8	11.2	10.7	11.6	13.0	16.8	18.5	19.5	29.2	30.9
85–	24.3	7.6	8.9	14.9	19.1	16.3	22.7	20.0	21.0	33.7	37.4
Female											
0–4	0.0	0.0	0.0	0.1	0.0	0.0	0.0	0.0	0.0	0.0	0.0
5–9	0.0	0.0	0.0	0.0	0.1	0.0	0.0	0.0	0.0	0.0	0.0
10–14	0.0	0.0	0.0	0.0	0.0	0.0	0.0	0.0	0.0	0.0	0.0
15–19	0.0	0.1	0.0	0.0	0.1	0.0	0.0	0.0	0.1	0.0	0.0
20–24	0.1	0.1	0.2	0.2	0.1	0.0	0.1	0.0	0.0	0.1	0.1
25–29	0.1	0.0	0.1	0.1	0.1	0.2	0.2	0.1	0.1	0.2	0.2
30–34	0.2	0.1	0.2	0.2	0.2	0.2	0.2	0.1	0.1	0.1	0.2
35–39	0.3	0.3	0.2	0.3	0.4	0.3	0.4	0.2	0.2	0.2	0.5
40–44	0.6	0.5	0.5	0.3	0.5	0.5	0.4	0.6	0.5	0.4	0.7
45–49	1.1	0.6	1.1	0.6	0.6	0.8	0.8	0.8	0.7	0.8	0.9
50–54	1.8	1.6	0.7	1.0	1.1	1.3	1.1	0.9	1.0	1.5	1.6
55–59	1.5	1.6	1.7	2.2	1.6	1.8	1.9	1.9	1.3	1.7	1.7
60–64	2.7	2.0	1.3	2.2	2.6	3.3	2.2	1.8	2.3	3.2	3.0
65–69	5.0	2.9	2.9	2.8	2.8	3.3	3.5	3.2	3.1	3.2	3.5
70–74	4.5	3.8	3.0	4.7	4.6	4.1	4.3	3.8	4.1	5.3	5.7
75–79	5.3	4.3	5.0	5.7	6.1	7.2	7.1	6.5	5.1	6.6	7.7
80–84	9.4	7.4	10.2	8.8	5.4	6.8	9.3	8.2	9.5	11.7	12.4
85–	6.0	7.4	10.6	8.0	8.2	11.2	14.9	13.1	13.2	19.8	22.6

Mortality rates per 100,000 population.

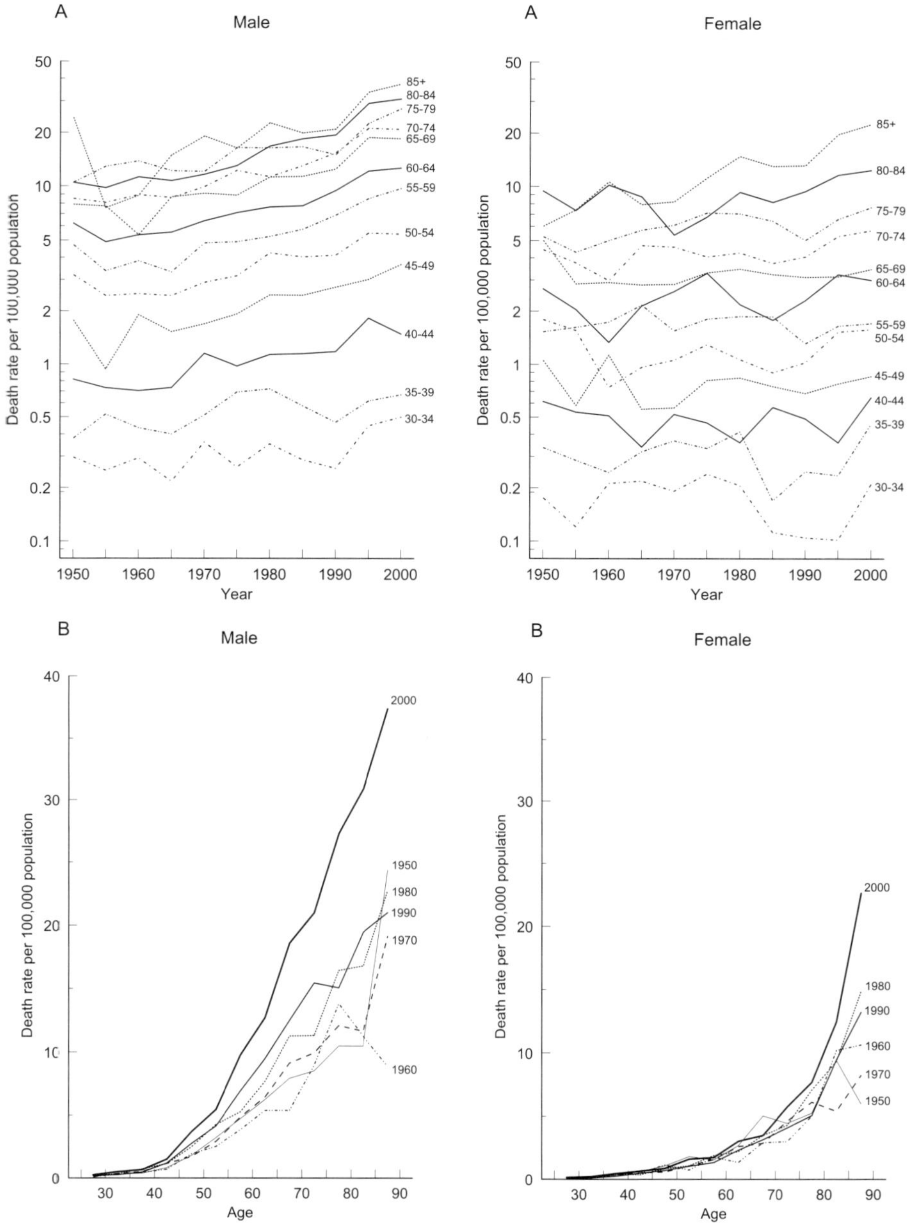

FIG. 3-2. Trends in the age- and sex-specific cancer mortality rate by age group (1950–2000) (A) and by year (1950, 1960, 1970, 1980, 1990, and 2000) (B) in Japan

Cancer of the buccal cavity and pharynx (ICD, 10th revision: C00–C14)

TABLE III-3. Age- and Sex-specific Cancer Mortality Rates in Japan (1950–2000)
Cancer of the esophagus (ICD, 10th revision: C15)

	1950	1955	1960	1965	1970	1975	1980	1985	1990	1995	2000
Male											
0–4	0.0	0.0	0.0	0.0	0.0	0.0	0.0	0.0	0.0	0.0	0.0
5–9	0.0	0.0	0.0	0.0	0.0	0.0	0.0	0.0	0.0	0.0	0.0
10–14	0.0	0.0	0.0	0.0	0.0	0.0	0.0	0.0	0.0	0.0	0.0
15–19	0.0	0.0	0.0	0.0	0.0	0.0	0.0	0.0	0.0	0.0	0.0
20–24	0.0	0.0	0.0	0.0	0.0	0.0	0.0	0.0	0.0	0.0	0.0
25–29	0.1	0.2	0.1	0.0	0.0	0.0	0.0	0.0	0.0	0.0	0.0
30–34	0.3	0.1	0.2	0.3	0.1	0.1	0.1	0.1	0.1	0.0	0.0
35–39	0.6	0.5	0.6	0.5	0.6	0.3	0.2	0.4	0.4	0.2	0.3
40–44	2.0	1.1	1.5	1.5	1.5	1.5	0.9	1.4	1.2	1.1	1.3
45–49	4.5	3.0	3.5	3.4	4.1	3.8	4.3	4.2	4.5	5.0	4.7
50–54	10.2	8.3	9.0	7.7	7.9	9.1	10.3	11.0	10.7	12.5	11.0
55–59	21.3	16.9	18.7	17.7	19.8	17.2	18.3	20.8	21.3	21.6	24.7
60–64	32.0	31.9	31.2	31.9	36.4	32.0	29.2	29.6	32.2	32.2	34.7
65–69	52.9	52.9	51.0	51.9	55.9	50.3	48.1	41.9	44.4	48.9	47.8
70–74	67.6	64.5	63.6	69.2	77.8	65.4	63.3	53.9	57.8	55.5	60.0
75–79	54.2	59.9	70.1	72.4	82.3	83.5	81.3	74.6	66.9	65.4	68.3
80–84	38.7	54.1	70.4	73.8	100.9	80.1	90.5	80.8	76.6	79.0	75.3
85–	27.8	42.8	23.0	70.4	76.5	67.8	91.5	80.6	70.2	79.7	78.1
Female											
0–4	0.0	0.0	0.0	0.0	0.0	0.0	0.0	0.0	0.0	0.0	0.0
5–9	0.0	0.0	0.0	0.0	0.0	0.0	0.0	0.0	0.0	0.0	0.0
10–14	0.0	0.0	0.0	0.0	0.0	0.0	0.0	0.0	0.0	0.0	0.0
15–19	0.0	0.0	0.0	0.0	0.0	0.0	0.0	0.0	0.0	0.0	0.0
20–24	0.0	0.0	0.1	0.0	0.0	0.0	0.0	0.0	0.0	0.0	0.0
25–29	0.1	0.0	0.2	0.1	0.0	0.0	0.0	0.0	0.0	0.0	0.0
30–34	0.2	0.2	0.0	0.1	0.1	0.0	0.0	0.0	0.1	0.0	0.0
35–39	0.6	0.5	0.4	0.3	0.3	0.1	0.0	0.0	0.2	0.1	0.1
40–44	1.4	1.3	0.9	0.4	0.5	0.5	0.4	0.1	0.2	0.2	0.3
45–49	2.4	1.8	1.5	1.2	1.2	0.7	0.3	0.5	0.6	0.5	0.8
50–54	4.4	2.9	3.0	2.8	2.0	1.9	1.3	1.0	1.3	1.2	1.3
55–59	6.3	5.9	5.2	5.6	4.4	3.4	2.6	1.9	2.3	2.2	2.4
60–64	11.2	9.5	8.4	7.8	6.5	5.7	5.2	3.4	2.9	2.5	3.6
65–69	15.8	14.4	14.7	13.5	13.0	9.4	8.7	6.7	4.8	4.5	4.7
70–74	18.2	18.9	19.9	22.4	19.4	14.7	14.5	9.5	8.4	6.5	5.7
75–79	17.9	25.5	26.1	27.3	25.8	20.5	19.5	15.5	13.8	11.6	7.9
80–84	14.4	21.3	29.0	26.1	31.7	27.8	26.5	21.0	15.3	18.3	15.3
85–	13.5	16.9	30.4	21.6	17.9	29.9	28.0	26.9	29.0	24.7	22.9

Mortality rates per 100,000 population.

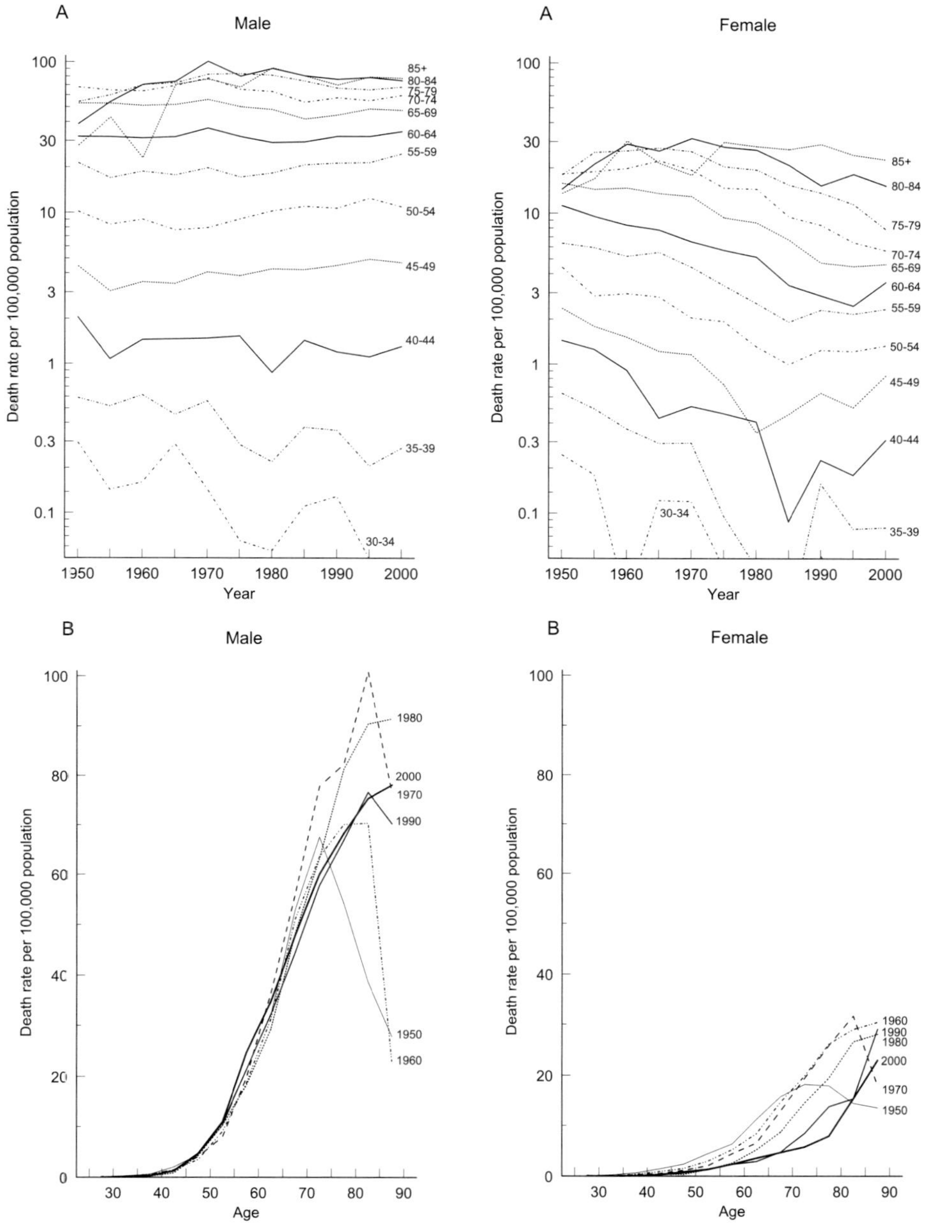

FIG. 3-3. Trends in the age- and sex-specific cancer mortality rate by age group (1950–2000) (A) and by year (1950, 1960, 1970, 1980, 1990, and 2000) (B) in Japan

Cancer of the esophagus (ICD, 10th revision: C15)

TABLE III-4. Age- and Sex-specific Cancer Mortality Rates in Japan (1950–2000)
Cancer of the stomach (ICD, 10th revision: C16)

	1950	1955	1960	1965	1970	1975	1980	1985	1990	1995	2000
Male											
0–4	0.1	0.0	0.0	0.0	0.0	0.0	0.0	0.0	0.0	0.0	0.0
5–9	0.1	0.0	0.0	0.0	0.0	0.0	0.0	0.0	0.0	0.0	0.0
10–14	0.2	0.0	0.0	0.0	0.0	0.0	0.0	0.0	0.0	0.0	0.0
15–19	0.2	0.2	0.3	0.3	0.4	0.2	0.1	0.1	0.2	0.1	0.1
20–24	0.7	0.7	1.1	1.6	1.5	1.3	0.7	0.5	0.4	0.4	0.4
25–29	2.3	2.8	3.1	3.8	3.6	3.0	2.3	2.2	1.2	1.1	0.6
30–34	7.0	7.0	8.0	8.5	8.3	6.7	5.7	4.3	2.6	1.9	1.6
35–39	15.1	17.0	17.0	16.4	15.3	13.4	11.5	8.4	7.0	5.3	3.5
40–44	35.8	36.7	34.7	28.6	27.5	24.4	19.3	15.9	12.1	11.0	7.8
45–49	69.6	73.4	67.2	58.8	52.2	45.0	39.4	29.2	24.6	19.4	16.3
50–54	128.3	128.0	121.9	110.5	93.0	74.0	69.8	56.3	44.4	37.0	31.0
55–59	219.3	211.3	206.2	189.9	158.4	139.5	105.5	95.8	79.1	66.7	57.6
60–64	324.6	336.2	317.8	307.2	265.6	218.3	186.4	146.6	131.8	112.1	91.1
65–69	435.3	456.4	467.2	449.8	409.0	341.1	289.0	230.6	186.4	174.4	156.2
70–74	463.6	546.2	597.8	568.1	545.5	489.1	417.0	330.8	273.5	252.1	225.3
75–79	397.1	509.3	607.6	666.1	651.7	602.0	560.7	463.8	385.5	364.4	299.7
80–84	273.0	359.6	490.1	553.1	604.4	650.8	632.4	605.3	517.5	495.7	435.5
85–	219.1	234.4	329.5	362.9	391.4	499.1	545.8	607.5	611.7	662.4	605.2
Female											
0–4	0.0	0.0	0.0	0.0	0.0	0.0	0.0	0.0	0.0	0.0	0.0
5–9	0.1	0.0	0.0	0.0	0.0	0.0	0.0	0.0	0.0	0.0	0.0
10–14	0.0	0.0	0.0	0.0	0.0	0.0	0.0	0.0	0.0	0.0	0.0
15–19	0.2	0.2	0.2	0.2	0.5	0.2	0.1	0.1	0.0	0.1	0.1
20–24	1.0	1.0	1.3	1.4	1.6	1.4	1.1	0.5	0.6	0.2	0.2
25–29	3.4	3.1	3.7	4.7	5.1	4.6	4.0	3.2	1.9	1.5	1.0
30–34	8.5	8.7	10.3	10.5	9.1	10.1	8.1	6.6	4.7	3.2	2.3
35–39	15.5	17.7	18.2	17.9	16.0	15.0	13.5	10.6	8.7	6.2	4.1
40–44	29.7	29.9	31.2	26.5	25.6	21.4	17.9	15.2	12.8	10.1	8.0
45–49	45.4	44.0	45.0	42.2	37.5	31.2	24.8	21.1	15.8	15.8	13.5
50–54	69.8	69.3	64.7	63.9	54.2	45.1	35.6	28.0	23.0	18.4	17.1
55–59	108.7	104.8	96.7	88.6	82.4	64.0	52.9	39.7	30.0	26.6	22.3
60–64	158.3	153.6	142.1	128.9	119.1	97.2	80.9	63.1	45.2	37.2	32.5
65–69	219.4	223.0	208.7	192.9	175.0	145.6	116.5	88.1	68.6	56.4	43.8
70–74	235.0	264.2	282.8	275.0	254.4	211.3	173.0	131.8	98.1	85.3	66.1
75–79	229.4	284.1	321.3	316.1	321.2	279.0	250.9	194.6	150.0	125.8	103.6
80–84	169.8	253.9	307.2	315.1	332.0	319.1	307.7	268.6	225.9	202.1	166.2
85–	133.5	162.0	237.2	230.0	239.6	258.1	293.5	316.7	297.7	295.7	270.9

Mortality rates per 100,000 population.

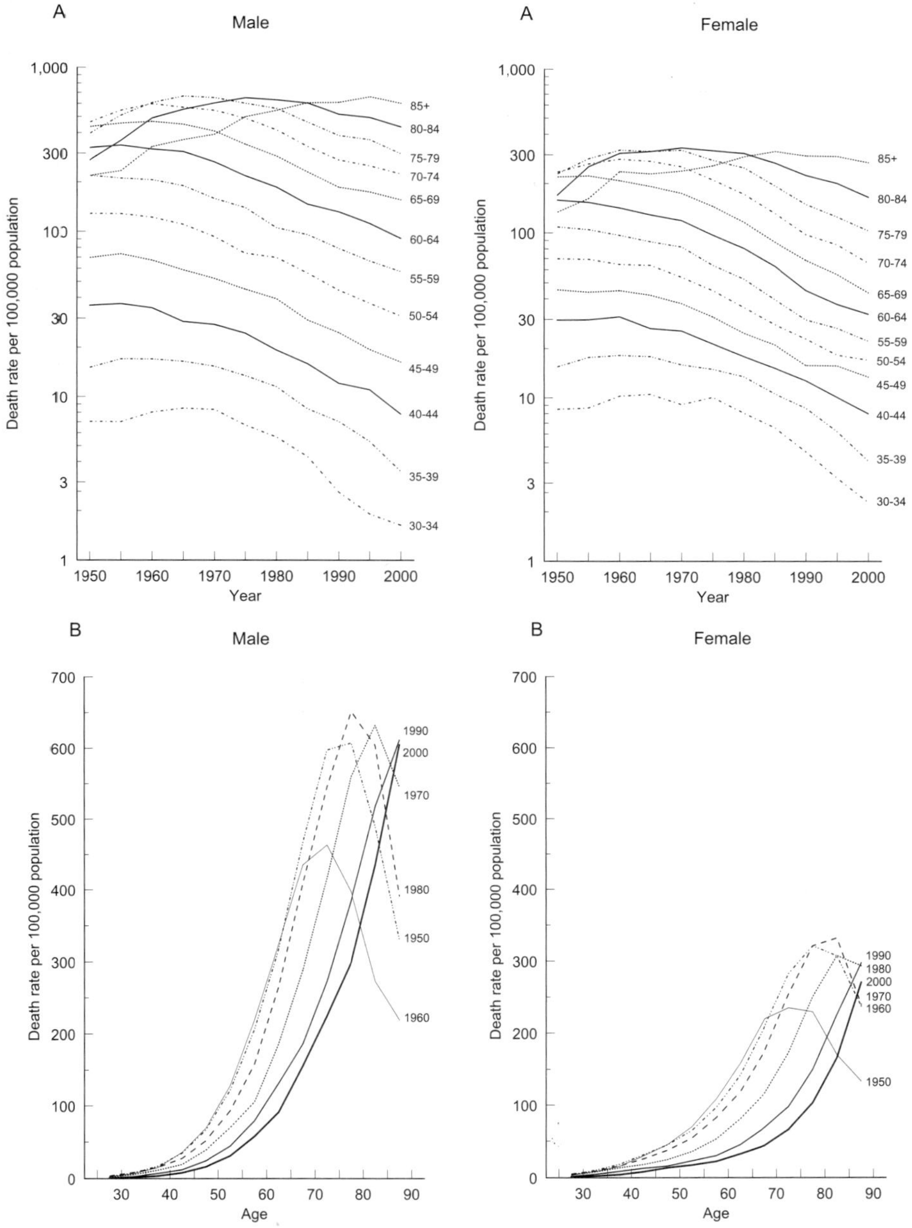

FIG. 3-4. Trends in the age- and sex-specific cancer mortality rate by age group (1950–2000) (A) and by year (1950, 1960, 1970, 1980, 1990, and 2000) (B) in Japan

Cancer of the stomach (ICD, 10th revision: C16)

TABLE III-5. Age- and Sex-specific Cancer Mortality Rates in Japan (1950–2000)
Cancer of the colon (ICD, 10th revision: C18)

	1950	1955	1960	1965	1970	1975	1980	1985	1990	1995	2000
Male											
0–4	0.1	0.0	0.0	0.0	0.0	0.0	0.0	0.0	0.0	0.0	0.0
5–9	0.0	0.0	0.0	0.0	0.0	0.0	0.0	0.0	0.0	0.0	0.0
10–14	0.0	0.0	0.0	0.1	0.0	0.0	0.0	0.0	0.0	0.0	0.0
15–19	0.1	0.1	0.1	0.2	0.1	0.1	0.1	0.0	0.1	0.0	0.1
20–24	0.1	0.1	0.2	0.2	0.5	0.3	0.1	0.3	0.3	0.2	0.1
25–29	0.2	0.3	0.4	0.6	0.8	0.6	0.6	0.5	0.4	0.4	0.4
30–34	0.3	0.4	0.5	0.8	1.1	0.8	1.2	1.1	0.8	1.1	0.8
35–39	0.8	0.9	0.8	1.1	1.5	1.9	2.2	1.3	1.6	1.5	1.3
40–44	1.4	1.2	1.2	1.9	2.3	3.1	2.7	3.0	3.2	2.8	2.9
45–49	1.9	2.7	2.2	2.8	3.5	4.0	5.0	5.4	6.2	5.7	5.2
50–54	3.5	3.0	3.4	4.8	5.1	6.7	7.4	10.0	11.1	12.1	10.8
55–59	5.9	5.0	6.0	7.2	9.2	11.9	13.4	18.2	21.6	21.3	20.7
60–64	10.0	10.1	9.4	11.1	11.8	16.5	20.6	26.4	35.1	35.9	34.8
65–69	13.1	12.9	14.3	16.7	22.7	26.8	33.0	36.0	47.5	56.6	53.7
70–74	15.0	19.5	21.1	25.7	27.4	36.5	50.6	59.9	66.0	81.3	82.5
75–79	17.9	16.4	24.4	28.5	40.7	53.0	67.9	86.6	90.7	115.5	111.0
80–84	15.7	16.5	24.8	30.0	40.3	64.5	93.4	117.1	145.8	165.8	163.2
85–	13.9	20.2	39.0	29.8	27.0	67.0	79.8	130.0	187.5	239.2	252.4
Female											
0–4	0.0	0.0	0.1	0.0	0.0	0.0	0.0	0.0	0.0	0.0	0.0
5–9	0.0	0.0	0.0	0.1	0.0	0.0	0.0	0.0	0.0	0.0	0.0
10–14	0.0	0.0	0.0	0.0	0.0	0.0	0.0	0.0	0.0	0.0	0.0
15–19	0.0	0.0	0.1	0.0	0.0	0.1	0.1	0.0	0.0	0.0	0.1
20–24	0.1	0.2	0.1	0.4	0.2	0.1	0.3	0.2	0.3	0.0	0.2
25–29	0.3	0.2	0.3	0.3	0.6	0.5	0.5	0.6	0.3	0.2	0.3
30–34	0.5	0.5	0.5	0.8	0.8	1.1	0.9	0.8	0.9	0.6	0.8
35–39	0.9	0.9	1.3	0.9	1.4	1.8	1.7	1.7	1.6	1.9	1.2
40–44	1.9	1.7	1.5	1.7	2.2	2.8	2.5	3.4	3.2	3.1	2.5
45–49	2.2	2.2	2.3	3.1	3.3	4.0	4.5	5.4	5.9	5.8	4.7
50–54	4.0	3.8	3.4	5.3	5.2	6.8	7.9	9.5	9.1	10.4	9.7
55–59	7.4	5.6	6.4	6.5	7.6	9.8	11.4	13.3	15.5	15.2	15.1
60–64	11.6	9.1	9.4	10.7	11.7	13.3	17.1	19.5	22.0	23.0	20.9
65–69	15.6	14.7	14.2	15.1	18.3	20.8	24.8	28.0	32.0	31.9	31.2
70–74	18.1	19.5	22.1	26.7	29.3	34.1	37.5	42.0	47.7	48.3	48.2
75–79	16.3	19.7	24.7	34.9	42.4	44.9	56.1	61.8	67.9	70.1	68.2
80–84	16.6	16.8	28.4	31.9	44.9	56.8	68.6	89.0	100.3	112.1	106.9
85–	10.5	15.9	23.6	30.7	30.6	45.2	71.5	92.2	131.1	171.1	179.7

Mortality rates per 100,000 population.

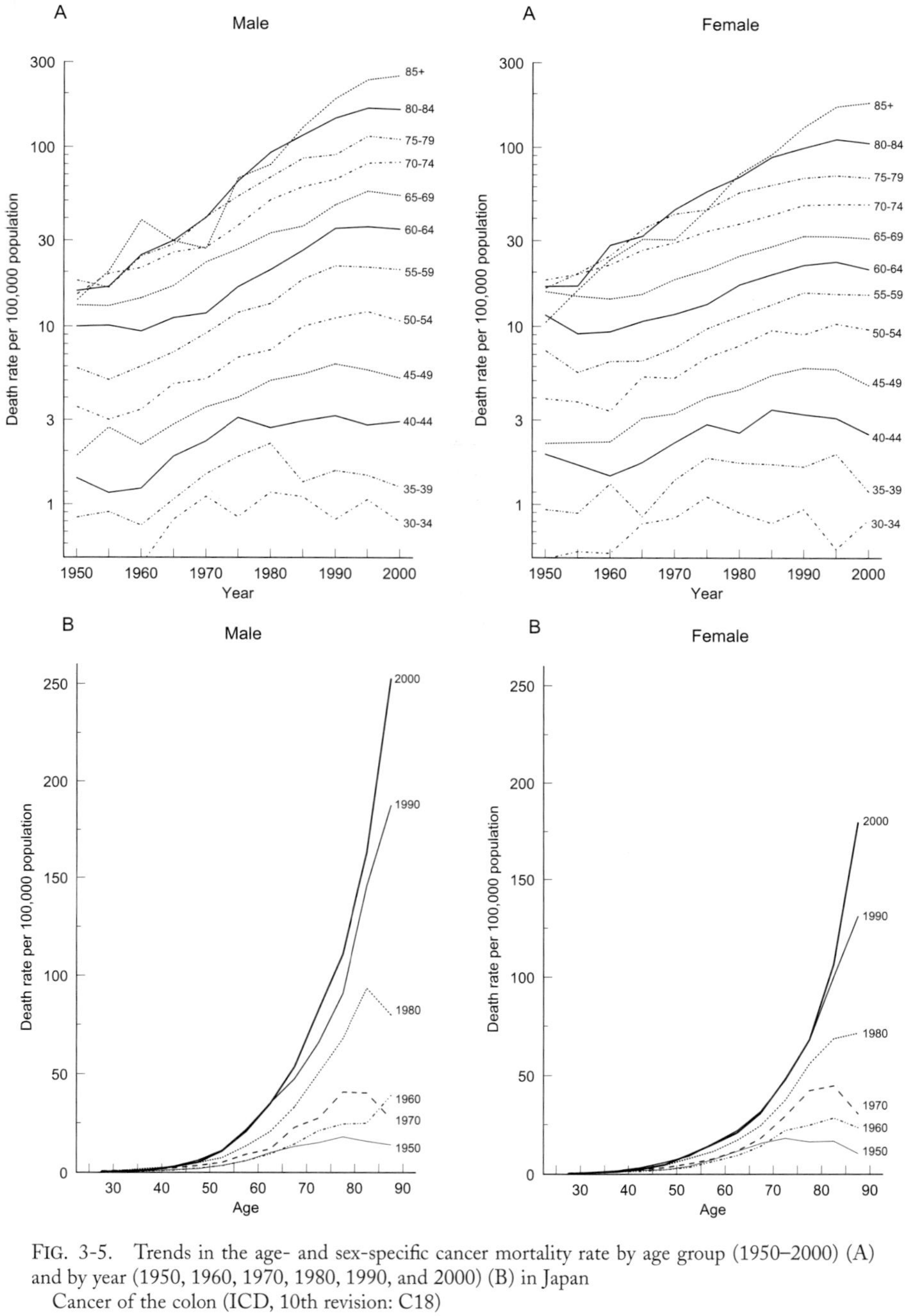

FIG. 3-5. Trends in the age- and sex-specific cancer mortality rate by age group (1950–2000) (A) and by year (1950, 1960, 1970, 1980, 1990, and 2000) (B) in Japan

Cancer of the colon (ICD, 10th revision: C18)

TABLE III-6. Age- and Sex-specific Cancer Mortality Rates in Japan (1950–2000)
Cancer of the rectum (ICD, 10th revision: C19–C21)

	1950	1955	1960	1965	1970	1975	1980	1985	1990	1995	2000
Male											
0–4	0.0	0.0	0.0	0.0	0.0	0.0	0.0	0.0	0.0	0.0	0.0
5–9	0.0	0.0	0.0	0.0	0.0	0.0	0.0	0.0	0.0	0.0	0.0
10–14	0.0	0.0	0.0	0.0	0.0	0.0	0.0	0.0	0.0	0.0	0.0
15–19	0.1	0.0	0.1	0.1	0.1	0.0	0.0	0.0	0.0	0.0	0.0
20–24	0.1	0.1	0.2	0.6	0.4	0.2	0.1	0.1	0.0	0.0	0.2
25–29	0.6	0.3	0.1	0.5	1.1	0.6	0.4	0.3	0.1	0.2	0.2
30–34	0.8	0.6	0.7	0.9	1.2	1.5	0.9	0.6	0.6	0.4	0.5
35–39	1.3	1.2	0.6	1.0	2.1	2.2	2.1	1.6	1.4	1.1	0.7
40–44	1.9	2.3	2.0	1.9	2.8	3.2	3.6	3.3	2.9	2.2	2.3
45–49	4.8	3.8	2.7	4.2	4.4	4.9	6.0	5.5	5.9	5.4	5.2
50–54	7.0	4.9	4.9	6.4	7.1	6.4	9.1	10.3	10.4	11.0	10.5
55–59	11.5	9.6	8.9	10.7	12.0	12.2	12.0	16.1	17.3	19.5	18.7
60–64	17.8	17.2	17.4	17.7	19.2	19.9	20.0	20.9	25.1	29.7	27.9
65–69	25.0	25.8	23.6	29.3	30.5	32.2	32.1	31.7	33.5	41.4	40.6
70–74	34.4	39.2	41.1	39.5	44.1	47.2	51.4	46.6	44.5	49.0	49.8
75–79	38.5	46.2	44.6	52.9	59.5	65.6	69.3	67.4	60.2	58.4	57.9
80–84	20.9	38.3	46.7	71.7	70.6	84.0	90.2	93.2	93.0	91.0	82.9
85–	13.9	32.8	46.1	56.9	66.4	69.4	101.9	97.1	110.8	115.5	107.1
Female											
0–4	0.0	0.0	0.0	0.0	0.0	0.0	0.0	0.0	0.0	0.0	0.0
5–9	0.0	0.0	0.0	0.0	0.0	0.0	0.0	0.0	0.0	0.0	0.0
10–14	0.0	0.0	0.0	0.0	0.0	0.0	0.0	0.0	0.0	0.0	0.0
15–19	0.0	0.1	0.1	0.0	0.0	0.0	0.0	0.0	0.0	0.0	0.0
20–24	0.1	0.2	0.1	0.4	0.1	0.1	0.1	0.1	0.0	0.0	0.1
25–29	0.4	0.3	0.3	0.6	0.9	0.4	0.3	0.2	0.1	0.1	0.2
30–34	1.0	0.3	0.5	0.9	1.3	1.3	0.8	0.5	0.5	0.5	0.3
35–39	1.7	1.1	1.1	1.2	1.6	2.0	1.7	0.9	1.0	0.7	0.7
40–44	3.0	2.9	2.0	2.3	2.3	2.6	2.8	2.4	1.6	2.1	1.4
45–49	4.5	3.5	4.0	3.9	3.3	4.3	3.9	4.0	4.3	3.6	3.1
50–54	6.9	6.7	6.0	5.6	7.0	6.1	6.0	5.8	6.5	5.6	5.7
55–59	10.2	10.1	9.6	9.2	8.3	9.6	7.9	8.1	8.2	7.9	8.3
60–64	12.6	13.5	13.3	11.6	11.9	12.3	11.4	11.3	11.3	10.9	12.1
65–69	18.2	17.1	18.5	19.9	19.4	18.8	15.7	15.6	14.7	15.6	14.1
70–74	18.6	21.8	29.0	28.5	27.1	30.8	26.2	23.7	20.2	19.2	20.7
75–79	15.3	27.2	33.7	36.5	41.8	41.0	40.4	32.3	29.5	28.5	24.9
80–84	16.1	25.3	29.6	41.6	44.4	54.6	53.5	45.7	42.1	42.6	35.5
85–	15.0	16.9	24.3	28.4	38.3	50.8	53.8	62.5	61.1	59.6	56.8

Mortality rates per 100,000 population.

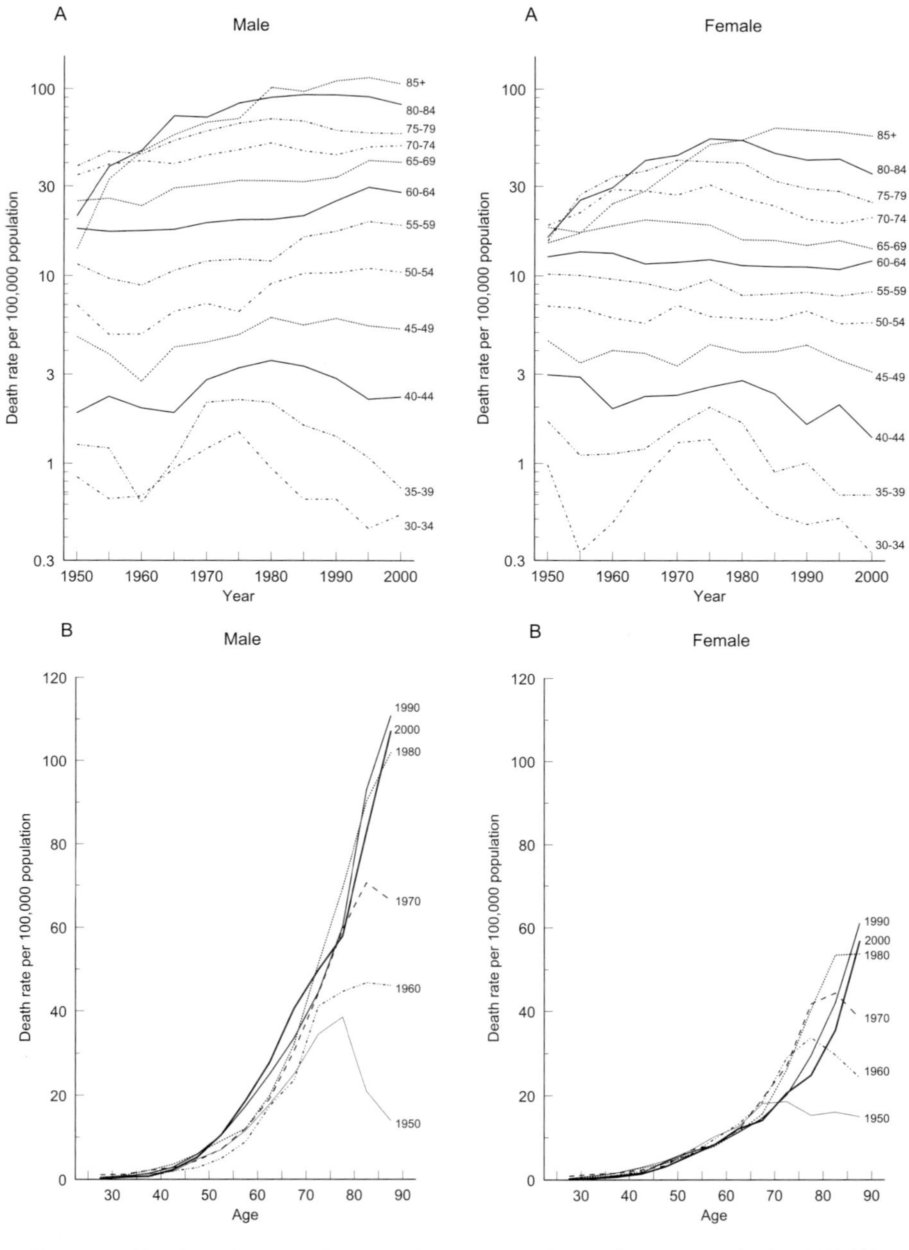

FIG. 3-6. Trends in the age- and sex-specific cancer mortality rate by age group (1950–2000) (A) and by year (1950, 1960, 1970, 1980, 1990, and 2000) (B) in Japan

Cancer of the rectum (ICD, 10th revision: C19–C21)

TABLE III-7. Age- and Sex-specific Cancer Mortality Rates in Japan (1950–2000)
Cancer of the liver (ICD, 10th revision: C22)

	1950	1955	1960	1965	1970	1975	1980	1985	1990	1995	2000
Male											
0–4			0.2	0.3	0.4	0.5	0.3	0.4	0.2	0.2	0.2
5–9			0.1	0.1	0.2	0.1	0.1	0.0	0.0	0.2	0.1
10–14			0.1	0.1	0.1	0.0	0.1	0.1	0.0	0.1	0.1
15–19			0.2	0.1	0.0	0.1	0.1	0.1	0.1	0.2	0.1
20–24			0.4	0.2	0.3	0.3	0.2	0.1	0.1	0.1	0.1
25–29			0.5	0.5	0.4	0.4	0.4	0.3	0.2	0.4	0.4
30–34			1.1	0.9	0.9	1.4	1.3	1.0	0.7	0.6	0.7
35–39			2.4	2.8	3.1	2.6	2.9	3.6	2.7	2.2	1.5
40–44			6.3	6.3	6.4	6.9	6.3	7.3	7.2	6.6	4.8
45–49			12.5	13.1	12.4	13.5	20.7	17.5	15.4	15.8	12.4
50–54			28.6	20.5	23.6	23.4	37.3	50.9	35.0	33.9	27.6
55–59			42.6	33.0	37.2	38.9	50.0	72.8	94.7	65.0	51.3
60–64			64.1	53.3	50.6	51.0	69.6	87.1	114.9	141.8	89.4
65–69			83.9	71.7	76.7	74.1	79.6	98.4	118.4	159.6	164.8
70–74			115.3	90.0	94.5	92.3	107.2	114.7	127.7	163.4	173.0
75–79			127.2	114.9	117.6	101.0	113.6	133.1	137.5	169.2	172.4
80–84			87.5	125.2	115.8	113.6	132.0	146.3	157.4	180.5	186.9
85–			76.2	81.2	106.8	107.0	107.2	130.0	154.5	175.3	173.6
Female											
0–4			0.3	0.4	0.3	0.3	0.2	0.3	0.2	0.2	0.1
5–9			0.0	0.0	0.1	0.1	0.0	0.0	0.0	0.1	0.0
10–14			0.0	0.1	0.0	0.1	0.0	0.1	0.0	0.0	0.0
15–19			0.1	0.1	0.1	0.0	0.0	0.0	0.0	0.0	0.0
20–24			0.3	0.2	0.2	0.2	0.0	0.0	0.1	0.1	0.1
25–29			0.3	0.3	0.3	0.3	0.1	0.2	0.2	0.0	0.2
30–34			0.7	0.9	0.7	0.3	0.3	0.4	0.3	0.2	0.3
35–39			2.0	1.5	1.3	1.2	1.0	0.7	0.4	0.3	0.5
40–44			4.3	3.0	2.7	2.4	1.9	1.4	0.9	1.0	0.7
45–49			7.9	6.5	5.3	4.5	3.2	3.3	2.1	2.2	1.6
50–54			13.1	10.9	9.4	7.8	6.0	6.4	4.9	5.0	4.2
55–59			20.8	18.0	15.7	13.1	12.1	13.0	12.8	11.6	9.1
60–64			36.7	28.3	23.9	20.9	19.0	22.2	24.2	30.3	21.4
65–69			49.7	45.4	37.1	32.9	30.5	30.7	37.0	45.8	45.3
70–74			70.0	57.5	54.3	47.5	45.3	43.8	49.0	60.3	64.5
75–79			80.3	74.8	72.5	59.6	60.9	59.3	57.9	74.4	77.8
80–84			71.4	65.1	61.8	65.8	69.8	70.2	70.8	79.7	89.9
85–			64.6	51.7	60.1	56.0	62.5	72.5	86.0	91.0	95.4

Mortality rates per 100,000 population.

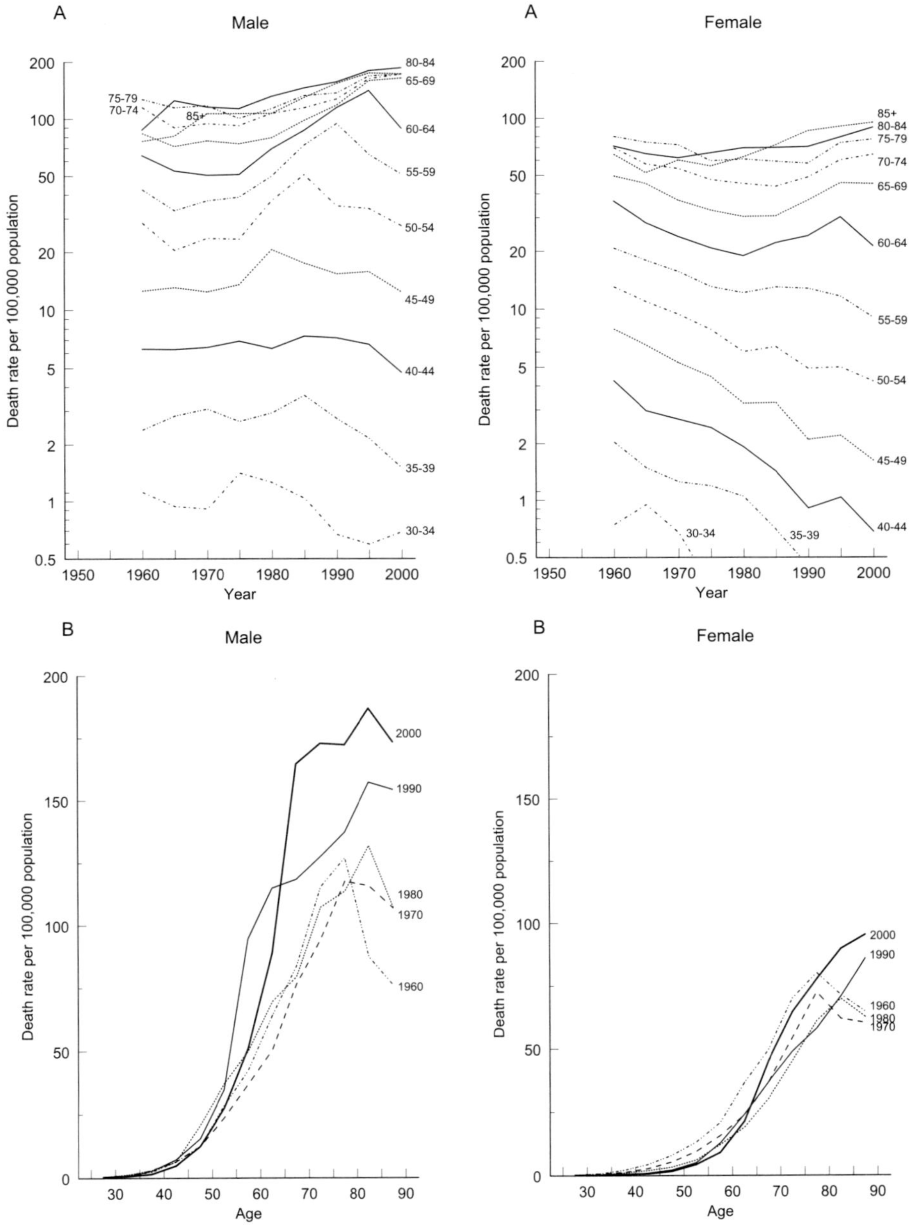

FIG. 3-7. Trends in the age- and sex-specific cancer mortality rate by age group (1960–2000) (A) and by year (1960, 1970, 1980, 1990, and 2000) (B) in Japan
Cancer of the liver (ICD, 10th revision: C22)

TABLE III-8. Age- and Sex-specific Cancer Mortality Rates in Japan (1950–2000)
Cancer of the biliary passages (ICD, 10th revision: C23, C24)

	1950	1955	1960	1965	1970	1975	1980	1985	1990	1995	2000
Male											
0–4			0.0	0.0	0.0	0.0	0.0	0.0	0.0	0.0	0.0
5–9			0.0	0.0	0.0	0.0	0.0	0.0	0.0	0.0	0.0
10–14			0.0	0.0	0.0	0.0	0.0	0.0	0.0	0.0	0.0
15–19			0.0	0.0	0.0	0.0	0.0	0.0	0.0	0.0	0.0
20–24			0.0	0.0	0.1	0.0	0.1	0.0	0.0	0.0	0.0
25–29			0.0	0.1	0.0	0.1	0.1	0.1	0.1	0.0	0.0
30–34			0.0	0.1	0.1	0.2	0.1	0.2	0.2	0.2	0.3
35–39			0.3	0.3	0.4	0.5	0.4	0.5	0.6	0.4	0.4
40–44			0.5	0.7	0.8	0.8	0.8	1.3	1.1	0.9	0.9
45–49			1.0	1.8	2.1	2.6	2.5	2.6	2.7	2.3	1.8
50–54			2.6	4.0	4.3	4.3	4.9	4.1	4.9	4.9	4.2
55–59			4.9	6.2	7.9	8.8	9.7	9.0	10.3	9.2	8.6
60–64			7.4	10.8	12.0	12.6	15.9	17.9	19.2	18.3	17.6
65–69			9.6	16.3	19.9	23.3	29.5	34.6	31.4	33.1	29.3
70–74			15.0	21.8	24.8	34.0	42.5	49.6	56.6	52.2	45.9
75–79			11.7	23.2	31.1	42.0	54.5	75.8	80.0	87.1	77.5
80–84			7.1	23.0	29.9	41.0	64.3	90.3	102.1	113.7	116.3
85–			8.9	8.1	14.6	35.9	60.0	95.5	119.8	155.3	154.4
Female											
0–4			0.0	0.0	0.0	0.0	0.0	0.0	0.0	0.0	0.0
5–9			0.0	0.0	0.0	0.0	0.0	0.0	0.0	0.0	0.0
10–14			0.0	0.0	0.0	0.0	0.0	0.0	0.0	0.0	0.0
15–19			0.0	0.0	0.1	0.0	0.0	0.0	0.0	0.0	0.1
20–24			0.1	0.0	0.0	0.1	0.1	0.0	0.1	0.0	0.1
25–29			0.0	0.0	0.1	0.1	0.1	0.1	0.1	0.1	0.0
30–34			0.1	0.2	0.2	0.2	0.2	0.3	0.2	0.2	0.2
35–39			0.1	0.3	0.4	0.5	0.4	0.6	0.5	0.4	0.6
40–44			0.7	0.8	1.1	1.2	1.3	1.5	1.0	1.1	1.3
45–49			1.3	1.3	2.2	2.4	2.6	3.1	2.8	1.9	3.0
50–54			2.6	3.7	4.4	4.6	5.9	5.8	5.2	4.5	4.6
55–59			4.3	6.8	8.3	10.4	10.7	10.9	9.3	7.9	8.5
60–64			6.3	10.7	16.7	15.1	18.5	17.7	16.5	14.2	15.6
65–69			10.1	13.5	21.6	25.1	29.3	31.2	29.0	25.8	25.6
70–74			9.7	16.3	27.2	35.4	43.4	51.0	49.2	41.8	41.1
75–79			9.9	21.3	26.3	43.7	56.5	73.7	73.1	64.3	57.4
80–84			7.6	18.8	24.5	35.0	59.3	89.5	109.0	102.0	85.9
85–			9.9	9.1	13.1	27.6	41.5	84.1	116.9	136.0	101.5

Mortality rates per 100,000 population.

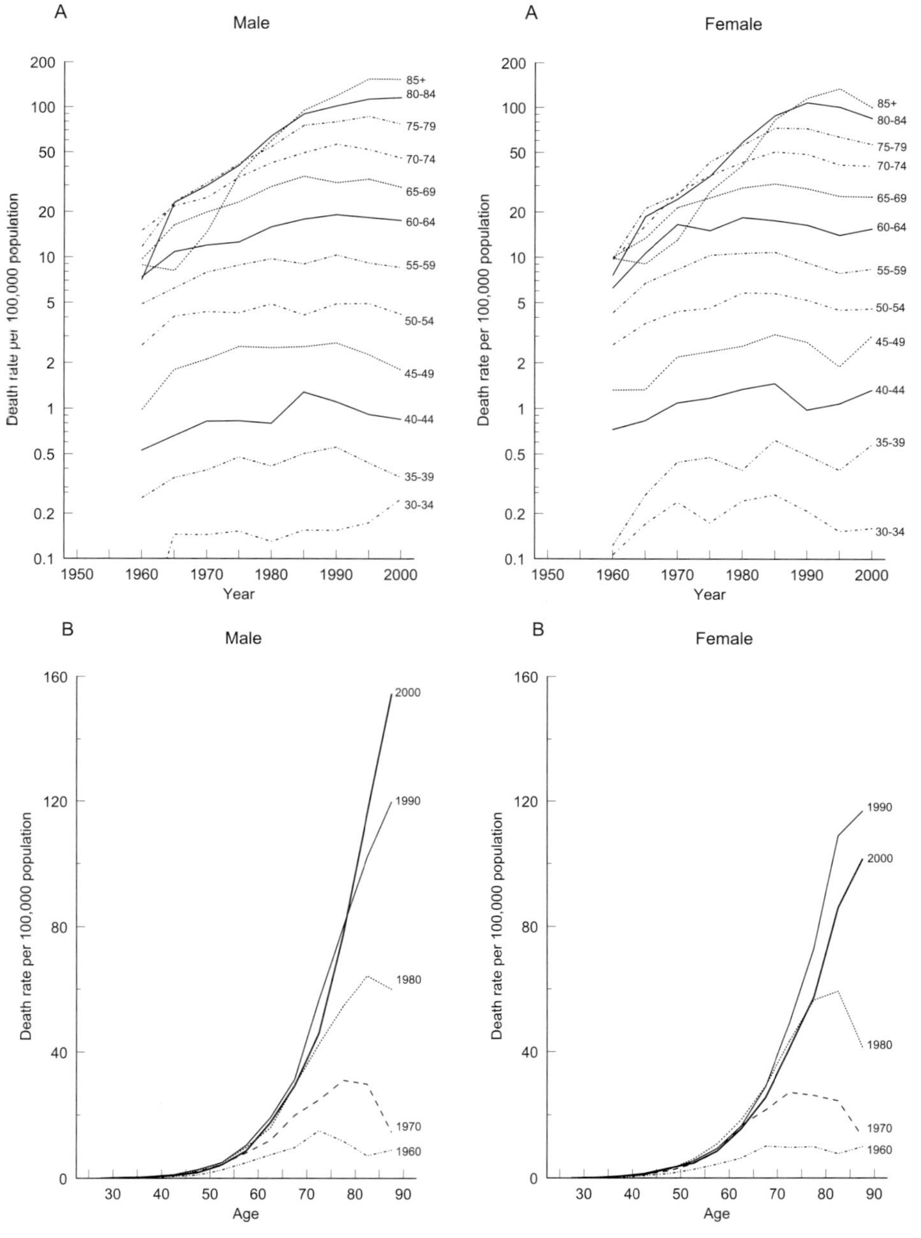

FIG. 3-8. Trends in the age- and sex-specific cancer mortality rate by age group (1960–2000) (A) and by year (1960, 1970, 1980, 1990, and 2000) (B) in Japan

Cancer of the biliary passages (ICD, 10th revision: C23, C24)

TABLE III-9. Age- and Sex-specific Cancer Mortality Rates in Japan (1950–2000)
Cancer of the pancreas (ICD, 10th revision: C25)

	1950	1955	1960	1965	1970	1975	1980	1985	1990	1995	2000
Male											
0–4	0.0	0.0	0.0	0.0	0.0	0.0	0.0	0.0	0.0	0.0	0.0
5–9	0.0	0.0	0.0	0.0	0.0	0.0	0.0	0.0	0.0	0.0	0.0
10–14	0.0	0.0	0.0	0.0	0.1	0.0	0.0	0.0	0.0	0.0	0.0
15–19	0.0	0.0	0.0	0.1	0.0	0.0	0.0	0.0	0.0	0.0	0.0
20–24	0.1	0.0	0.1	0.1	0.2	0.1	0.1	0.0	0.0	0.1	0.0
25–29	0.0	0.1	0.2	0.2	0.2	0.3	0.3	0.0	0.0	0.1	0.1
30–34	0.3	0.3	0.3	0.6	0.6	0.4	0.4	0.4	0.3	0.4	0.5
35–39	0.6	0.6	0.9	0.9	1.4	1.1	1.4	0.9	1.3	1.0	0.9
40–44	1.4	1.5	1.9	1.9	2.4	2.2	3.1	2.8	2.8	2.8	2.5
45–49	1.7	2.3	4.4	4.5	4.1	5.2	6.1	6.3	6.3	5.9	6.1
50–54	2.7	5.0	6.6	9.1	10.1	9.7	10.9	11.5	11.0	12.0	11.9
55–59	4.7	7.0	11.1	13.4	18.1	17.0	19.1	20.8	18.5	20.7	21.2
60–64	6.2	9.3	13.9	20.6	25.5	26.6	32.3	31.9	33.0	33.0	33.5
65–69	4.0	11.8	20.4	25.5	36.7	38.8	45.2	51.4	49.0	53.2	50.0
70–74	3.7	9.9	17.3	30.2	42.7	47.6	57.6	69.6	71.5	71.3	71.4
75–79	1.5	5.6	19.6	28.5	35.8	52.0	71.2	89.5	99.5	100.9	95.7
80–84	2.1	2.3	10.1	23.0	34.0	41.7	67.9	92.7	115.1	130.8	122.0
85–	3.5	2.5	5.3	13.5	28.1	31.9	54.8	92.4	126.5	134.1	142.8
Female											
0–4	0.0	0.0	0.0	0.0	0.0	0.0	0.0	0.0	0.0	0.0	0.0
5–9	0.0	0.0	0.0	0.0	0.0	0.0	0.0	0.0	0.0	0.0	0.0
10–14	0.0	0.0	0.0	0.0	0.0	0.0	0.0	0.0	0.0	0.0	0.0
15–19	0.0	0.0	0.0	0.0	0.0	0.0	0.0	0.0	0.0	0.0	0.0
20–24	0.1	0.0	0.0	0.0	0.1	0.1	0.0	0.1	0.0	0.0	0.0
25–29	0.1	0.1	0.1	0.2	0.2	0.1	0.2	0.2	0.1	0.1	0.1
30–34	0.2	0.2	0.4	0.3	0.5	0.3	0.3	0.3	0.4	0.2	0.2
35–39	0.3	0.7	0.4	0.5	0.8	0.6	0.5	0.6	1.0	0.4	0.5
40–44	0.6	1.5	1.3	1.7	1.5	1.4	1.3	1.6	1.2	1.2	1.4
45–49	1.0	1.8	2.6	3.0	2.9	3.5	3.0	3.0	2.8	2.7	3.2
50–54	1.1	2.6	5.0	5.3	6.0	6.6	5.9	4.9	5.0	5.5	5.6
55–59	3.0	5.0	7.4	10.3	9.4	10.0	9.3	9.4	9.7	8.6	10.7
60–64	3.3	5.4	8.2	14.0	15.5	15.5	17.7	17.2	16.1	17.5	16.1
65–69	2.4	8.1	12.7	17.2	21.0	23.2	26.7	26.0	27.5	24.4	27.3
70–74	1.6	5.8	11.6	15.9	27.4	31.0	40.3	43.5	42.2	41.1	40.9
75–79	1.4	5.1	9.5	18.5	27.2	36.6	42.1	54.4	63.3	60.0	61.6
80–84	0.6	2.9	7.3	11.4	17.7	29.0	43.6	62.5	82.7	85.6	81.2
85–	3.0	3.2	0.8	5.7	10.2	16.4	32.0	58.3	97.4	103.4	115.2

Mortality rates per 100,000 population.

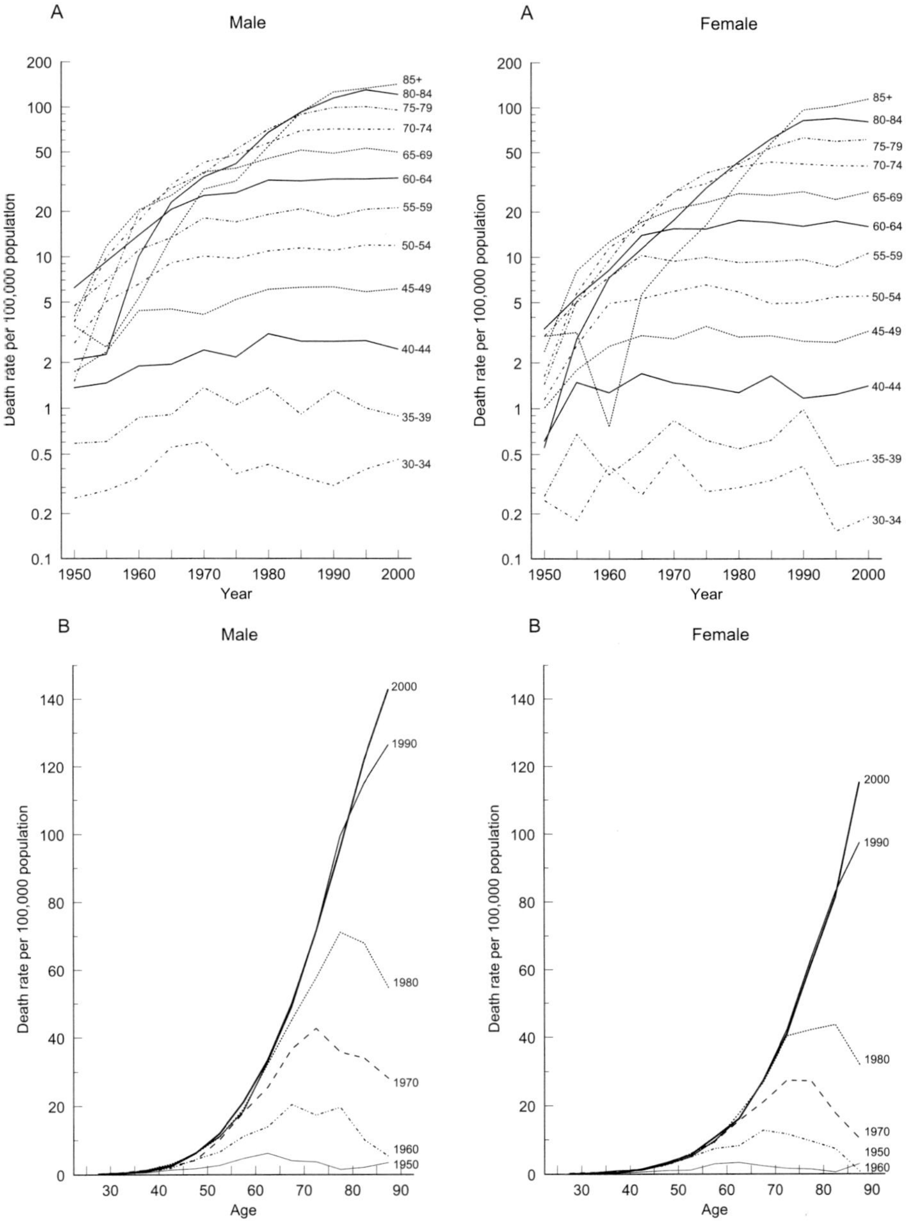

FIG. 3-9. Trends in the age- and sex-specific cancer mortality rate by age group (1950–2000) (A) and by year (1950, 1960, 1970, 1980, 1990, and 2000) (B) in Japan
Cancer of the pancreas (ICD, 10th revision: C25)

TABLE III-10. Age- and Sex-specific Cancer Mortality Rates in Japan (1950–2000)
Cancer of the larynx (ICD, 10th revision: C32)

	1950	1955	1960	1965	1970	1975	1980	1985	1990	1995	2000
Male											
0–4	0.0	0.0	0.0	0.0	0.0	0.0	0.0	0.0	0.0	0.0	0.0
5–9	0.0	0.0	0.0	0.0	0.0	0.0	0.0	0.0	0.0	0.0	0.0
10–14	0.0	0.0	0.0	0.0	0.0	0.0	0.0	0.0	0.0	0.0	0.0
15–19	0.0	0.0	0.0	0.0	0.0	0.0	0.0	0.0	0.0	0.0	0.0
20–24	0.0	0.0	0.0	0.0	0.0	0.0	0.0	0.0	0.0	0.0	0.0
25–29	0.0	0.0	0.0	0.0	0.0	0.0	0.0	0.0	0.0	0.0	0.0
30–34	0.1	0.0	0.0	0.0	0.0	0.0	0.0	0.0	0.0	0.0	0.0
35–39	0.5	0.0	0.2	0.0	0.0	0.0	0.0	0.0	0.0	0.0	0.0
40–44	0.7	0.4	0.3	0.4	0.3	0.1	0.1	0.2	0.1	0.1	0.1
45–49	1.9	1.1	0.8	0.4	0.6	0.6	0.6	0.3	0.3	0.3	0.3
50–54	3.7	2.7	2.0	1.6	1.3	1.0	1.0	0.7	0.8	0.8	0.6
55–59	7.8	5.4	4.4	3.3	3.1	2.6	2.6	2.5	2.3	1.3	1.6
60–64	8.2	8.8	8.0	7.6	7.8	5.4	3.8	3.6	3.2	2.9	2.5
65–69	13.7	10.7	10.8	12.0	12.6	9.9	7.0	6.1	5.5	4.6	4.7
70–74	17.4	17.5	12.0	15.3	16.2	12.8	11.7	10.0	8.2	7.9	7.1
75–79	11.6	12.0	15.1	16.4	21.3	20.7	16.1	13.2	9.4	11.3	9.8
80–84	8.4	7.5	18.9	18.2	20.8	21.8	21.6	16.5	15.2	15.5	13.5
85–	7.0	5.0	10.6	9.5	22.5	9.8	19.2	16.4	16.5	21.1	19.0
Female											
0–4	0.0	0.0	0.0	0.0	0.0	0.0	0.0	0.0	0.0	0.0	0.0
5–9	0.0	0.0	0.0	0.0	0.0	0.0	0.0	0.0	0.0	0.0	0.0
10–14	0.0	0.0	0.0	0.0	0.0	0.0	0.0	0.0	0.0	0.0	0.0
15–19	0.0	0.0	0.0	0.0	0.0	0.0	0.0	0.0	0.0	0.0	0.0
20–24	0.0	0.0	0.0	0.0	0.0	0.0	0.0	0.0	0.0	0.0	0.0
25–29	0.1	0.0	0.0	0.0	0.0	0.0	0.0	0.0	0.0	0.0	0.0
30–34	0.0	0.1	0.0	0.0	0.0	0.0	0.0	0.0	0.0	0.0	0.0
35–39	0.1	0.1	0.1	0.0	0.0	0.0	0.0	0.0	0.0	0.0	0.0
40–44	0.5	0.3	0.3	0.1	0.2	0.0	0.0	0.0	0.0	0.0	0.0
45–49	0.8	0.5	0.4	0.1	0.1	0.1	0.0	0.0	0.0	0.0	0.1
50–54	1.4	0.7	0.5	0.5	0.2	0.3	0.2	0.1	0.1	0.0	0.1
55–59	2.2	1.0	1.4	1.0	1.0	0.3	0.3	0.1	0.1	0.0	0.1
60–64	3.5	2.0	1.7	1.7	1.4	0.6	0.7	0.3	0.1	0.1	0.2
65–69	4.2	3.2	2.3	2.2	1.8	0.9	0.9	0.5	0.2	0.3	0.3
70–74	4.6	4.3	2.8	2.9	2.4	1.5	1.6	0.7	0.7	0.6	0.3
75–79	2.2	4.1	5.2	3.6	3.5	2.0	1.4	0.9	1.1	0.6	0.5
80–84	2.8	3.3	4.8	3.8	2.5	4.2	2.8	2.3	1.0	1.4	0.9
85–	4.5	2.1	3.0	2.3	2.4	3.7	3.4	1.3	1.4	1.6	1.4

Mortality rates per 100,000 population.

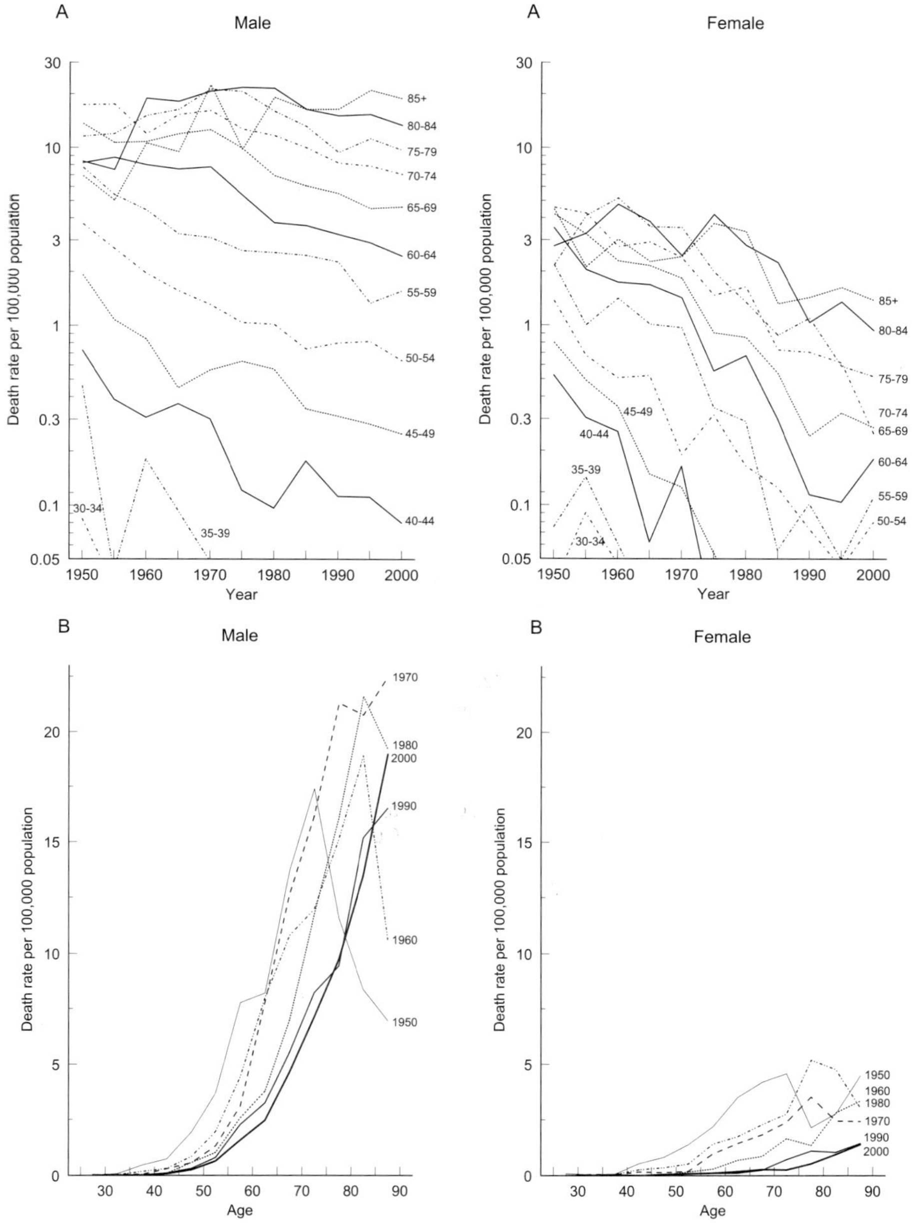

FIG. 3-10. Trends in the age- and sex-specific cancer mortality rate by age group (1950–2000) (A) and by year (1950, 1960, 1970, 1980, 1990, and 2000) (B) in Japan

Cancer of the larynx (ICD, 10th revision: C32)

TABLE III-11. Age- and Sex-specific Cancer Mortality Rates in Japan (1950–2000)
Cancer of the trachea, bronchus, and lung (ICD, 10th revision: C33, C34)

	1950	1955	1960	1965	1970	1975	1980	1985	1990	1995	2000
Male											
0–4	0.0	0.0	0.0	0.0	0.0	0.0	0.0	0.0	0.0	0.0	0.0
5–9	0.0	0.0	0.0	0.0	0.0	0.0	0.0	0.0	0.0	0.0	0.0
10–14	0.1	0.1	0.0	0.1	0.0	0.0	0.0	0.0	0.0	0.0	0.0
15–19	0.2	0.1	0.2	0.1	0.1	0.0	0.1	0.0	0.0	0.1	0.1
20–24	0.1	0.2	0.2	0.4	0.2	0.2	0.1	0.1	0.1	0.1	0.1
25–29	0.2	0.3	0.4	0.5	0.4	0.4	0.5	0.3	0.4	0.3	0.2
30–34	0.1	0.5	0.7	0.8	0.8	0.9	0.9	1.0	1.0	1.2	1.3
35–39	0.4	0.8	1.1	1.8	1.6	1.9	2.5	2.9	3.3	2.6	2.4
40–44	0.9	2.0	2.7	3.6	4.6	4.9	5.0	6.1	6.8	6.4	7.4
45–49	2.1	4.9	7.7	8.5	8.5	11.4	11.2	11.1	12.9	14.3	14.3
50–54	4.9	10.1	15.8	18.7	20.1	20.8	26.4	25.2	23.0	25.9	28.3
55–59	7.7	15.5	30.5	32.0	40.7	43.9	48.8	53.5	53.4	47.1	51.7
60–64	13.7	29.5	46.5	66.3	71.5	79.7	96.0	98.2	113.0	104.5	89.6
65–69	21.9	43.2	71.4	93.1	125.0	139.4	157.2	179.1	190.2	202.3	173.1
70–74	20.4	51.5	86.9	118.5	156.6	210.5	252.7	282.5	300.3	316.1	307.2
75–79	21.3	36.3	81.8	126.1	160.9	238.3	329.1	396.4	419.7	454.6	451.9
80–84	8.4	27.0	62.1	105.9	127.0	191.7	321.4	435.4	515.0	575.6	596.2
85–	3.5	15.1	37.2	39.3	77.6	127.4	242.3	391.5	497.8	599.5	637.4
Female											
0–4	0.0	0.0	0.0	0.0	0.0	0.0	0.0	0.0	0.0	0.0	0.0
5–9	0.0	0.1	0.0	0.0	0.0	0.0	0.0	0.0	0.0	0.0	0.0
10–14	0.1	0.0	0.0	0.0	0.0	0.0	0.0	0.0	0.0	0.0	0.0
15–19	0.1	0.1	0.1	0.1	0.1	0.0	0.0	0.0	0.0	0.0	0.0
20–24	0.0	0.1	0.2	0.2	0.1	0.0	0.1	0.1	0.0	0.1	0.0
25–29	0.1	0.2	0.1	0.3	0.2	0.3	0.3	0.2	0.2	0.1	0.2
30–34	0.2	0.6	0.8	0.9	0.8	0.7	0.8	0.4	0.7	0.9	0.7
35–39	0.4	1.1	1.3	1.8	1.2	1.7	1.7	1.8	2.0	1.7	1.9
40–44	0.8	1.9	1.8	2.7	2.9	2.4	2.9	3.3	3.1	3.8	3.8
45–49	1.1	3.0	4.9	3.9	5.2	5.4	5.1	5.3	5.7	7.2	5.9
50–54	2.7	4.4	6.4	9.3	8.0	9.4	9.6	9.3	10.4	12.3	12.8
55–59	3.6	6.6	10.5	14.1	14.2	15.9	15.9	16.4	15.7	18.2	18.2
60–64	4.1	9.4	16.7	20.7	24.5	23.3	27.4	28.0	25.3	26.5	26.9
65–69	5.0	13.2	22.1	27.8	32.0	35.8	42.1	43.4	42.7	41.8	42.9
70–74	5.9	14.1	23.3	35.9	41.3	51.1	63.7	65.9	69.3	64.4	62.6
75–79	4.5	9.4	25.4	41.8	46.7	58.5	84.4	94.6	99.6	109.0	97.6
80–84	3.3	6.5	19.8	31.7	47.6	55.2	90.4	119.3	119.8	142.9	144.6
85–	1.5	4.2	16.0	17.0	25.7	51.2	67.8	114.2	150.2	172.9	195.5

Mortality rates per 100,000 population.

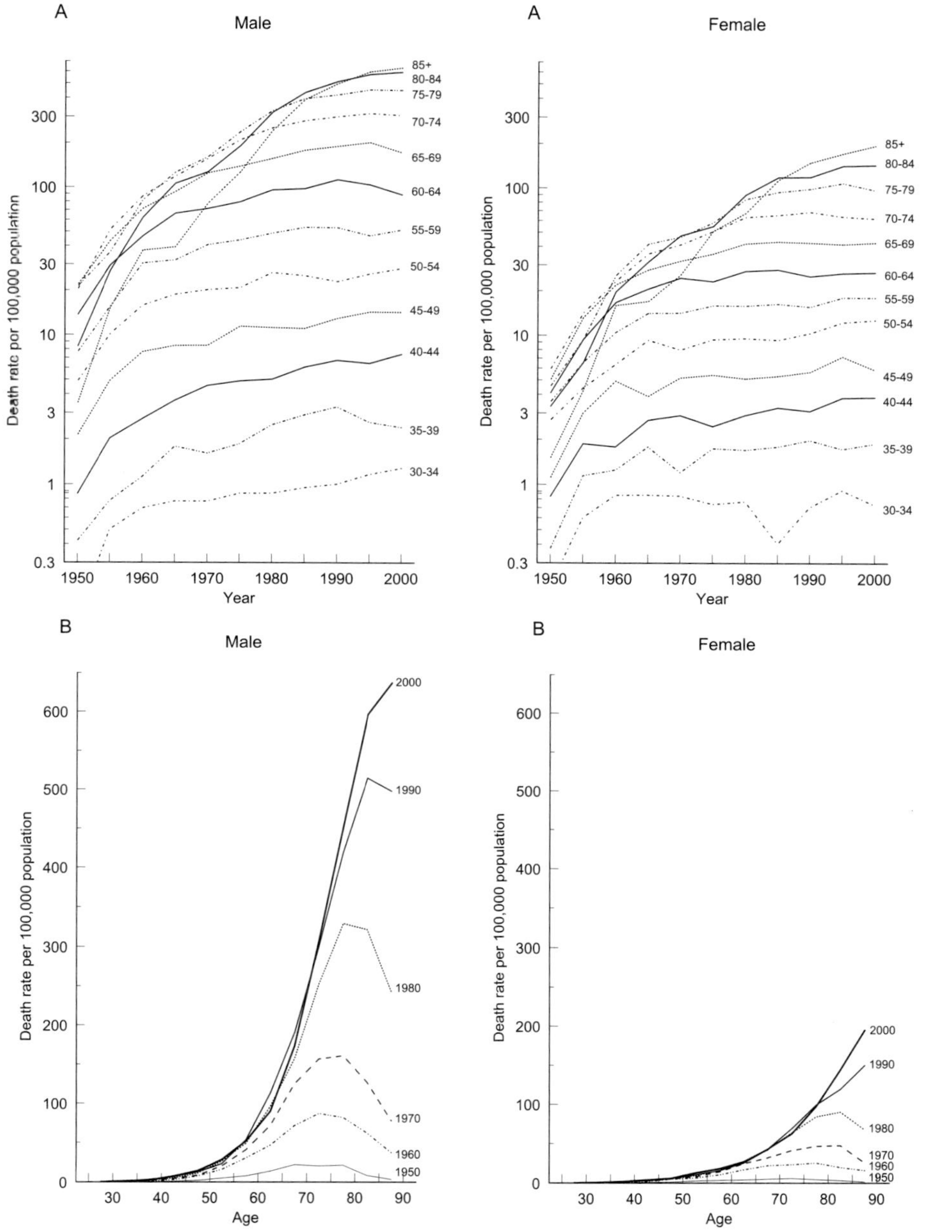

FIG. 3-11. Trends in the age- and sex-specific cancer mortality rate by age group (1950–2000) (A) and by year (1950, 1960, 1970, 1980, 1990, and 2000) (B) in Japan

Cancer of the trachea, bronchus, and lung (ICD, 10th revision: C33, C34)

TABLE III-12. Age- and Sex-specific Cancer Mortality Rates in Japan (1950–2000)
Cancer of the bone (ICD, 10th revision: C40, C41)

	1950	1955	1960	1965	1970	1975	1980	1985	1990	1995	2000
Male											
0–4	0.1	0.1	0.0	0.2	0.1	0.0	0.1	0.0	0.1	0.0	0.0
5–9	0.0	0.1	0.1	0.2	0.2	0.1	0.1	0.1	0.1	0.2	0.0
10–14	0.2	0.3	0.4	0.5	0.6	0.6	0.4	0.4	0.3	0.3	0.1
15–19	0.3	0.4	0.9	0.8	1.2	0.7	0.6	1.0	0.9	0.4	0.5
20–24	0.1	0.3	0.3	0.4	0.7	0.7	0.4	0.3	0.4	0.5	0.4
25–29	0.1	0.2	0.2	0.3	0.4	0.3	0.2	0.2	0.2	0.3	0.2
30–34	0.1	0.5	0.3	0.3	0.2	0.4	0.2	0.1	0.1	0.1	0.1
35–39	0.4	0.6	1.0	0.4	0.4	0.1	0.2	0.1	0.2	0.3	0.3
40–44	0.6	0.6	1.5	0.8	0.4	0.2	0.2	0.2	0.2	0.3	0.1
45–49	0.7	1.6	1.5	1.0	1.3	0.4	0.3	0.3	0.2	0.2	0.4
50–54	1.5	2.5	2.8	2.1	1.4	1.0	0.5	0.4	0.3	0.2	0.4
55–59	2.0	3.2	4.0	3.4	2.1	1.5	0.8	0.5	0.6	0.3	0.4
60–64	2.9	6.0	6.5	4.9	3.6	2.2	1.4	0.6	0.7	0.5	0.6
65–69	3.4	6.9	7.1	8.0	4.9	3.3	1.4	1.2	0.9	0.6	0.7
70–74	3.1	9.1	7.2	9.1	6.6	5.4	3.5	1.7	1.1	0.5	0.8
75–79	4.5	8.2	7.7	10.8	5.5	5.4	3.1	2.8	1.4	1.8	1.1
80–84	4.2	8.3	6.5	7.0	9.1	3.9	1.9	4.3	2.7	1.5	0.6
85–	0.0	2.5	1.8	5.4	5.6	8.2	3.5	1.6	2.5	1.9	1.2
Female											
0–4	0.1	0.1	0.0	0.2	0.1	0.0	0.1	0.1	0.0	0.0	0.0
5–9	0.0	0.1	0.0	0.1	0.2	0.2	0.1	0.1	0.1	0.0	0.0
10–14	0.1	0.2	0.4	0.4	0.5	0.3	0.5	0.5	0.4	0.3	0.5
15–19	0.2	0.3	0.4	0.4	0.6	0.3	0.6	0.4	0.3	0.4	0.3
20–24	0.1	0.1	0.2	0.3	0.2	0.3	0.4	0.2	0.2	0.1	0.3
25–29	0.1	0.4	0.1	0.2	0.2	0.1	0.2	0.1	0.2	0.0	0.2
30–34	0.1	0.2	0.4	0.3	0.2	0.1	0.2	0.1	0.2	0.1	0.1
35–39	0.4	0.5	0.5	0.3	0.3	0.1	0.1	0.1	0.1	0.1	0.1
40–44	0.5	0.8	0.8	0.6	0.4	0.4	0.1	0.1	0.1	0.1	0.1
45–49	0.7	1.3	1.8	0.7	0.7	0.4	0.3	0.1	0.2	0.2	0.2
50–54	1.0	1.8	1.5	1.6	0.9	0.5	0.3	0.4	0.1	0.2	0.2
55–59	2.0	2.0	3.2	1.7	1.7	1.1	0.4	0.2	0.2	0.2	0.2
60–64	1.5	3.0	3.3	3.8	1.8	1.0	0.7	0.5	0.5	0.2	0.3
65–69	1.7	2.5	3.4	3.2	2.3	1.8	1.1	0.7	0.6	0.4	0.3
70–74	2.3	4.9	4.7	5.1	3.3	1.8	1.1	0.9	0.7	0.4	0.3
75–79	3.8	4.9	6.2	5.1	4.1	2.9	0.8	2.1	1.0	0.8	0.6
80–84	3.3	5.3	4.5	7.3	5.6	4.2	1.5	2.0	1.3	0.5	0.8
85–	0.0	5.3	3.8	2.3	4.4	2.6	2.0	1.9	1.3	1.2	1.2

Mortality rates per 100,000 population.

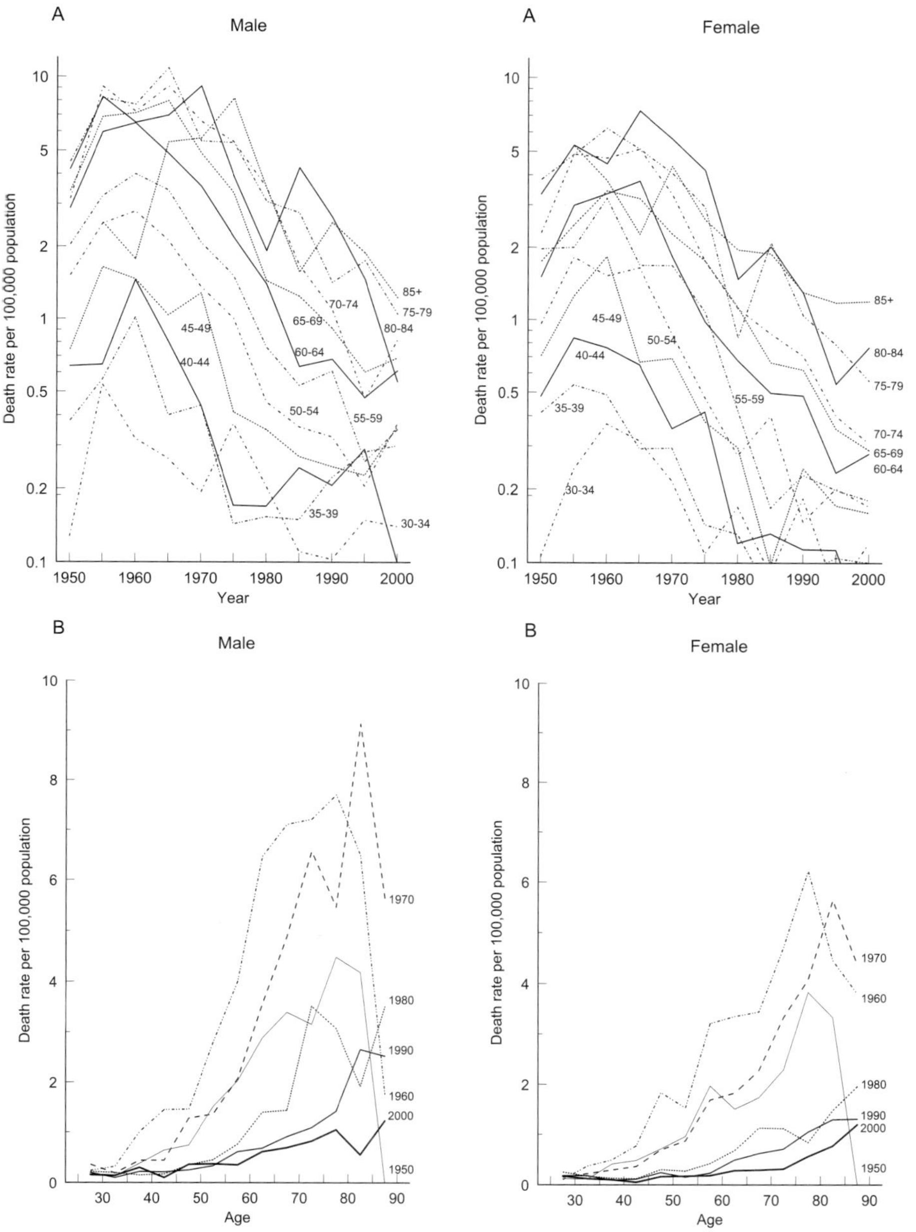

FIG. 3-12. Trends in the age- and sex-specific cancer mortality rate by age group (1950–2000) (A) and by year (1950, 1960, 1970, 1980, 1990, and 2000) (B) in Japan

Cancer of the bone (ICD, 10th revision: C40, C41)

TABLE III-13. Age- and Sex-specific Cancer Mortality Rates in Japan (1950–2000)
Cancer of the skin (ICD, 10th revision: C43, C44)

	1950	1955	1960	1965	1970	1975	1980	1985	1990	1995	2000
Male											
0–4	0.1	0.1	0.1	0.1	0.1	0.0	0.0	0.0	0.0	0.0	0.0
5–9	0.1	0.1	0.0	0.0	0.0	0.0	0.0	0.0	0.0	0.0	0.0
10–14	0.1	0.1	0.1	0.0	0.1	0.0	0.0	0.0	0.0	0.0	0.0
15–19	0.1	0.0	0.0	0.1	0.0	0.0	0.0	0.1	0.0	0.0	0.1
20–24	0.1	0.1	0.0	0.0	0.1	0.1	0.0	0.0	0.0	0.0	0.1
25–29	0.1	0.1	0.1	0.1	0.1	0.1	0.1	0.1	0.0	0.1	0.1
30–34	0.1	0.2	0.1	0.2	0.2	0.0	0.2	0.1	0.1	0.1	0.2
35–39	0.3	0.3	0.2	0.2	0.2	0.3	0.2	0.2	0.0	0.2	0.3
40–44	0.5	0.5	0.1	0.6	0.3	0.3	0.3	0.4	0.2	0.2	0.2
45–49	1.0	0.6	0.8	0.7	0.7	0.6	0.4	0.3	0.3	0.5	0.2
50–54	1.3	1.5	1.0	1.2	0.9	0.9	0.9	0.8	0.6	0.8	0.4
55–59	1.8	1.9	1.7	1.1	2.0	1.2	1.0	1.1	1.0	0.8	0.6
60–64	2.8	3.3	2.5	1.8	2.4	2.3	1.6	1.2	1.3	1.0	1.5
65–69	7.2	5.1	5.7	4.3	3.5	3.8	1.6	2.3	1.9	1.9	1.9
70–74	7.4	6.7	4.9	4.8	5.1	5.2	3.8	3.5	2.7	2.6	2.9
75–79	9.3	9.4	9.0	12.0	10.0	7.3	5.3	4.5	4.5	5.4	3.0
80–84	17.8	13.5	21.9	16.0	15.4	10.1	8.6	7.4	6.6	6.0	6.8
85–	24.3	17.6	14.2	17.6	32.6	18.8	18.6	14.1	15.4	14.9	14.4
Female											
0–4	0.1	0.1	0.1	0.1	0.0	0.0	0.0	0.0	0.0	0.0	0.0
5–9	0.0	0.1	0.0	0.0	0.0	0.0	0.0	0.0	0.0	0.0	0.0
10–14	0.0	0.0	0.1	0.0	0.1	0.0	0.0	0.0	0.0	0.0	0.0
15–19	0.0	0.1	0.0	0.0	0.1	0.1	0.0	0.0	0.0	0.0	0.0
20–24	0.1	0.0	0.1	0.1	0.0	0.0	0.0	0.0	0.0	0.0	0.0
25–29	0.1	0.1	0.1	0.0	0.1	0.1	0.0	0.0	0.0	0.1	0.1
30–34	0.1	0.2	0.1	0.2	0.1	0.1	0.1	0.1	0.1	0.1	0.1
35–39	0.4	0.3	0.3	0.1	0.1	0.2	0.2	0.1	0.2	0.1	0.2
40–44	0.6	0.2	0.3	0.2	0.2	0.2	0.2	0.2	0.2	0.3	0.1
45–49	0.9	0.7	0.6	0.5	0.4	0.4	0.2	0.2	0.3	0.3	0.5
50–54	1.0	1.4	0.9	0.7	0.6	0.3	0.6	0.5	0.2	0.5	0.4
55–59	1.5	1.3	1.5	0.8	1.1	0.7	0.6	0.4	0.3	0.8	0.5
60–64	2.3	1.9	1.9	1.7	1.4	1.4	0.6	0.7	0.6	0.9	0.4
65–69	3.9	2.9	2.4	2.6	2.1	2.3	1.2	1.3	0.8	1.2	1.0
70–74	3.8	5.0	4.0	4.9	3.2	3.1	2.1	1.9	1.2	1.1	1.2
75–79	4.5	6.2	9.9	5.0	7.3	6.2	3.0	3.0	1.8	1.9	2.0
80–84	3.9	12.3	10.5	13.8	12.0	7.2	6.5	5.0	3.8	3.8	3.2
85–	15.0	11.6	22.0	22.2	20.9	17.2	18.5	13.1	12.3	11.5	12.7

Mortality rates per 100,000 population.

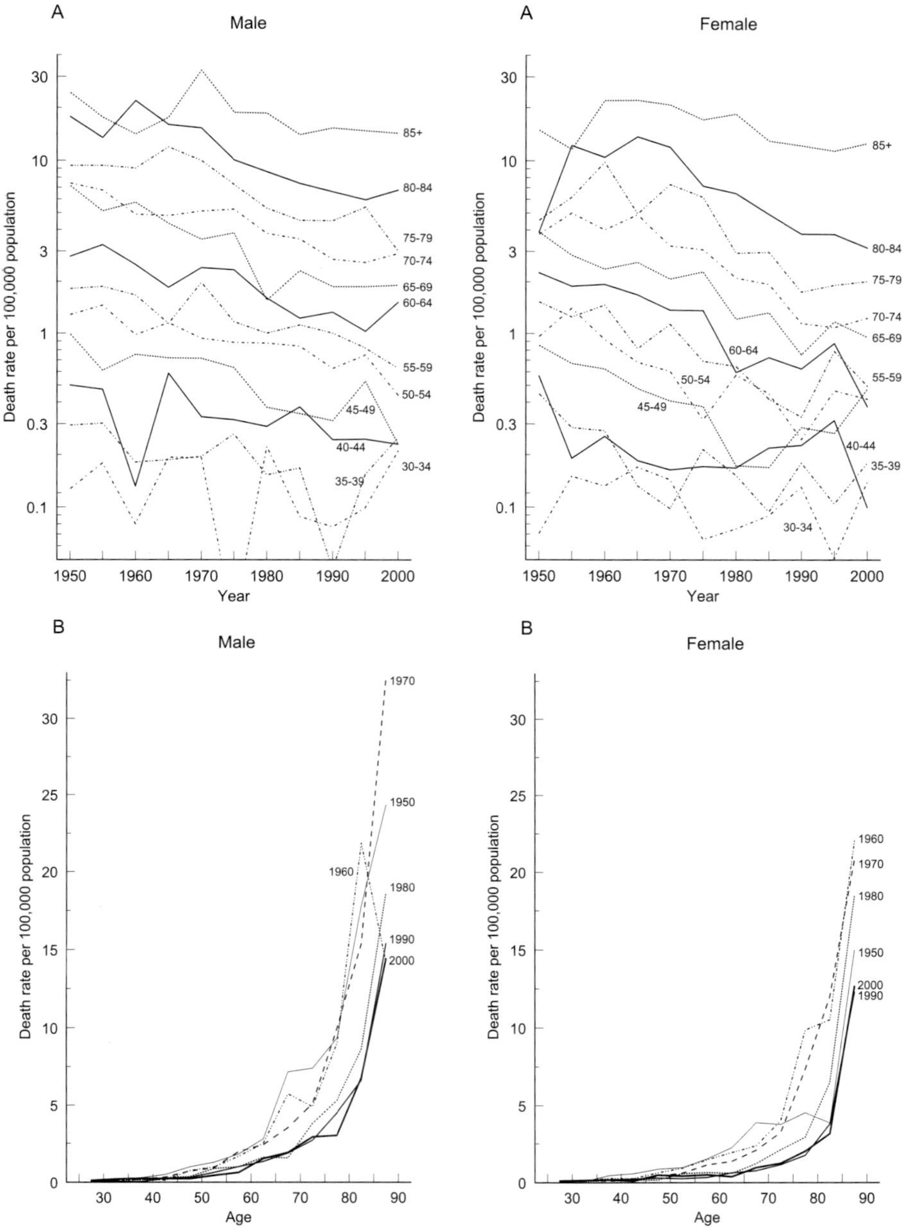

FIG. 3-13. Trends in the age- and sex-specific cancer mortality rate by age group (1950–2000) (A) and by year (1950, 1960, 1970, 1980, 1990, and 2000) (B) in Japan
Cancer of the skin (ICD, 10th revision: C43, C44)

TABLE III-14. Age- and Sex-specific Cancer Mortality Rates in Japan (1950–2000)
Cancer of the breast (ICD, 10th revision: C50)

	1950	1955	1960	1965	1970	1975	1980	1985	1990	1995	2000
Female											
0–4	0.0	0.0	0.0	0.0	0.0	0.0	0.0	0.0	0.0	0.0	0.0
5–9	0.0	0.0	0.0	0.0	0.0	0.0	0.0	0.0	0.0	0.0	0.0
10–14	0.0	0.0	0.0	0.0	0.0	0.0	0.0	0.0	0.0	0.0	0.0
15–19	0.0	0.0	0.0	0.0	0.0	0.0	0.0	0.0	0.0	0.0	0.0
20–24	0.1	0.1	0.0	0.0	0.1	0.2	0.1	0.2	0.0	0.1	0.1
25–29	0.4	0.5	0.4	0.5	0.6	0.5	1.0	0.8	0.8	0.6	0.5
30–34	1.8	1.8	1.6	1.7	2.0	2.3	2.5	3.0	2.6	2.4	2.3
35–39	3.6	4.3	4.1	4.0	4.2	4.6	5.5	5.5	6.4	7.3	7.3
40–44	7.0	6.4	6.4	6.8	7.2	8.6	8.6	9.5	10.8	12.4	12.5
45–49	9.0	8.7	9.5	9.4	10.6	12.3	13.3	13.1	15.8	18.6	20.2
50–54	10.9	10.1	9.6	12.6	13.2	17.1	17.2	17.9	19.2	26.6	28.4
55–59	13.6	11.6	11.5	12.6	14.2	16.4	19.9	20.7	22.5	25.3	29.9
60–64	15.2	13.6	10.3	11.9	14.0	15.8	17.2	19.9	20.2	24.0	26.5
65–69	15.0	14.7	11.9	12.9	12.5	14.6	18.2	19.1	19.6	25.0	26.3
70–74	14.8	16.9	15.6	12.6	15.3	14.8	18.0	19.7	20.1	22.0	24.7
75–79	17.0	18.4	17.8	12.7	14.4	15.4	18.2	17.6	18.5	24.7	27.8
80–84	15.5	18.0	21.7	17.0	23.3	18.2	20.2	19.5	20.9	26.4	27.9
85–	15.0	23.3	28.1	20.4	30.1	24.3	23.3	26.3	23.3	32.8	37.1

Mortality rates per 100,000 population.

TABLE III-15. Age- and Sex-specific Cancer Mortality Rates in Japan (1950–2000)
Cancer of the uterus (ICD, 10th revision: C53–C55, C58)

	1950	1955	1960	1965	1970	1975	1980	1985	1990	1995	2000
0–4	0.0	0.0	0.0	0.0	0.0	0.0	0.0	0.0	0.0	0.0	0.0
5–9	0.0	0.0	0.0	0.0	0.0	0.0	0.0	0.0	0.0	0.0	0.0
10–14	0.0	0.1	0.0	0.1	0.0	0.0	0.0	0.0	0.0	0.0	0.0
15–19	0.1	0.1	0.2	0.1	0.2	0.0	0.0	0.0	0.0	0.0	0.0
20–24	0.8	0.5	0.8	0.6	0.2	0.3	0.2	0.2	0.3	0.0	0.2
25–29	3.0	2.3	2.3	1.7	1.2	0.5	0.6	0.5	0.5	0.5	0.6
30–34	8.8	5.1	4.5	3.8	2.6	1.7	1.1	1.3	1.0	1.7	1.8
35–39	23.5	12.4	9.9	7.3	5.6	2.9	2.2	1.9	2.4	2.4	3.6
40–44	43.8	27.0	19.0	13.7	11.9	7.1	4.7	3.9	3.2	3.8	4.1
45–49	62.7	43.7	34.5	23.5	19.5	14.8	9.5	7.1	5.4	6.0	7.1
50–54	76.8	58.8	46.9	36.5	26.8	22.1	14.9	10.8	7.9	8.3	9.1
55–59	80.3	65.6	55.7	46.6	37.1	28.7	21.0	14.2	12.3	11.1	12.5
60–64	84.1	70.2	64.7	57.0	49.3	36.9	27.8	20.5	14.3	13.5	12.1
65–69	85.5	71.9	68.0	63.3	52.5	47.5	35.7	26.7	20.0	16.1	13.8
70–74	72.2	79.9	71.9	65.5	61.9	57.0	43.8	32.6	25.2	21.7	18.5
75–79	53.6	65.8	71.6	70.2	62.3	59.5	54.2	41.2	34.1	27.2	23.6
80–84	52.2	50.3	51.9	66.2	59.4	56.6	64.5	56.4	47.2	39.2	32.8
85–	22.5	39.2	43.3	39.2	48.0	52.3	53.5	52.6	51.8	56.1	46.1

Mortality rates per 100,000 population.

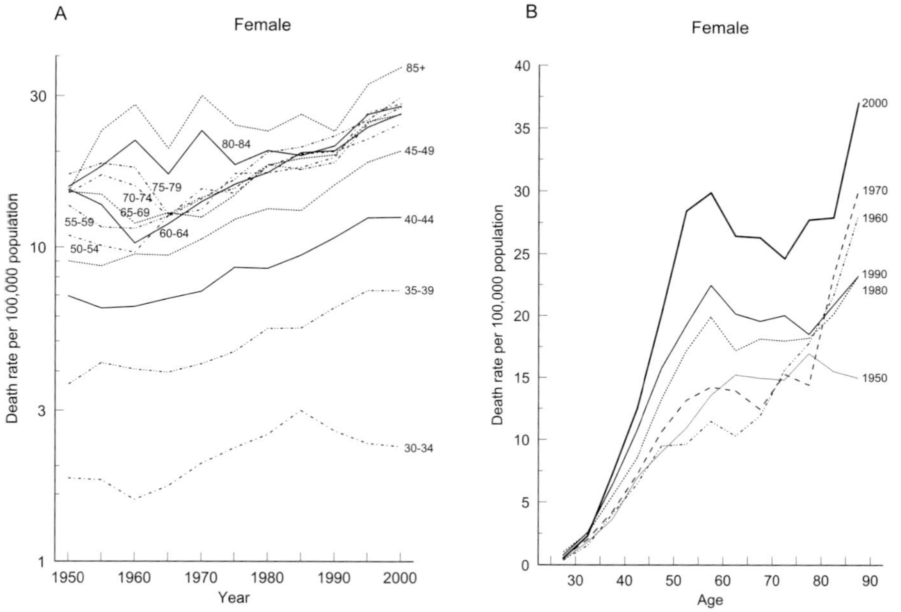

FIG. 3-14. Trends in the age- and sex-specific cancer mortality rate by age group (1950–2000) (A) and by year (1950, 1960, 1970, 1980, 1990, and 2000) (B) in Japan
Cancer of the breast (ICD, 10th revision: C50)

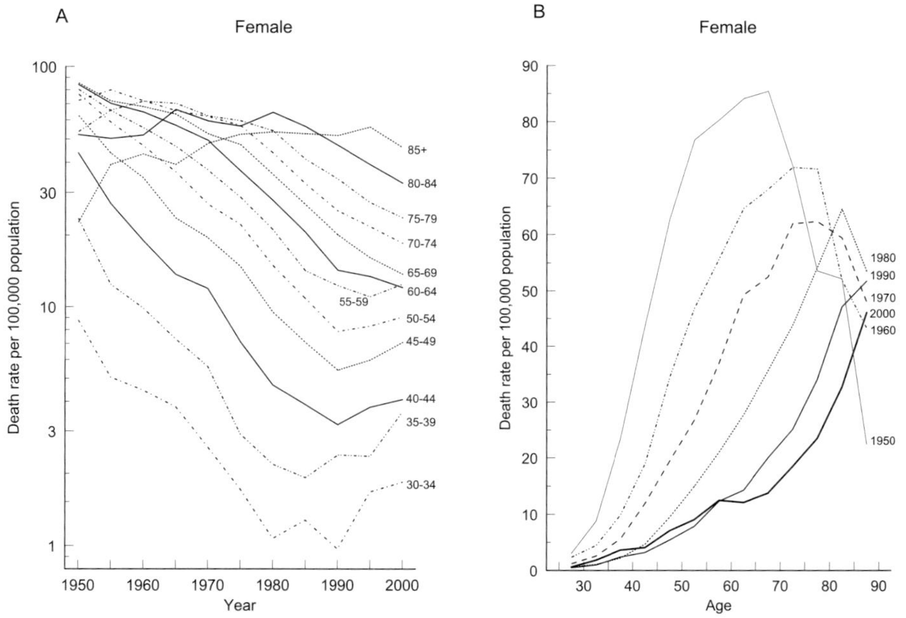

FIG. 3-15. Trends in the age- and sex-specific cancer mortality rate by age group (1950–2000) (A) and by year (1950, 1960, 1970, 1980, 1990, and 2000) (B) in Japan
Cancer of the uterus (ICD, 10th revision: C53–C55, C58)

TABLE III-16. Age- and Sex-specific Cancer Mortality Rates in Japan (1950–2000)
Cancer of the ovary (ICD, 10th revision: C56)

	1950	1955	1960	1965	1970	1975	1980	1985	1990	1995	2000
0–4	0.0	0.0	0.0	0.0	0.1	0.1	0.0	0.0	0.0	0.1	0.0
5–9	0.0	0.0	0.1	0.1	0.1	0.1	0.1	0.0	0.0	0.0	0.0
10–14	0.1	0.2	0.4	0.3	0.2	0.3	0.3	0.2	0.0	0.1	0.1
15–19	0.4	0.2	0.6	0.4	0.7	0.5	0.3	0.4	0.1	0.3	0.2
20–24	0.6	0.5	0.5	0.7	1.0	0.6	0.8	0.5	0.4	0.4	0.3
25–29	0.7	0.7	0.7	0.8	0.9	0.8	0.8	0.5	0.6	0.4	0.4
30–34	0.6	0.8	0.7	1.0	1.2	1.0	1.1	1.2	0.9	0.9	0.8
35–39	1.0	1.5	1.9	1.6	1.4	1.7	1.5	1.9	2.0	1.7	1.8
40–44	1.2	1.8	1.9	2.4	2.5	3.4	3.4	4.1	3.8	3.7	3.5
45–49	2.2	3.0	3.1	4.5	4.2	4.7	5.7	5.9	7.4	7.2	7.0
50–54	2.8	3.4	3.7	4.8	4.9	7.7	9.3	10.3	9.3	9.9	9.6
55–59	2.2	3.9	4.1	4.5	6.1	7.1	8.8	10.1	11.2	10.7	11.0
60–64	2.5	2.6	4.4	5.2	6.0	8.2	9.6	10.7	11.9	12.9	10.0
65–69	2.7	2.5	3.6	4.4	7.0	7.9	10.9	10.9	11.3	14.1	12.2
70–74	2.3	2.5	3.7	4.4	5.9	7.0	11.2	12.9	15.0	15.6	14.0
75–79	3.1	3.2	2.9	3.1	7.5	7.2	11.6	14.3	17.1	18.2	16.6
80–84	1.1	0.8	4.1	3.8	4.4	7.0	9.5	13.8	16.9	19.0	19.2
85–	0.0	1.1	0.8	2.8	3.4	3.4	5.3	12.1	20.9	24.1	23.6

Mortality rates per 100,000 population.

TABLE III-17. Age- and Sex-specific Cancer Mortality Rates in Japan (1950–2000)
Cancer of the prostate (ICD, 10th revision: C61)

	1950	1955	1960	1965	1970	1975	1980	1985	1990	1995	2000
0–4	0.0	0.0	0.0	0.0	0.0	0.0	0.0	0.0	0.0	0.0	0.0
5–9	0.0	0.0	0.0	0.0	0.0	0.0	0.0	0.0	0.0	0.0	0.0
10–14	0.0	0.0	0.0	0.0	0.0	0.0	0.0	0.0	0.0	0.0	0.0
15–19	0.0	0.0	0.0	0.0	0.0	0.0	0.0	0.0	0.0	0.0	0.0
20–24	0.0	0.0	0.0	0.0	0.0	0.0	0.0	0.0	0.0	0.0	0.0
25–29	0.0	0.0	0.0	0.0	0.0	0.1	0.0	0.0	0.1	0.0	0.0
30–34	0.0	0.0	0.1	0.1	0.1	0.0	0.0	0.0	0.1	0.0	0.0
35–39	0.0	0.0	0.1	0.1	0.0	0.0	0.0	0.0	0.0	0.0	0.0
40–44	0.0	0.0	0.0	0.1	0.1	0.1	0.1	0.0	0.1	0.2	0.1
45–49	0.1	0.1	0.4	0.1	0.2	0.2	0.1	0.2	0.1	0.2	0.3
50–54	0.3	0.7	0.5	0.9	0.7	0.6	0.8	0.6	0.6	0.7	0.9
55–59	0.9	1.5	1.4	2.1	1.9	2.0	2.1	2.3	2.4	3.0	3.3
60–64	0.8	3.4	4.2	4.0	4.9	5.5	5.8	5.2	7.6	8.3	8.6
65–69	2.5	6.5	8.5	10.3	11.3	11.0	12.5	13.6	13.4	20.7	22.5
70–74	2.8	11.1	16.7	20.4	19.8	27.5	27.4	32.3	35.2	41.8	49.5
75–79	3.7	11.7	26.8	32.5	36.0	45.3	53.1	67.2	65.4	83.9	81.9
80–84	6.3	14.3	32.5	44.9	49.0	64.5	80.4	109.5	118.1	150.7	173.6
85–	3.5	2.5	23.0	32.5	77.6	74.3	98.5	158.5	183.6	255.1	305.9

Mortality rates per 100,000 population.

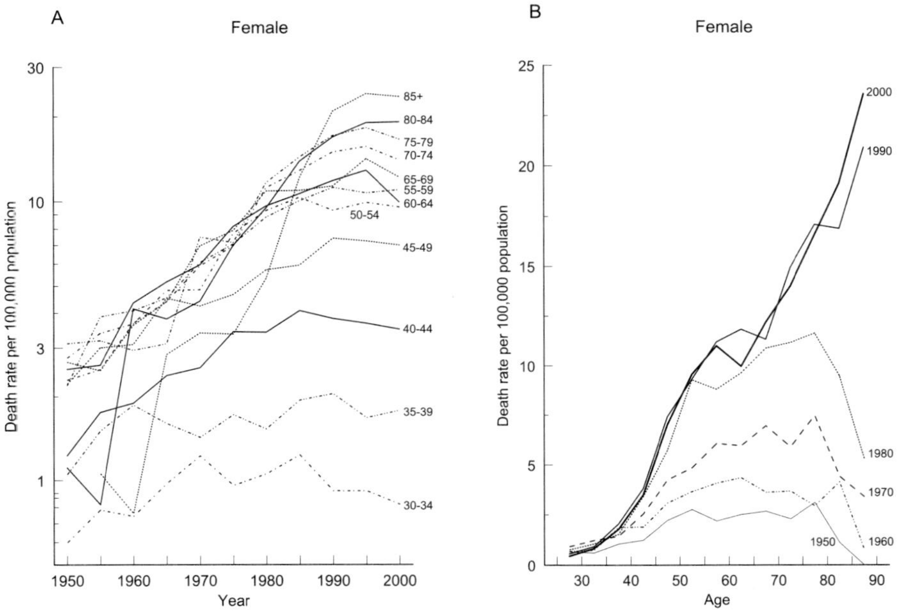

FIG. 3-16. Trends in the age- and sex-specific cancer mortality rate by age group (1950–2000) (A) and by year (1950, 1960, 1970, 1980, 1990, and 2000) (B) in Japan
Cancer of the ovary (ICD, 10th revision: C56)

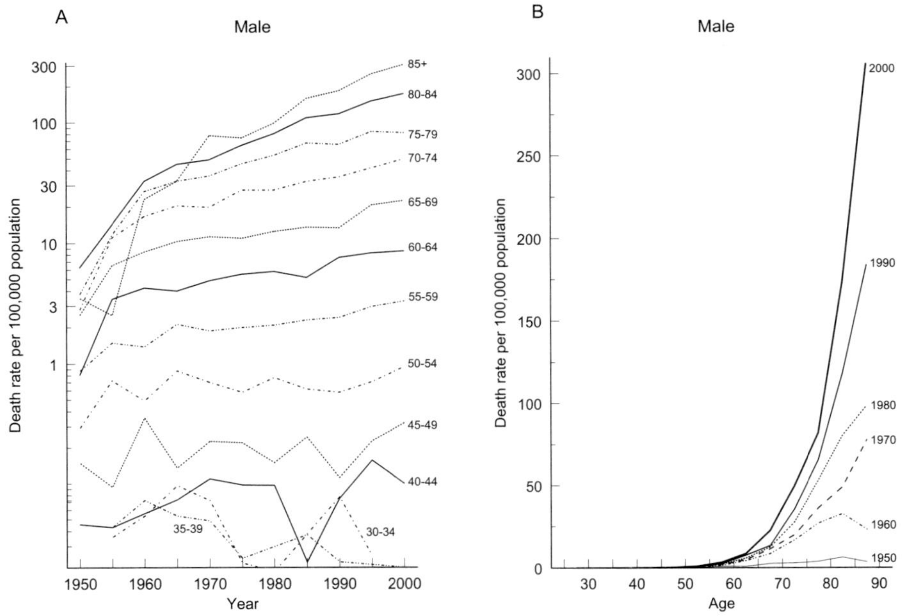

FIG. 3-17. Trends in the age- and sex-specific cancer mortality rate by age group (1950–2000) (A) and by year (1950, 1960, 1970, 1980, 1990, and 2000) (B) in Japan
Cancer of the prostate (ICD, 10th revision: C61)

TABLE III-18. Age- and Sex-specific Cancer Mortality Rates in Japan (1950–2000)
Cancer of the urinary bladder (ICD, 10th revision: C67)

	1950	1955	1960	1965	1970	1975	1980	1985	1990	1995	2000
Male											
0–4	0.0	0.0	0.0	0.0	0.0	0.1	0.0	0.0	0.0	0.0	0.0
5–9	0.0	0.0	0.0	0.0	0.0	0.0	0.0	0.0	0.0	0.0	0.0
10–14	0.0	0.0	0.0	0.0	0.0	0.0	0.0	0.0	0.0	0.0	0.0
15–19	0.1	0.0	0.0	0.0	0.0	0.0	0.0	0.0	0.0	0.0	0.0
20–24	0.0	0.0	0.0	0.0	0.0	0.0	0.0	0.0	0.0	0.0	0.0
25–29	0.0	0.0	0.0	0.0	0.0	0.0	0.0	0.0	0.0	0.0	0.0
30–34	0.1	0.2	0.0	0.1	0.0	0.1	0.0	0.1	0.1	0.0	0.0
35–39	0.1	0.2	0.1	0.2	0.3	0.0	0.0	0.1	0.0	0.1	0.1
40–44	0.2	0.4	0.2	0.5	0.4	0.4	0.4	0.3	0.3	0.5	0.3
45–49	0.7	1.0	0.6	1.1	0.8	0.8	0.8	0.6	0.7	0.8	0.6
50–54	1.2	1.8	1.7	2.0	2.0	1.2	1.8	1.2	1.2	1.3	1.7
55–59	2.1	3.1	3.7	3.4	4.2	4.3	4.0	3.8	3.1	2.8	2.9
60–64	4.6	5.0	6.8	6.4	8.2	6.3	6.9	5.7	6.1	5.0	5.4
65–69	8.7	12.2	12.5	12.6	13.6	12.0	14.4	11.3	10.3	11.1	9.9
70–74	9.8	18.0	20.8	21.4	22.3	23.4	21.7	20.3	20.6	19.7	21.5
75–79	12.7	20.2	26.8	31.0	31.5	29.9	40.0	36.5	34.9	38.0	35.3
80–84	19.9	31.5	34.3	37.4	40.7	50.1	63.1	54.2	55.4	65.0	56.7
85–	13.9	25.2	35.4	47.4	41.6	51.5	69.9	70.9	100.2	117.8	112.6
Female											
0–4	0.0	0.0	0.0	0.0	0.0	0.0	0.0	0.0	0.0	0.0	0.0
5–9	0.0	0.0	0.0	0.0	0.0	0.0	0.0	0.0	0.0	0.0	0.0
10–14	0.0	0.0	0.0	0.0	0.0	0.0	0.0	0.0	0.0	0.0	0.0
15–19	0.0	0.0	0.0	0.0	0.0	0.0	0.0	0.0	0.0	0.0	0.0
20–24	0.0	0.0	0.0	0.0	0.0	0.0	0.0	0.0	0.0	0.0	0.0
25–29	0.1	0.1	0.0	0.0	0.0	0.1	0.0	0.0	0.0	0.0	0.0
30–34	0.0	0.0	0.0	0.1	0.0	0.0	0.0	0.0	0.0	0.1	0.0
35–39	0.0	0.0	0.0	0.2	0.1	0.0	0.1	0.0	0.0	0.1	0.0
40–44	0.5	0.5	0.3	0.2	0.2	0.0	0.1	0.2	0.1	0.0	0.1
45–49	0.7	0.7	0.6	0.5	0.8	0.4	0.4	0.3	0.2	0.2	0.1
50–54	1.4	1.2	1.1	1.4	0.6	0.6	0.5	0.5	0.3	0.4	0.5
55–59	1.3	1.9	1.7	2.3	1.1	1.4	1.2	1.0	0.5	0.5	0.9
60–64	3.3	3.4	6.0	3.5	3.2	3.0	2.3	1.9	1.5	1.2	1.3
65–69	3.8	5.4	7.1	5.0	6.3	5.2	4.0	4.1	2.9	2.6	2.7
70–74	3.9	7.6	7.9	8.0	8.5	8.8	7.8	7.0	5.3	5.1	4.7
75–79	4.5	8.2	10.9	12.1	15.8	13.8	13.1	13.9	10.8	10.9	9.5
80–84	2.8	5.7	10.8	12.9	14.5	21.4	22.1	17.2	18.8	19.8	20.5
85–	3.0	3.2	11.4	6.8	11.2	18.7	25.5	27.1	29.0	35.3	33.8

Mortality rates per 100,000 population.

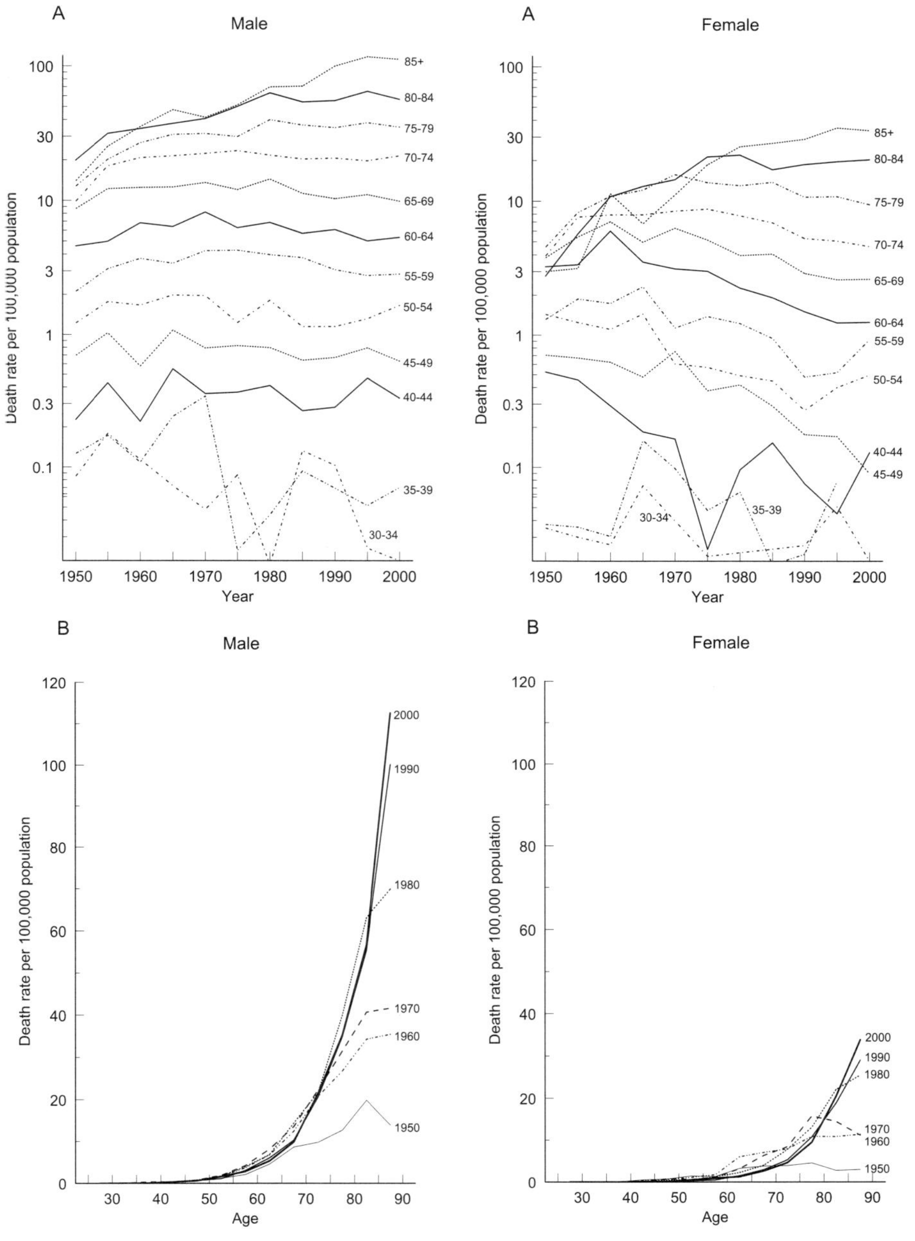

FIG. 3-18. Trends in the age- and sex-specific cancer mortality rate by age group (1950–2000) (A) and by year (1950, 1960, 1970, 1980, 1990, and 2000) (B) in Japan

Cancer of the urinary bladder (ICD, 10th revision: C67)

TABLE III-19. Age- and Sex-specific Cancer Mortality Rates in Japan (1950–2000)
Cancer of the kidney (ICD, 10th revision: C64, C65)

	1950	1955	1960	1965	1970	1975	1980	1985	1990	1995	2000
Male											
0–4	0.3	0.2	0.4	0.5	0.4	0.3	0.3	0.2	0.1	0.1	0.0
5–9	0.0	0.1	0.1	0.1	0.1	0.1	0.1	0.0	0.0	0.1	0.0
10–14	0.0	0.0	0.1	0.0	0.0	0.0	0.0	0.0	0.0	0.0	0.0
15–19	0.0	0.0	0.0	0.0	0.0	0.0	0.1	0.1	0.1	0.0	0.0
20–24	0.0	0.1	0.0	0.2	0.1	0.1	0.0	0.0	0.0	0.0	0.1
25–29	0.1	0.0	0.2	0.1	0.0	0.1	0.0	0.2	0.0	0.1	0.0
30–34	0.0	0.0	0.1	0.0	0.2	0.0	0.0	0.3	0.2	0.1	0.0
35–39	0.2	0.3	0.1	0.2	0.1	0.2	0.1	0.2	0.3	0.3	0.4
40–44	0.6	0.2	0.4	0.2	0.4	0.6	0.7	0.5	0.7	0.6	0.7
45–49	0.4	0.5	0.9	0.9	0.9	0.6	1.5	1.5	1.3	1.6	1.4
50–54	0.6	0.7	1.2	1.8	1.8	1.9	2.7	3.0	3.0	2.5	3.0
55–59	0.7	1.1	2.4	2.4	2.3	4.2	4.2	4.9	5.3	5.2	4.4
60–64	1.4	2.5	3.3	3.7	4.7	5.0	6.8	7.9	8.5	9.1	8.1
65–69	1.6	1.8	3.9	4.5	6.0	7.7	9.0	12.8	12.0	13.2	13.8
70–74	1.1	3.2	3.6	4.8	6.5	9.0	10.1	14.0	16.6	18.7	18.2
75–79	0.7	1.5	4.8	3.8	5.7	7.6	14.3	16.9	22.6	22.6	23.3
80–84	2.1	0.0	3.0	2.7	4.6	8.1	15.4	16.5	24.2	30.6	28.5
85–	0.0	2.5	1.8	2.7	3.4	4.1	12.8	16.4	23.5	35.6	37.4
Female											
0–4	0.1	0.2	0.5	0.6	0.4	0.1	0.3	0.1	0.2	0.0	0.1
5–9	0.1	0.1	0.2	0.1	0.1	0.0	0.1	0.1	0.0	0.0	0.1
10–14	0.0	0.0	0.0	0.0	0.0	0.0	0.0	0.1	0.0	0.0	0.0
15–19	0.1	0.0	0.0	0.0	0.0	0.1	0.1	0.0	0.0	0.0	0.1
20–24	0.1	0.0	0.1	0.0	0.0	0.0	0.0	0.0	0.0	0.0	0.1
25–29	0.1	0.1	0.1	0.0	0.1	0.0	0.0	0.2	0.1	0.0	0.1
30–34	0.0	0.1	0.1	0.1	0.1	0.0	0.0	0.1	0.1	0.1	0.1
35–39	0.2	0.1	0.2	0.1	0.1	0.2	0.2	0.1	0.1	0.2	0.1
40–44	0.3	0.4	0.3	0.1	0.2	0.1	0.2	0.3	0.4	0.4	0.4
45–49	0.2	0.3	0.4	0.5	0.4	0.3	0.3	0.3	0.4	0.7	0.6
50–54	0.5	0.9	0.7	0.8	0.7	0.6	0.9	0.8	0.9	0.9	0.7
55–59	0.4	0.5	0.9	0.8	1.0	1.4	1.3	1.4	1.8	1.4	1.4
60–64	0.5	0.9	1.3	1.6	1.8	2.1	2.4	3.0	2.4	2.6	2.5
65–69	1.4	1.1	1.3	2.0	2.5	3.7	3.2	3.7	3.7	3.8	3.6
70–74	1.5	1.3	2.5	2.9	3.8	3.4	4.6	4.6	5.6	6.4	5.7
75–79	1.4	1.5	2.6	3.1	2.0	4.0	4.7	7.2	8.2	7.7	8.5
80–84	0.6	1.6	1.3	2.1	1.7	3.0	2.7	8.1	10.9	12.6	13.0
85–	1.5	1.1	2.3	0.6	1.9	4.1	4.2	6.8	11.8	14.2	16.7

Mortality rates per 100,000 population.

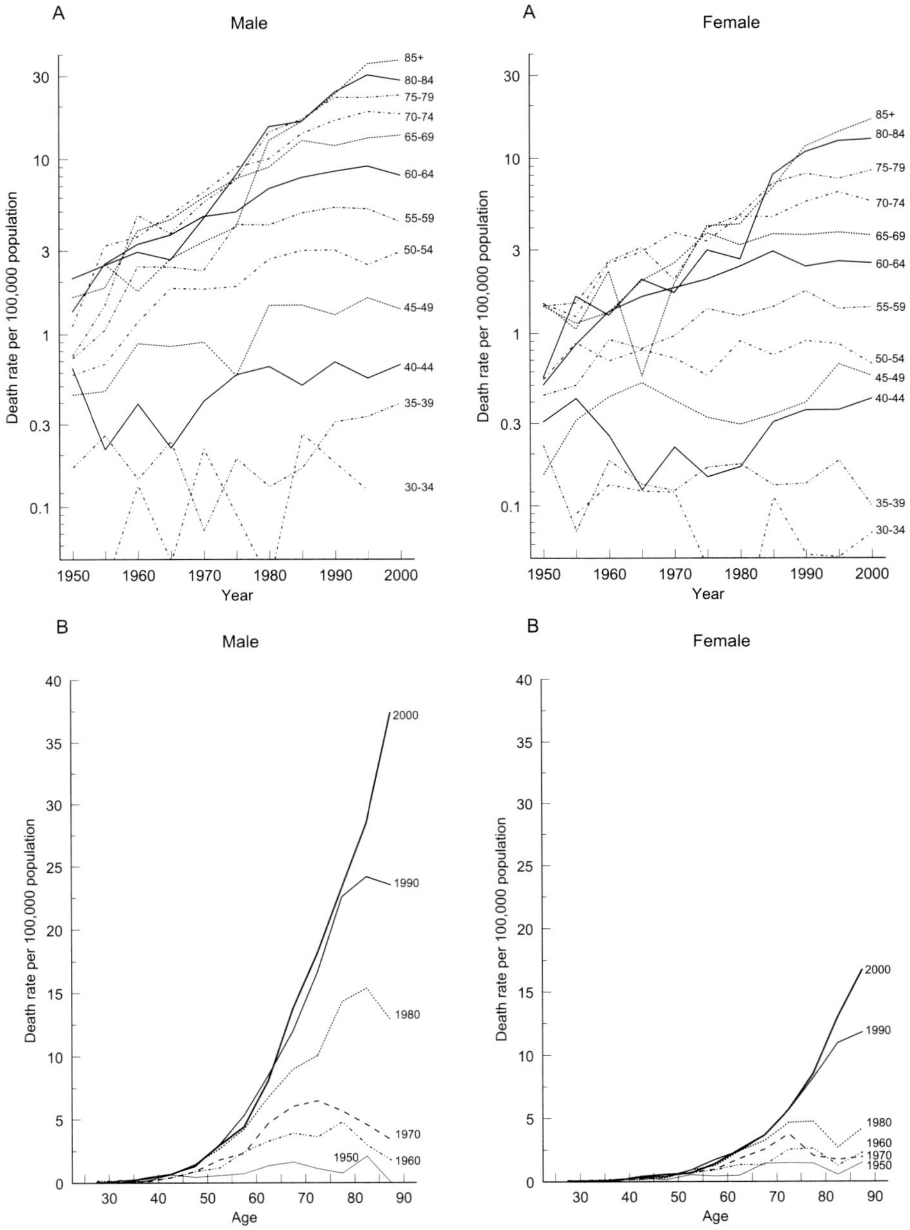

FIG. 3-19. Trends in the age- and sex-specific cancer mortality rate by age group (1950–2000) (A) and by year (1950, 1960, 1970, 1980, 1990, and 2000) (B) in Japan

Cancer of the kidney (ICD, 10th revision: C64, C65)

TABLE III-20. Age- and Sex-specific Cancer Mortality Rates in Japan (1950–2000)
Cancer of the lymphatic and hematopoietic systems other than leukemia (ICD, 10th revision: C81–C90, C96)

	1950	1955	1960	1965	1970	1975	1980	1985	1990	1995	2000
Male											
0–4	0.7	0.5	0.7	0.7	0.4	0.6	0.6	0.7	0.3	0.2	0.1
5–9	0.4	0.4	0.7	0.8	0.5	0.5	0.6	0.5	0.5	0.3	0.2
10–14	0.2	0.4	0.6	0.6	0.9	0.9	0.7	0.7	0.4	0.3	0.3
15–19	0.3	0.8	0.6	0.8	0.8	1.1	1.3	1.0	0.6	0.6	0.4
20–24	0.5	0.3	0.7	0.7	1.0	1.0	0.8	0.6	0.8	0.6	0.6
25–29	0.5	0.8	0.6	1.0	1.0	0.9	1.0	0.7	1.0	0.9	0.7
30–34	0.7	1.0	1.1	1.3	1.3	1.0	1.0	0.7	1.1	0.9	1.0
35–39	1.1	1.4	1.6	1.7	1.6	1.9	1.8	1.8	1.2	1.6	1.4
40–44	1.1	1.7	2.2	2.7	2.6	3.0	2.7	2.1	2.2	2.5	2.3
45–49	2.1	3.4	3.2	3.3	3.7	4.9	5.1	4.0	4.0	3.6	4.2
50–54	2.7	4.0	5.1	5.3	5.4	6.7	8.1	6.6	5.5	7.0	5.5
55–59	3.8	5.0	7.1	6.9	9.6	11.2	11.1	11.0	12.2	10.3	11.3
60–64	4.7	7.0	9.0	11.7	13.6	15.2	16.6	16.9	19.1	18.6	16.0
65–69	6.4	7.1	8.6	14.1	16.8	21.9	23.4	23.9	23.8	27.5	27.9
70–74	5.4	8.9	10.4	14.1	19.7	24.8	32.2	38.2	38.5	41.7	43.5
75–79	5.6	7.6	8.8	12.6	19.0	26.7	38.5	49.1	53.2	55.9	62.5
80–84	4.2	4.5	7.7	10.7	16.6	27.7	38.4	59.4	61.9	80.6	79.5
85–	0.0	7.6	12.4	14.9	19.1	21.2	40.2	52.1	64.1	84.9	105.1
Female											
0–4	0.4	0.7	0.3	0.5	0.4	0.4	0.4	0.4	0.3	0.2	0.1
5–9	0.3	0.4	0.4	0.5	0.2	0.2	0.2	0.2	0.2	0.2	0.1
10–14	0.0	0.2	0.3	0.3	0.3	0.5	0.2	0.3	0.1	0.2	0.1
15–19	0.3	0.3	0.3	0.5	0.3	0.4	0.5	0.4	0.3	0.4	0.3
20–24	0.1	0.3	0.3	0.5	0.5	0.4	0.4	0.3	0.5	0.1	0.4
25–29	0.3	0.3	0.5	0.5	0.3	0.6	0.7	0.5	0.3	0.4	0.5
30–34	0.4	0.7	0.6	0.8	0.7	0.8	0.7	0.6	0.7	0.4	0.6
35–39	0.8	0.6	0.7	0.7	1.2	1.0	0.9	0.9	1.0	1.0	1.0
40–44	1.2	0.6	0.8	1.2	1.1	1.1	1.5	1.2	1.5	1.4	1.7
45–49	1.6	1.3	2.0	2.0	2.2	2.3	2.3	2.1	2.2	2.0	2.2
50–54	1.1	1.9	2.6	2.8	3.5	4.0	4.0	3.4	3.3	3.5	4.0
55–59	2.8	3.4	3.0	4.6	5.7	6.1	7.0	5.7	6.0	5.6	6.1
60–64	2.3	3.6	3.8	4.8	8.1	8.2	9.3	8.8	9.5	8.8	9.3
65–69	3.4	4.1	4.9	7.7	9.1	12.2	12.3	14.5	13.5	16.1	15.5
70–74	3.0	3.9	7.0	6.2	9.4	12.8	18.1	19.6	21.2	23.6	24.0
75–79	1.7	3.7	5.7	7.1	11.6	15.7	21.9	27.4	29.0	33.0	35.2
80–84	3.9	4.5	8.0	5.3	5.4	13.0	19.9	27.0	39.1	47.1	46.7
85–	3.0	3.2	6.8	5.1	4.9	11.6	15.1	28.4	30.1	45.3	52.7

Mortality rates per 100,000 population.

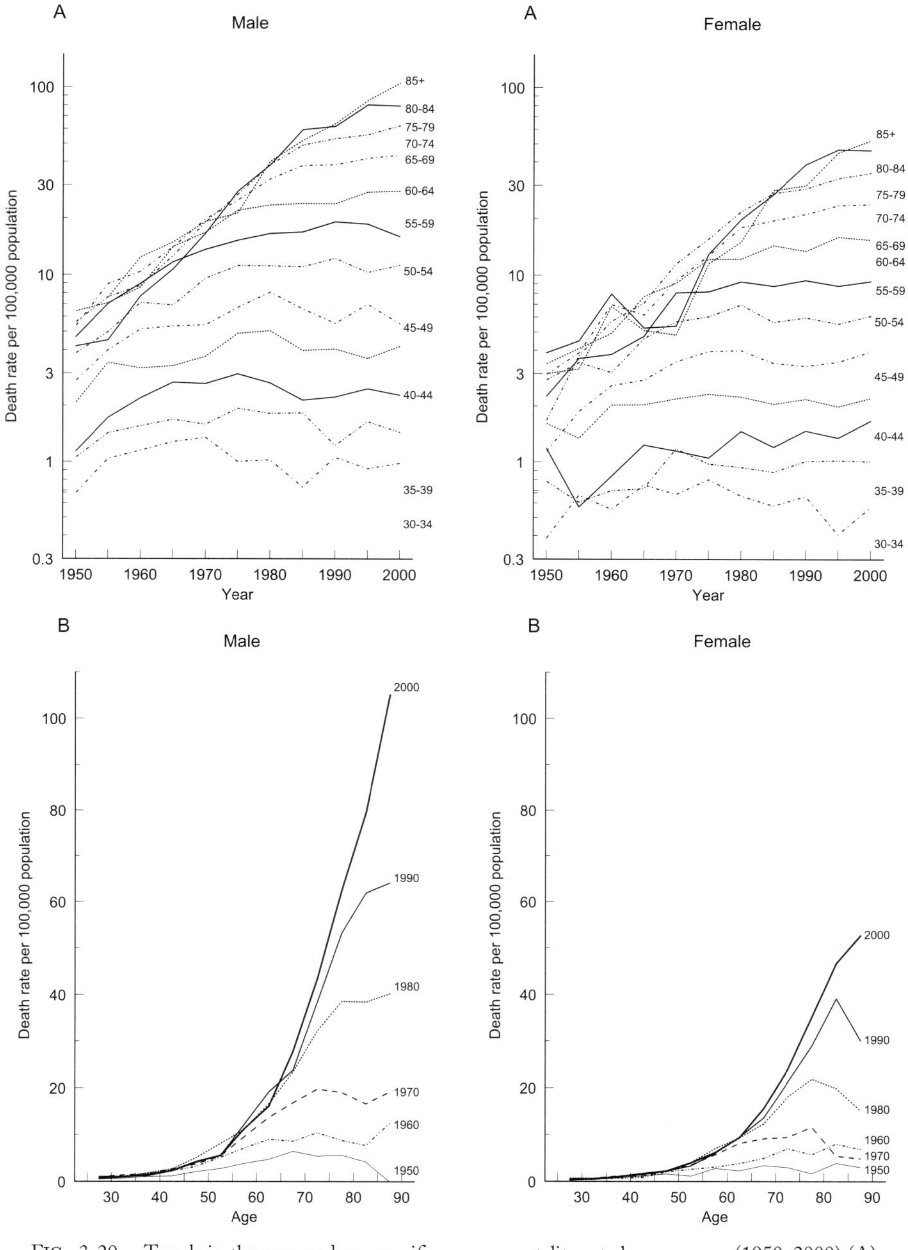

FIG. 3-20. Trends in the age- and sex-specific cancer mortality rate by age group (1950–2000) (A) and by year (1950, 1960, 1970, 1980, 1990, and 2000) (B) in Japan

Cancer of the lymphatic and hematopoietic systems other than leukemia (ICD, 10th revision: C81–C90, C96)

TABLE III-21. Age- and Sex-specific Cancer Mortality Rates in Japan (1950–2000)
Leukemia (ICD, 10th revision: C91–C95)

	1950	1955	1960	1965	1970	1975	1980	1985	1990	1995	2000
Male											
0–4	2.4	4.1	4.5	4.4	4.6	3.9	2.8	1.3	1.4	1.1	1.0
5–9	1.5	2.8	2.9	3.7	3.5	3.5	3.3	2.6	1.4	1.5	1.0
10–14	1.5	2.3	2.8	3.0	2.2	2.3	2.6	2.2	2.0	1.5	0.9
15–19	1.7	2.5	2.8	3.3	3.2	2.8	2.5	2.6	2.2	2.4	1.2
20–24	1.2	2.1	2.4	2.7	2.5	2.6	2.0	2.2	2.3	1.8	1.3
25–29	1.3	2.3	2.2	2.6	2.7	2.4	2.8	2.1	2.1	1.9	1.6
30–34	1.7	2.2	2.4	2.4	2.9	3.4	2.4	2.8	2.2	1.9	1.5
35–39	1.7	2.6	2.5	3.2	3.5	3.5	3.5	3.4	3.1	2.4	2.6
40–44	1.9	3.4	3.5	3.0	3.8	4.0	4.0	3.7	3.5	3.5	3.3
45–49	2.1	3.0	3.7	4.6	5.0	4.9	4.9	4.8	4.3	4.1	4.0
50–54	2.3	2.8	4.0	4.9	5.1	5.6	5.7	5.8	6.0	5.4	5.9
55–59	1.9	3.3	5.4	5.2	6.2	6.4	7.1	7.5	8.3	8.2	6.9
60–64	2.5	3.2	4.6	7.1	7.4	8.5	8.4	10.1	11.9	11.0	10.8
65–69	2.0	3.0	5.0	7.0	8.9	10.2	12.5	14.6	13.2	16.4	17.2
70–74	0.7	2.9	5.6	5.2	9.7	11.7	16.8	20.2	18.2	21.1	21.8
75–79	1.9	1.8	3.2	5.1	8.1	13.1	19.6	25.4	24.5	27.7	28.8
80–84	1.0	0.8	4.1	2.1	4.2	10.4	21.1	25.9	33.0	33.7	35.9
85–	0.0	0.0	1.8	2.7	3.4	6.5	17.5	23.1	31.3	45.2	42.0
Female											
0–4	2.0	2.7	3.7	3.5	3.6	3.1	2.0	1.4	1.4	1.2	0.9
5–9	1.0	1.8	2.2	2.7	2.8	2.7	2.3	1.7	1.4	0.9	0.7
10–14	1.1	1.8	2.1	2.4	2.3	1.9	1.9	1.6	1.2	0.9	0.4
15–19	1.0	1.4	2.0	2.6	2.3	2.2	2.2	1.7	1.2	0.9	1.0
20–24	1.0	1.4	2.1	1.8	2.0	2.0	1.7	1.3	1.2	1.3	1.1
25–29	1.1	1.9	1.7	2.0	1.8	2.1	1.5	1.5	1.3	1.0	1.0
30–34	0.7	1.2	2.6	2.1	1.6	2.5	2.2	2.0	1.6	1.4	1.1
35–39	1.3	1.7	2.4	2.8	2.7	2.4	2.5	2.3	2.5	1.8	1.3
40–44	1.0	2.3	2.6	2.9	3.0	3.1	3.4	3.0	2.6	2.3	2.1
45–49	1.5	2.2	3.3	3.3	4.2	3.5	3.3	3.6	3.7	3.0	2.9
50–54	1.6	1.9	2.3	3.7	3.0	4.1	4.5	4.6	4.3	3.7	3.6
55–59	1.2	2.3	2.9	4.1	5.6	5.6	4.3	5.4	5.6	5.3	4.5
60–64	1.4	1.9	2.9	4.6	5.0	5.4	6.0	6.4	6.5	5.8	6.2
65–69	1.1	1.7	3.3	3.8	5.2	6.8	7.1	7.5	8.2	6.9	8.9
70–74	0.8	1.3	1.8	3.3	5.6	6.4	8.4	9.9	10.6	11.3	11.3
75–79	0.0	0.4	2.2	3.1	2.6	8.6	9.4	12.6	12.0	13.9	14.3
80–84	0.0	0.0	1.0	1.2	3.4	4.6	8.7	12.6	17.9	15.8	17.6
85–	0.0	0.0	0.0	0.0	0.0	3.7	5.9	11.9	13.6	18.6	20.5

Mortality rates per 100,000 population.

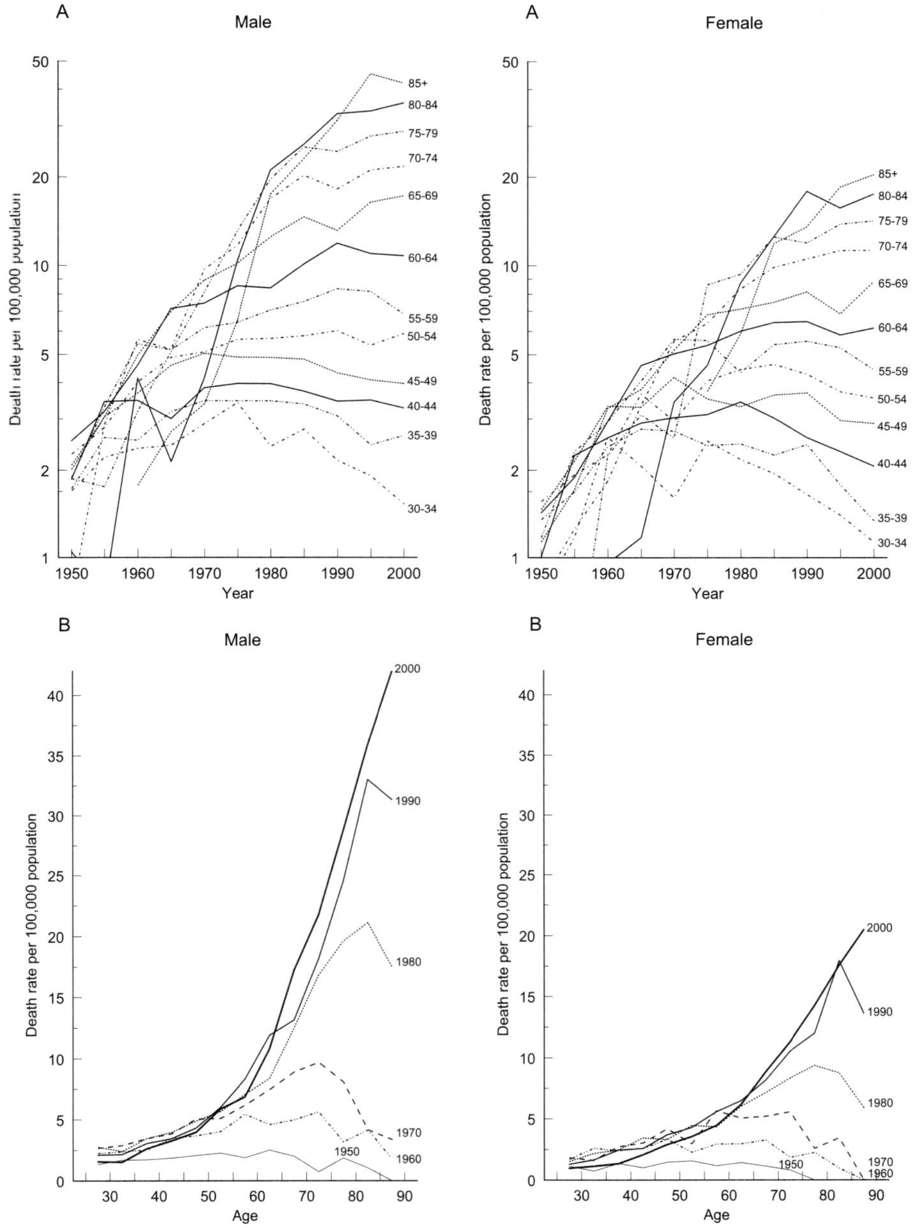

FIG. 3-21. Trends in the age- and sex-specific cancer mortality rate by age group (1950–2000) (A) and by year (1950, 1960, 1970, 1980, 1990, and 2000) (B) in Japan
Leukemia (ICD, 10th revision: C91–C95)

TABLE IV-1. Standardized Mortality Ratio (SMR) of Cancer in Japan by Prefecture (2000)

		A. Cancer of all sites (ICD, 10th revision: C00–C97)		B. Cancer of the buccal cavity and pharynx (ICD, 10th revision: C00–C14)	
		Male	Female	Male	Female
1	Hokkaido	103.6	101.2	110.1	107.7
2	Aomori	111.2	97.7	134.6	103.0
3	Iwate	94.5	92.1	113.5	57.2
4	Miyagi	97.5	98.6	90.1	103.1
5	Akita	111.4	104.7	152.2	120.7
6	Yamagata	101.8	103.1	91.7	78.4
7	Fukushima	97.3	97.2	86.1	110.3
8	Ibaraki	99.7	99.8	86.3	103.4
9	Tochigi	99.0	98.9	79.2	120.0
10	Gunma	90.4	97.5	74.9	83.2
11	Saitama	98.0	102.8	96.8	101.0
12	Chiba	95.1	97.1	89.5	105.6
13	Tokyo	99.3	107.8	120.7	120.0
14	Kanagawa	97.9	100.0	96.0	98.0
15	Niigata	102.1	96.5	96.0	87.5
16	Toyama	93.9	92.6	87.0	96.2
17	Ishikawa	98.4	97.9	63.9	66.9
18	Fukui	89.6	100.0	66.6	98.8
19	Yamanashi	92.3	91.9	74.1	52.5
20	Nagano	83.8	88.5	71.8	88.5
21	Gifu	95.9	100.8	57.5	121.3
22	Shizuoka	93.4	90.6	101.5	89.0
23	Aichi	95.1	100.9	87.4	104.4
24	Mie	96.4	94.1	52.3	95.8
25	Shiga	98.2	97.0	106.5	124.4
26	Kyoto	102.8	106.1	105.6	117.5
27	Osaka	114.4	114.0	108.8	116.6
28	Hyogo	107.5	105.0	107.1	120.4
29	Nara	101.6	97.1	66.8	67.6
30	Wakayama	105.6	100.3	79.6	73.9
31	Tottori	101.8	101.2	103.2	211.6
32	Shimane	104.0	86.3	101.3	89.6
33	Okayama	92.6	92.5	114.7	114.1
34	Hiroshima	100.5	92.2	81.5	66.8
35	Yamaguchi	103.1	101.0	96.2	71.1
36	Tokushima	98.4	98.1	90.3	135.6
37	Kagawa	96.5	96.2	83.0	84.9
38	Ehime	97.3	95.5	88.6	61.8
39	Kochi	90.1	93.0	138.9	70.6
40	Fukuoka	108.6	108.4	111.2	72.2
41	Saga	113.2	100.9	115.9	149.0
42	Nagasaki	109.3	99.3	118.0	86.1
43	Kumamoto	90.4	91.5	83.9	91.1
44	Oita	95.1	93.2	112.8	110.0
45	Miyazaki	98.0	87.3	124.2	81.7
46	Kagoshima	98.2	93.6	142.1	94.5
47	Okinawa	90.0	83.1	169.5	52.8

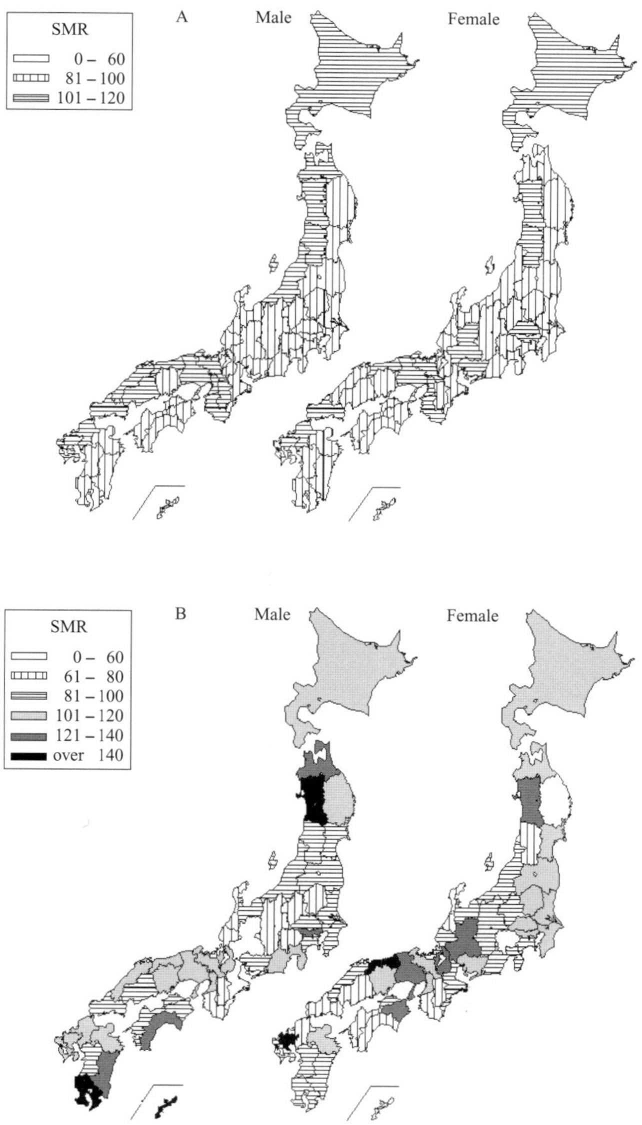

FIG. 4-1. Maps of the standardized mortality ratio (SMR) of cancer in Japan by prefecture (2000)
A: cancer of all sites (ICD, 10th revision: C00–C97)
B: cancer of the buccal cavity and pharynx (ICD, 10th revision: C00–C14)

TABLE IV-2. Standardized Mortality Ratio (SMR) of Cancer in Japan by Prefecture (2000)

		A. Cancer of the esophagus (ICD, 10th revision: C15)		B. Cancer of the stomach (ICD, 10th revision: C16)	
		Male	Female	Male	Female
1	Hokkaido	112.7	92.7	94.8	89.5
2	Aomori	123.6	106.4	116.3	105.4
3	Iwate	110.7	121.2	90.4	85.4
4	Miyagi	124.9	136.6	96.6	94.9
5	Akita	162.5	139.0	130.0	133.9
6	Yamagata	115.0	141.3	129.1	129.0
7	Fukushima	101.0	58.5	97.4	111.0
8	Ibaraki	101.4	111.7	112.7	109.7
9	Tochigi	102.7	133.9	120.4	102.3
10	Gunma	98.7	97.5	102.8	93.4
11	Saitama	100.7	115.5	107.9	110.5
12	Chiba	97.2	109.5	103.3	101.1
13	Tokyo	127.4	130.3	97.7	100.4
14	Kanagawa	119.8	114.5	100.1	95.5
15	Niigata	140.5	95.5	118.6	106.1
16	Toyama	84.5	78.0	105.2	105.9
17	Ishikawa	61.4	81.7	107.9	101.3
18	Fukui	63.1	42.1	79.8	106.6
19	Yamanashi	98.2	73.9	91.9	91.1
20	Nagano	79.6	104.3	89.4	88.6
21	Gifu	65.8	49.3	100.6	117.0
22	Shizuoka	79.2	79.3	87.0	88.6
23	Aichi	72.3	77.6	96.9	116.6
24	Mie	70.5	40.8	105.1	103.9
25	Shiga	74.6	58.7	95.4	99.7
26	Kyoto	80.7	125.2	97.0	112.7
27	Osaka	108.4	121.3	110.8	109.8
28	Hyogo	107.4	126.7	108.8	104.6
29	Nara	71.7	81.0	117.2	100.9
30	Wakayama	83.4	138.3	116.7	115.8
31	Tottori	100.1	62.6	104.2	119.3
32	Shimane	100.2	91.1	103.1	90.4
33	Okayama	80.2	114.1	82.5	100.9
34	Hiroshima	77.4	70.6	93.4	90.0
35	Yamaguchi	96.3	111.9	95.6	103.3
36	Tokushima	82.1	95.2	94.3	77.2
37	Kagawa	60.9	72.9	97.6	111.6
38	Ehime	59.1	66.7	100.9	99.7
39	Kochi	88.5	51.3	85.9	84.7
40	Fukuoka	101.9	83.7	97.0	97.3
41	Saga	84.6	85.4	102.0	91.5
42	Nagasaki	97.5	85.1	95.3	97.5
43	Kumamoto	69.3	71.1	69.6	70.6
44	Oita	60.1	108.2	82.1	75.7
45	Miyazaki	104.8	76.5	86.2	80.1
46	Kagoshima	117.1	77.8	74.0	68.6
47	Okinawa	116.9	64.6	54.4	45.0

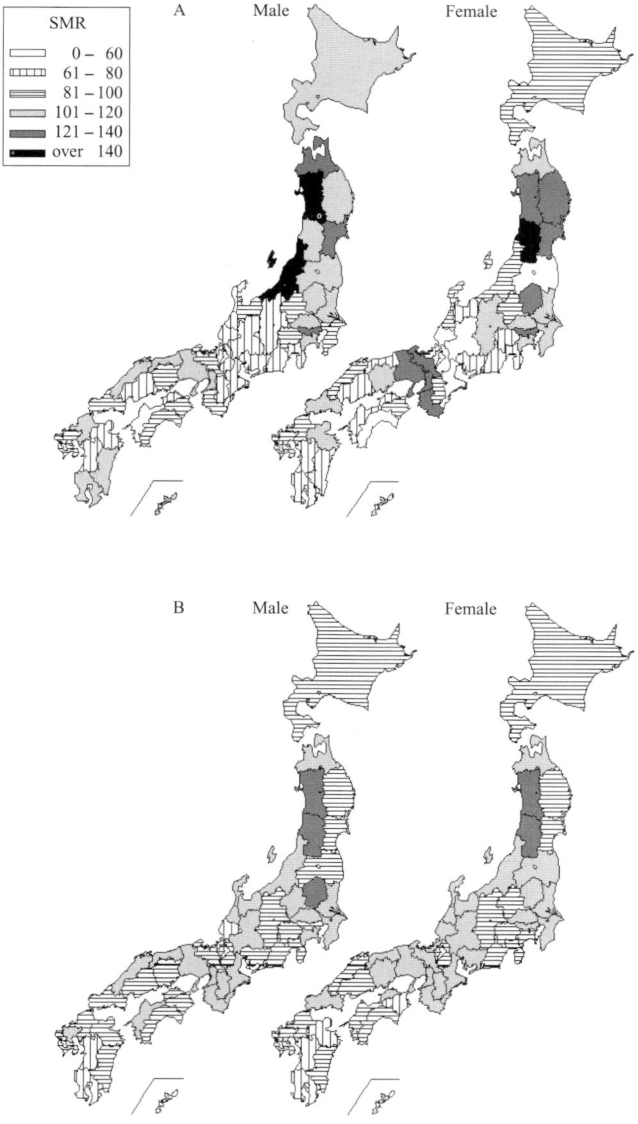

FIG. 4-2. Maps of the standardized mortality ratio (SMR) of cancer in Japan by prefecture (2000)
A: cancer of the esophagus (ICD, 10th revision: C15)
B: cancer of the stomach (ICD, 10th revision: C16)

TABLE IV-3. Standardized Mortality Ratio (SMR) of Cancer in Japan by Prefecture (2000)

		A. Cancer of the colon (ICD, 10th revision: C18)		B. Cancer of the rectum (ICD, 10th revision: C19–C21)	
		Male	Female	Male	Female
1	Hokkaido	117.5	107.6	101.5	106.2
2	Aomori	117.2	107.3	125.6	119.9
3	Iwate	100.0	110.0	112.1	125.7
4	Miyagi	108.6	102.0	112.3	95.5
5	Akita	134.2	129.1	106.2	129.6
6	Yamagata	93.5	115.2	109.0	129.4
7	Fukushima	96.7	96.3	104.3	93.8
8	Ibaraki	90.0	97.9	98.1	100.0
9	Tochigi	94.5	102.9	102.2	96.4
10	Gunma	83.5	93.4	96.7	112.4
11	Saitama	106.4	107.7	102.9	93.8
12	Chiba	99.1	104.6	108.3	97.2
13	Tokyo	110.8	109.9	109.8	105.9
14	Kanagawa	110.7	106.0	112.0	108.7
15	Niigata	99.8	107.0	102.5	127.2
16	Toyama	93.4	91.7	95.4	100.5
17	Ishikawa	104.5	96.1	78.1	121.6
18	Fukui	107.5	83.3	92.4	84.8
19	Yamanashi	88.8	85.7	89.1	107.5
20	Nagano	88.1	89.3	81.6	97.9
21	Gifu	102.5	112.5	102.8	86.3
22	Shizuoka	88.8	91.6	108.6	96.9
23	Aichi	94.2	108.3	97.8	101.3
24	Mie	87.3	95.5	88.0	89.4
25	Shiga	79.8	105.2	95.6	90.6
26	Kyoto	96.9	113.2	103.3	89.2
27	Osaka	114.1	109.7	104.2	97.6
28	Hyogo	97.4	90.8	101.2	112.0
29	Nara	90.7	107.1	78.6	78.0
30	Wakayama	99.3	96.9	94.9	111.4
31	Tottori	87.7	107.1	109.7	102.0
32	Shimane	98.5	89.0	114.3	98.0
33	Okayama	80.8	91.2	95.6	86.2
34	Hiroshima	102.0	86.7	87.7	81.9
35	Yamaguchi	99.9	81.7	70.7	105.8
36	Tokushima	83.0	85.9	104.0	95.8
37	Kagawa	72.7	81.6	79.3	75.6
38	Ehime	89.4	76.8	89.7	101.1
39	Kochi	77.0	86.1	82.3	66.9
40	Fukuoka	107.0	103.8	82.1	93.0
41	Saga	93.8	93.4	101.6	80.9
42	Nagasaki	95.3	77.4	105.2	97.3
43	Kumamoto	77.9	82.7	74.2	80.1
44	Oita	91.7	81.9	92.7	86.7
45	Miyazaki	74.0	89.9	85.9	110.0
46	Kagoshima	77.1	81.6	91.4	96.6
47	Okinawa	87.8	73.3	89.2	64.8

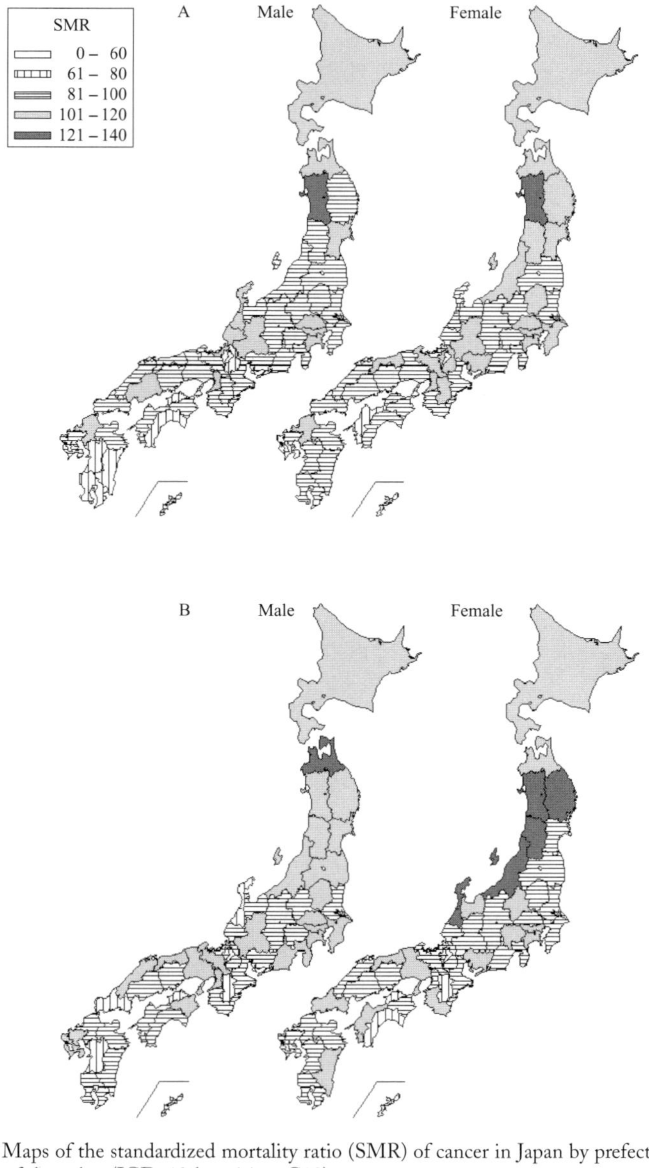

FIG. 4-3. Maps of the standardized mortality ratio (SMR) of cancer in Japan by prefecture (2000)
A: cancer of the colon (ICD, 10th revision: C18)
B: cancer of the rectum (ICD, 10th revision: C19–C21)

TABLE IV-4. Standardized Mortality Ratio (SMR) of Cancer in Japan by Prefecture (2000)

		A. Cancer of the liver (ICD, 10th revision: C22)		B. Cancer of the biliary passages (ICD, 10th revision: C23, C24)	
		Male	Female	Male	Female
1	Hokkaido	81.5	82.2	121.4	109.2
2	Aomori	70.7	81.7	127.9	101.7
3	Iwate	56.6	59.9	128.6	93.0
4	Miyagi	68.1	84.7	110.9	101.8
5	Akita	63.5	62.9	156.0	111.9
6	Yamagata	63.7	79.2	114.7	134.6
7	Fukushima	77.2	92.9	115.0	131.2
8	Ibaraki	91.5	79.2	104.8	115.0
9	Tochigi	87.5	90.8	94.1	107.9
10	Gunma	81.7	102.2	99.7	123.4
11	Saitama	85.9	86.7	99.0	107.2
12	Chiba	86.1	72.9	95.8	90.2
13	Tokyo	93.3	96.1	80.7	97.1
14	Kanagawa	89.7	95.0	83.5	85.1
15	Niigata	56.5	60.0	114.2	121.9
16	Toyama	73.3	80.2	83.4	120.2
17	Ishikawa	80.4	93.6	124.2	106.8
18	Fukui	84.6	91.6	110.3	150.5
19	Yamanashi	110.6	125.1	91.2	96.0
20	Nagano	61.0	76.3	103.7	95.8
21	Gifu	93.0	88.5	85.0	106.1
22	Shizuoka	103.5	92.9	97.9	94.6
23	Aichi	86.0	87.1	93.1	95.3
24	Mie	83.8	100.3	93.6	83.5
25	Shiga	76.2	78.5	97.9	96.3
26	Kyoto	105.8	114.6	106.4	100.3
27	Osaka	152.1	162.1	97.2	100.3
28	Hyogo	134.6	127.7	88.5	89.4
29	Nara	121.1	120.1	90.5	75.8
30	Wakayama	116.6	111.1	99.8	75.0
31	Tottori	110.6	83.4	105.5	114.8
32	Shimane	118.1	111.1	90.0	78.8
33	Okayama	103.3	91.8	106.9	80.4
34	Hiroshima	143.8	129.2	91.6	76.1
35	Yamaguchi	119.9	119.9	100.4	97.1
36	Tokushima	118.9	119.7	91.1	118.7
37	Kagawa	109.2	91.0	95.1	105.4
38	Ehime	132.1	109.9	99.1	79.9
39	Kochi	86.3	90.4	100.2	91.4
40	Fukuoka	158.9	145.2	96.3	99.7
41	Saga	151.4	149.4	120.0	113.1
42	Nagasaki	117.3	99.7	111.4	109.0
43	Kumamoto	113.3	96.3	102.4	96.4
44	Oita	110.5	117.8	126.5	93.2
45	Miyazaki	89.6	79.9	121.0	88.6
46	Kagoshima	101.4	104.2	107.2	117.2
47	Okinawa	53.7	43.3	109.4	105.7

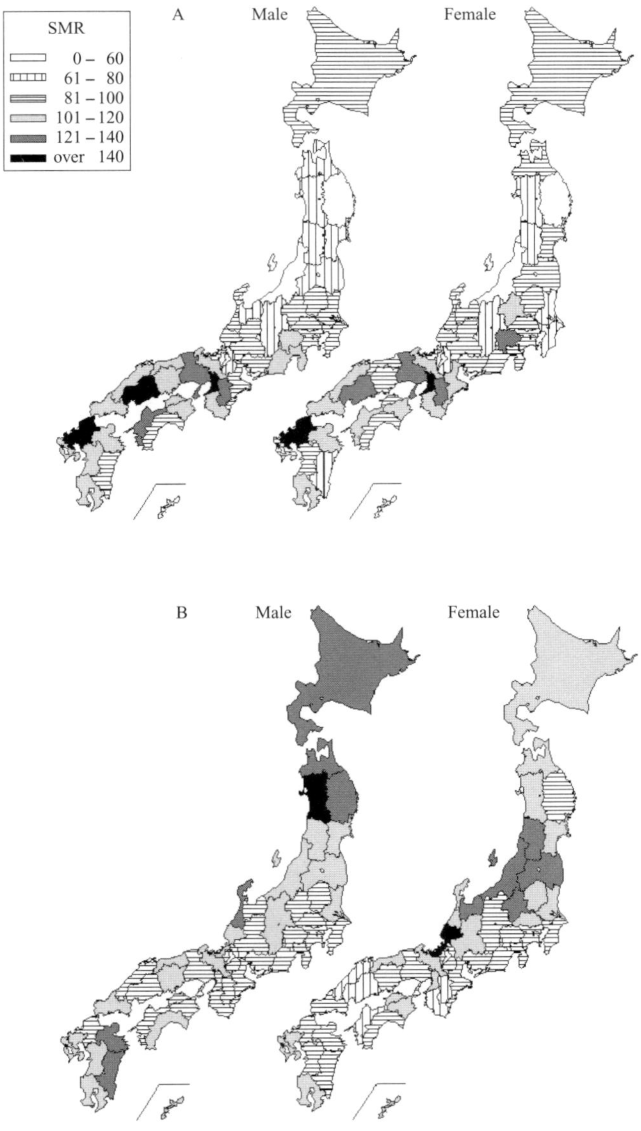

FIG. 4-4. Maps of the standardized mortality ratio (SMR) of cancer in Japan by prefecture (2000)
A: cancer of the liver (ICD, 10th revision: C22)
B: cancer of the biliary passages (ICD, 10th revision: C23, C24)

TABLE IV-5. Standardized Mortality Ratio (SMR) of Cancer in Japan by Prefecture (2000)

		A. Cancer of the pancreas (ICD, 10th revision: C25)		B. Cancer of the larynx (ICD, 10th revision: C32)	
		Male	Female	Male	Female
1	Hokkaido	128.3	113.8	126.0	198.4
2	Aomori	138.8	116.9	165.0	0.0
3	Iwate	96.0	91.9	120.6	85.3
4	Miyagi	104.7	112.2	68.7	190.3
5	Akita	110.3	111.0	142.8	94.1
6	Yamagata	115.1	100.1	85.4	91.7
7	Fukushima	106.2	82.5	133.7	120.9
8	Ibaraki	93.0	114.9	76.5	50.4
9	Tochigi	105.4	88.6	113.3	294.6
10	Gunma	98.8	87.0	43.2	68.5
11	Saitama	99.4	95.6	102.4	54.8
12	Chiba	92.7	98.0	94.0	0.0
13	Tokyo	93.4	102.4	101.4	133.2
14	Kanagawa	96.3	96.0	114.2	108.2
15	Niigata	112.2	102.7	81.8	47.7
16	Toyama	113.5	85.1	70.9	0.0
17	Ishikawa	117.4	103.8	106.4	0.0
18	Fukui	87.7	123.3	112.6	0.0
19	Yamanashi	83.0	107.3	93.2	0.0
20	Nagano	104.8	96.5	121.6	160.8
21	Gifu	109.4	108.4	106.4	0.0
22	Shizuoka	96.7	95.7	129.6	113.2
23	Aichi	96.6	97.3	100.5	171.8
24	Mie	112.4	86.1	86.8	71.7
25	Shiga	98.0	109.1	128.0	114.5
26	Kyoto	105.1	98.6	96.0	104.6
27	Osaka	96.7	106.2	96.2	151.1
28	Hyogo	101.1	105.0	103.6	106.4
29	Nara	108.2	86.0	84.9	612.0
30	Wakayama	92.1	127.6	74.5	0.0
31	Tottori	100.9	122.7	55.0	181.9
32	Shimane	114.6	118.4	116.6	132.1
33	Okayama	94.4	91.7	89.7	124.7
34	Hiroshima	85.5	92.5	47.6	0.0
35	Yamaguchi	94.2	101.1	128.9	217.5
36	Tokushima	77.7	109.0	40.5	0.0
37	Kagawa	110.3	98.4	44.0	0.0
38	Ehime	92.7	93.3	52.7	0.0
39	Kochi	94.3	104.5	167.0	127.9
40	Fukuoka	91.3	98.4	118.4	27.8
41	Saga	106.1	97.3	97.1	0.0
42	Nagasaki	97.9	99.3	126.0	156.9
43	Kumamoto	90.0	111.0	61.9	0.0
44	Oita	90.8	80.9	27.4	94.9
45	Miyazaki	106.6	90.2	112.4	0.0
46	Kagoshima	98.4	82.3	81.5	61.7
47	Okinawa	56.3	54.3	115.2	0.0

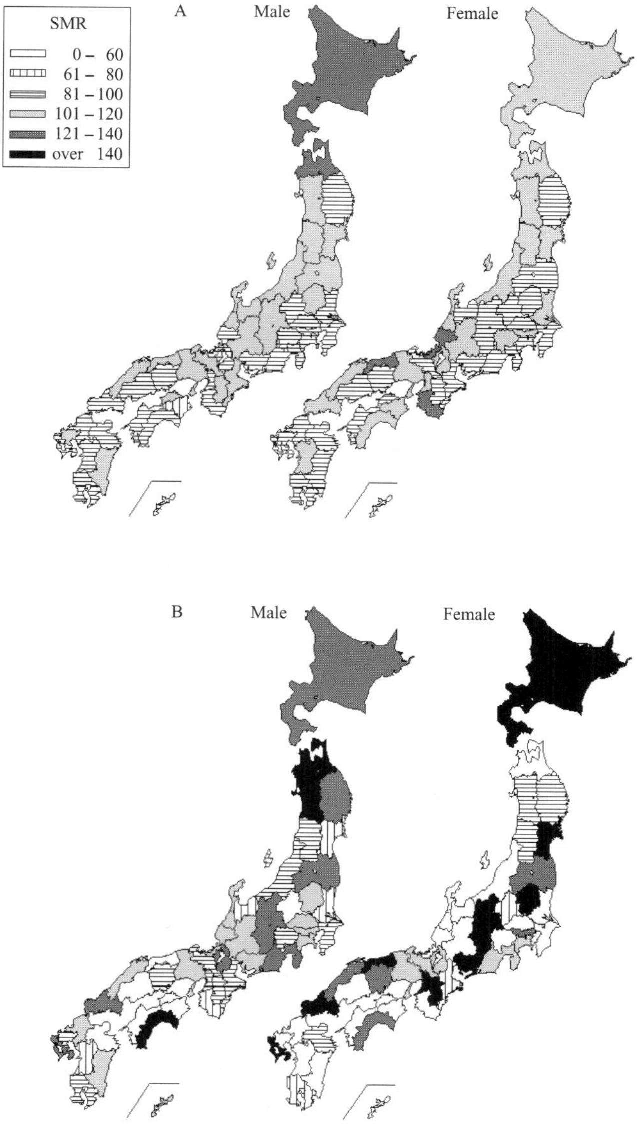

FIG. 4-5. Maps of the standardized mortality ratio (SMR) of cancer in Japan by prefecture (2000)
A: cancer of the pancreas (ICD, 10th revision: C25)
B: cancer of the larynx (ICD, 10th revision: C32)

TABLE IV-6. Standardized Mortality Ratio (SMR) of Cancer in Japan by Prefecture (2000)

		A. Cancer of the trachea, bronchus, and lung (ICD, 10th revision: C33, C34)		B. Cancer of the bone (ICD, 10th revision: C40, C41)	
		Male	Female	Male	Female
1	Hokkaido	104.0	106.8	151.3	178.1
2	Aomori	115.9	83.0	117.9	0.0
3	Iwate	99.5	86.0	157.4	0.0
4	Miyagi	101.3	98.1	97.8	33.7
5	Akita	99.5	89.3	137.2	178.5
6	Yamagata	102.7	81.2	174.9	114.9
7	Fukushima	98.1	89.9	53.0	35.4
8	Ibaraki	100.0	90.5	77.5	27.3
9	Tochigi	93.9	80.3	86.8	120.9
10	Gunma	84.1	85.8	113.5	117.4
11	Saitama	93.5	96.8	86.3	90.8
12	Chiba	90.5	94.1	109.1	88.3
13	Tokyo	94.1	114.2	72.5	127.3
14	Kanagawa	89.0	104.8	97.9	127.5
15	Niigata	106.2	81.6	89.4	29.4
16	Toyama	92.7	79.8	150.2	65.1
17	Ishikawa	101.3	84.8	245.1	128.5
18	Fukui	96.4	111.5	0.0	179.0
19	Yamanashi	84.0	74.2	128.0	171.3
20	Nagano	74.6	77.8	100.4	166.8
21	Gifu	98.2	95.2	136.9	74.7
22	Shizuoka	85.8	79.5	107.6	106.2
23	Aichi	102.1	101.6	102.3	86.6
24	Mie	107.8	90.4	155.5	124.5
25	Shiga	121.5	103.8	44.5	121.6
26	Kyoto	110.0	116.6	132.9	117.7
27	Osaka	117.3	128.7	75.6	67.7
28	Hyogo	108.9	108.1	107.7	115.5
29	Nara	95.4	95.7	81.7	109.3
30	Wakayama	113.6	105.1	158.7	0.0
31	Tottori	104.3	87.4	91.5	0.0
32	Shimane	94.6	78.0	0.0	0.0
33	Okayama	95.7	85.5	29.1	262.2
34	Hiroshima	101.9	84.8	140.9	53.1
35	Yamaguchi	113.5	111.4	145.8	137.8
36	Tokushima	116.1	90.1	0.0	172.2
37	Kagawa	102.1	79.5	109.5	142.2
38	Ehime	96.4	104.3	75.8	0.0
39	Kochi	92.0	113.2	0.0	166.7
40	Fukuoka	103.0	124.9	95.1	137.7
41	Saga	105.3	91.5	132.8	162.6
42	Nagasaki	120.8	107.6	76.5	47.1
43	Kumamoto	95.9	95.3	122.4	75.9
44	Oita	100.5	102.2	0.0	58.4
45	Miyazaki	94.6	86.6	98.7	61.6
46	Kagoshima	101.6	91.3	158.6	76.9
47	Okinawa	118.0	117.0	48.6	0.0

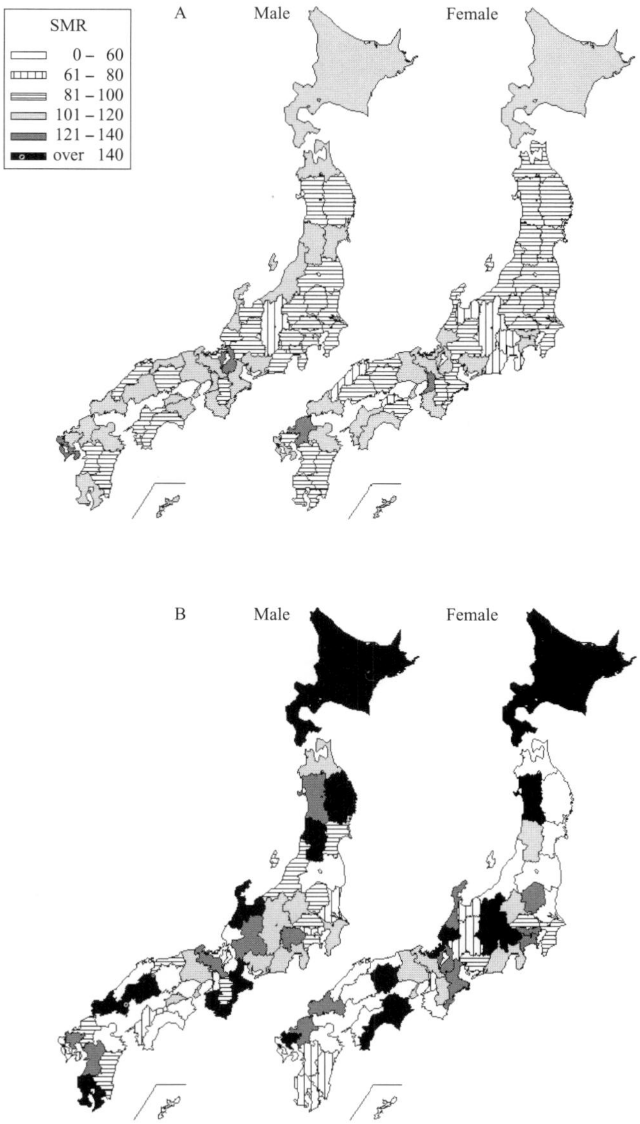

FIG. 4-6. Maps of the standardized mortality ratio (SMR) of cancer in Japan by prefecture (2000)
A: cancer of the trachea, bronchus, and lung (ICD, 10th revision: C33, C34)
B: cancer of the bone (ICD, 10th revision: C40, C41)

TABLE IV-7. Standardized Mortality Ratio (SMR) of Cancer in Japan by Prefecture (2000)

		A. Cancer of the skin (ICD, 10th revision: C43, C44)		B. Cancer of the breast (ICD, 10th revision: C50)	
		Male	Female	Male	Female
1	Hokkaido	123.8	114.6	0.0	108.3
2	Aomori	50.8	117.2	0.0	97.5
3	Iwate	78.6	142.1	0.0	82.4
4	Miyagi	110.0	128.3	71.4	117.5
5	Akita	106.0	141.5	0.0	89.9
6	Yamagata	50.3	168.8	210.5	95.2
7	Fukushima	141.3	122.4	69.0	79.1
8	Ibaraki	68.5	146.8	111.6	96.8
9	Tochigi	76.4	94.6	82.5	80.5
10	Gunma	71.1	187.2	0.0	101.7
11	Saitama	103.6	95.7	117.8	111.8
12	Chiba	99.8	139.8	32.0	106.9
13	Tokyo	109.1	129.3	160.0	126.8
14	Kanagawa	80.8	59.6	114.3	113.7
15	Niigata	150.1	103.8	55.8	87.5
16	Toyama	39.2	56.3	247.4	92.3
17	Ishikawa	143.3	118.2	129.7	106.9
18	Fukui	136.1	105.4	172.5	101.3
19	Yamanashi	204.4	103.1	162.4	98.1
20	Nagano	75.7	67.6	178.8	86.3
21	Gifu	148.2	61.2	73.4	96.9
22	Shizuoka	91.4	109.7	84.9	92.2
23	Aichi	120.4	89.8	80.8	100.4
24	Mie	115.9	91.1	166.7	104.5
25	Shiga	101.4	82.3	0.0	82.8
26	Kyoto	95.7	37.4	250.0	87.4
27	Osaka	94.2	90.2	65.7	103.1
28	Hyogo	99.0	91.8	61.8	97.1
29	Nara	54.1	73.6	0.0	81.5
30	Wakayama	124.9	39.8	132.0	72.0
31	Tottori	249.6	32.6	0.0	71.2
32	Shimane	50.7	47.4	0.0	66.9
33	Okayama	46.0	88.5	146.9	90.6
34	Hiroshima	107.2	49.1	105.6	90.1
35	Yamaguchi	69.9	52.3	264.0	79.9
36	Tokushima	79.3	99.6	0.0	94.5
37	Kagawa	170.4	83.0	269.0	87.8
38	Ehime	29.3	98.3	0.0	98.1
39	Kochi	75.6	68.5	0.0	95.4
40	Fukuoka	105.1	114.8	170.4	105.2
41	Saga	161.5	217.1	0.0	93.9
42	Nagasaki	138.2	113.8	0.0	98.5
43	Kumamoto	71.8	99.8	226.8	90.0
44	Oita	160.5	138.1	0.0	68.1
45	Miyazaki	99.4	18.7	125.9	73.3
46	Kagoshima	24.5	77.9	153.7	89.0
47	Okinawa	69.9	107.2	312.9	90.6

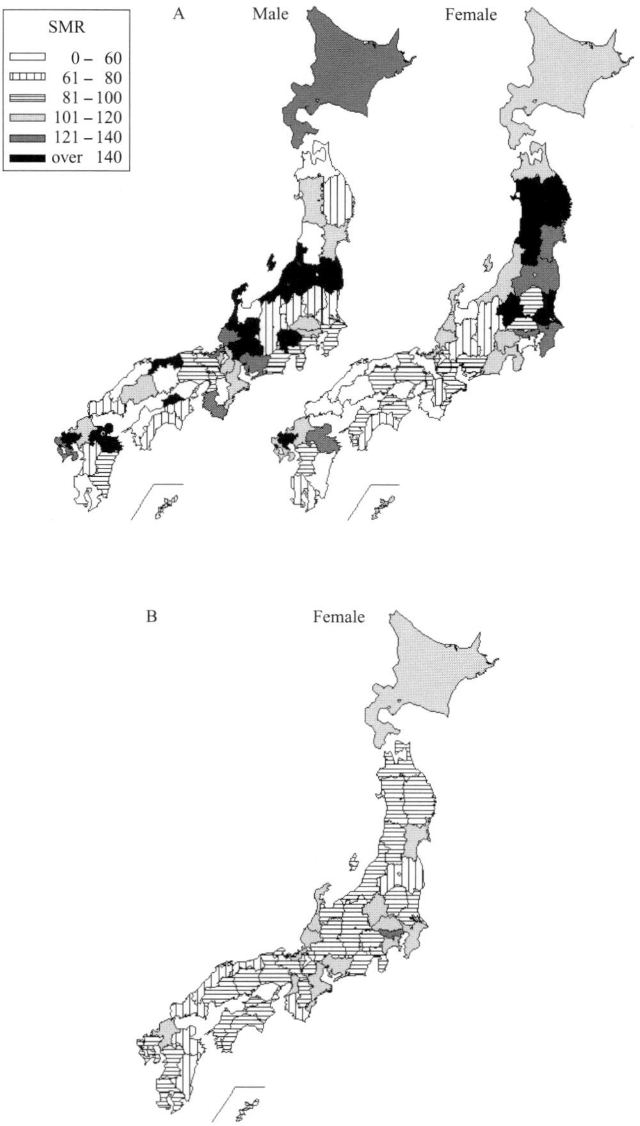

FIG. 4-7. Maps of the standardized mortality ratio (SMR) of cancer in Japan by prefecture (2000)
A: cancer of the skin (ICD, 10th revision: C43, C44)
B: cancer of the breast (ICD, 10th revision: C50)

TABLE IV-8. Standardized Mortality Ratio (SMR) of Cancer in Japan by Prefecture (2000)

		A. Cancer of the uterus (ICD, 10th revision: C53–C55, C58)	B. Cancer of the ovary (ICD, 10th revision: C56)
1	Hokkaido	96.2	99.0
2	Aomori	84.8	84.8
3	Iwate	69.0	128.9
4	Miyagi	66.8	100.8
5	Akita	83.2	85.7
6	Yamagata	59.5	79.4
7	Fukushima	75.3	96.8
8	Ibaraki	105.7	103.6
9	Tochigi	136.4	105.1
10	Gunma	98.8	91.1
11	Saitama	100.3	114.7
12	Chiba	110.1	122.2
13	Tokyo	117.9	124.1
14	Kanagawa	95.5	119.4
15	Niigata	83.1	98.3
16	Toyama	54.3	82.2
17	Ishikawa	82.8	89.1
18	Fukui	95.0	63.5
19	Yamanashi	89.6	68.4
20	Nagano	76.5	114.2
21	Gifu	108.7	96.1
22	Shizuoka	92.1	94.5
23	Aichi	95.7	97.8
24	Mie	98.0	89.9
25	Shiga	85.1	71.0
26	Kyoto	90.2	86.6
27	Osaka	110.8	99.6
28	Hyogo	104.3	100.6
29	Nara	99.9	79.2
30	Wakayama	117.3	98.7
31	Tottori	106.5	98.4
32	Shimane	64.6	64.0
33	Okayama	89.3	111.6
34	Hiroshima	101.3	95.8
35	Yamaguchi	108.5	92.3
36	Tokushima	102.3	89.9
37	Kagawa	97.4	74.5
38	Ehime	119.2	97.6
39	Kochi	96.6	79.3
40	Fukuoka	112.5	86.6
41	Saga	102.5	94.6
42	Nagasaki	104.4	81.4
43	Kumamoto	105.4	75.1
44	Oita	119.6	78.2
45	Miyazaki	105.7	79.7
46	Kagoshima	98.4	91.4
47	Okinawa	139.7	82.8

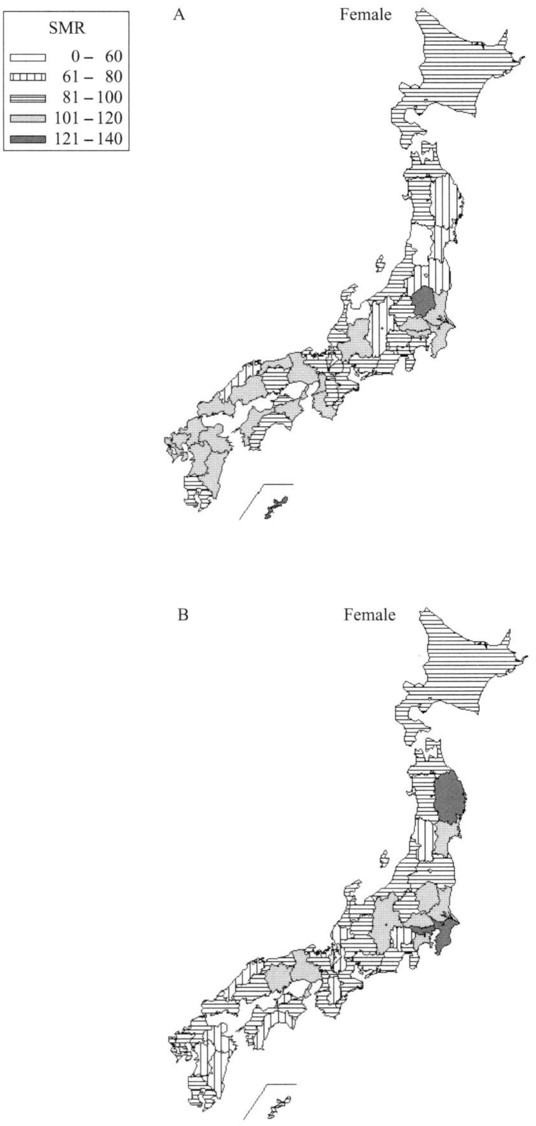

FIG. 4-8. Maps of the standardized mortality ratio (SMR) of cancer in Japan by prefecture (2000)
A: cancer of the uterus (ICD, 10th revision: C53–C55, C58)
B: cancer of the ovary (ICD, 10th revision: C56)

TABLE IV-9. Standardized Mortality Ratio (SMR) of Cancer in Japan by Prefecture (2000)

		A. Cancer of the prostate (ICD, 10th revision: C61)	B. Cancer of the urinary bladder (ICD, 10th revision: C67)	
		Male	Male	Female
1	Hokkaido	102.0	108.7	105.4
2	Aomori	111.1	140.2	116.9
3	Iwate	123.2	104.7	68.9
4	Miyagi	100.6	68.9	90.1
5	Akita	93.5	89.8	92.4
6	Yamagata	103.0	114.4	103.8
7	Fukushima	118.3	105.3	125.0
8	Ibaraki	109.0	103.0	94.6
9	Tochigi	91.8	126.2	121.0
10	Gunma	115.7	73.3	135.2
11	Saitama	90.9	92.7	114.3
12	Chiba	103.3	89.9	67.2
13	Tokyo	104.1	97.5	92.5
14	Kanagawa	107.0	102.3	101.2
15	Niigata	87.4	105.1	80.9
16	Toyama	68.9	88.7	95.1
17	Ishikawa	94.0	90.6	75.4
18	Fukui	80.1	102.6	74.5
19	Yamanashi	80.1	84.9	97.0
20	Nagano	117.3	81.2	93.1
21	Gifu	96.6	77.6	102.1
22	Shizuoka	103.9	106.7	84.1
23	Aichi	93.8	95.6	89.8
24	Mie	104.7	82.1	107.9
25	Shiga	83.8	100.0	106.5
26	Kyoto	93.8	97.7	117.8
27	Osaka	90.3	112.8	110.4
28	Hyogo	80.7	108.5	112.0
29	Nara	111.3	100.3	144.9
30	Wakayama	94.6	116.4	106.5
31	Tottori	92.3	79.6	81.0
32	Shimane	96.5	128.9	50.8
33	Okayama	96.1	106.0	112.4
34	Hiroshima	104.6	91.0	102.5
35	Yamaguchi	105.0	100.3	98.3
36	Tokushima	79.3	83.3	62.7
37	Kagawa	106.0	95.8	137.3
38	Ehime	84.4	89.6	66.4
39	Kochi	75.0	114.9	113.6
40	Fukuoka	105.3	114.9	106.9
41	Saga	126.3	105.3	68.6
42	Nagasaki	96.3	120.2	102.7
43	Kumamoto	114.9	92.7	115.0
44	Oita	97.0	93.0	140.6
45	Miyazaki	134.4	108.5	111.9
46	Kagoshima	106.5	94.5	96.2
47	Okinawa	102.9	76.0	64.5

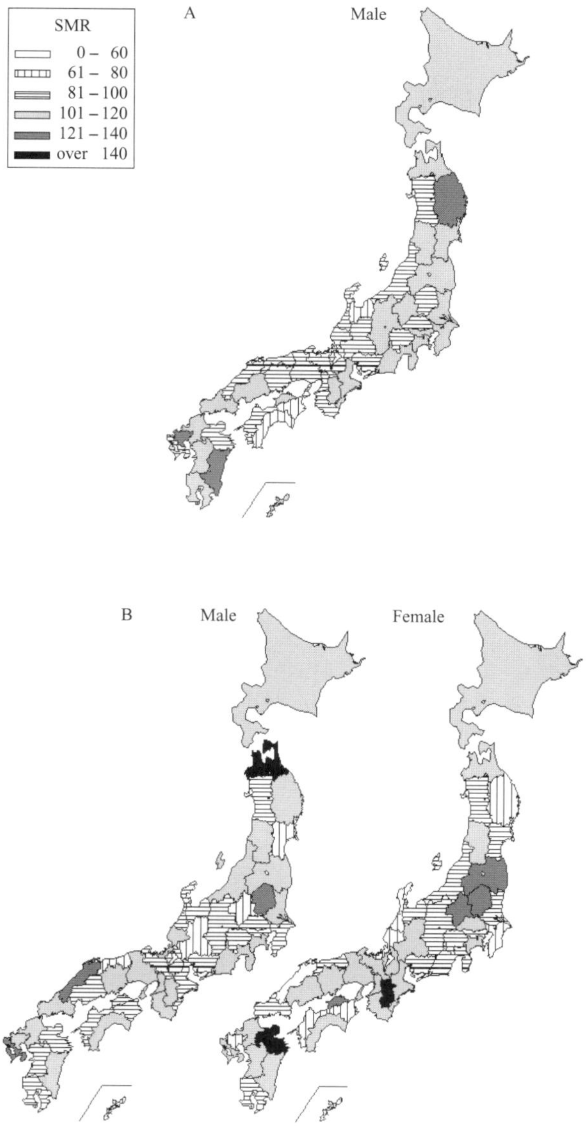

FIG. 4-9. Maps of the standardized mortality ratio (SMR) of cancer in Japan by prefecture (2000)
A: cancer of the prostate (ICD, 10th revision: C61)
B: cancer of the urinary bladder (ICD, 10th revision: C67)

TABLE IV-10. Standardized Mortality Ratio (SMR) of Cancer in Japan by Prefecture (2000)

		A. Cancer of the kidney (ICD, 10th revision: C64, C65)		B. Cancer of the lymphoid tissue (ICD, 10th revision: C81–C90, C96)	
		Male	Female	Male	Female
1	Hokkaido	118.6	117.3	104.0	100.6
2	Aomori	154.3	121.8	73.6	96.5
3	Iwate	93.9	40.7	77.5	94.3
4	Miyagi	106.1	120.7	99.8	100.2
5	Akita	87.7	76.6	113.9	83.7
6	Yamagata	65.0	99.6	95.9	90.0
7	Fukushima	67.1	114.9	101.0	88.8
8	Ibaraki	113.1	100.2	85.8	94.8
9	Tochigi	101.1	90.4	87.0	109.3
10	Gunma	78.5	98.8	100.1	100.4
11	Saitama	101.3	104.1	98.5	104.8
12	Chiba	92.7	111.9	93.6	89.9
13	Tokyo	108.2	119.9	99.4	100.2
14	Kanagawa	108.2	107.3	107.0	93.9
15	Niigata	111.7	85.1	87.0	95.8
16	Toyama	130.4	58.2	122.6	111.2
17	Ishikawa	160.1	83.6	101.8	100.2
18	Fukui	96.0	81.0	101.3	102.5
19	Yamanashi	60.6	49.4	132.2	102.4
20	Nagano	74.5	99.3	100.4	101.1
21	Gifu	83.9	137.5	108.7	87.0
22	Shizuoka	93.7	85.7	111.3	98.0
23	Aichi	101.1	92.9	101.3	94.5
24	Mie	84.8	83.8	89.4	94.0
25	Shiga	106.3	78.7	119.9	123.4
26	Kyoto	111.2	141.5	114.9	119.8
27	Osaka	110.0	105.6	101.5	97.7
28	Hyogo	102.0	133.7	98.1	105.1
29	Nara	90.5	77.5	92.4	88.4
30	Wakayama	84.4	106.1	96.4	96.0
31	Tottori	132.6	100.0	126.7	81.2
32	Shimane	84.9	36.4	110.7	87.9
33	Okayama	93.0	90.6	101.8	94.1
34	Hiroshima	104.3	110.9	81.6	95.7
35	Yamaguchi	89.8	110.2	99.3	98.8
36	Tokushima	66.4	76.4	103.7	131.1
37	Kagawa	100.3	96.0	120.0	134.7
38	Ehime	80.1	48.2	109.9	114.9
39	Kochi	98.2	88.3	87.4	119.4
40	Fukuoka	101.4	93.7	96.3	99.8
41	Saga	105.0	74.7	118.8	118.9
42	Nagasaki	98.1	86.0	103.6	102.8
43	Kumamoto	73.0	68.4	96.0	122.1
44	Oita	79.7	97.5	92.7	105.8
45	Miyazaki	69.2	91.9	103.1	76.8
46	Kagoshima	54.9	80.2	89.7	111.9
47	Okinawa	140.9	52.2	90.9	92.9

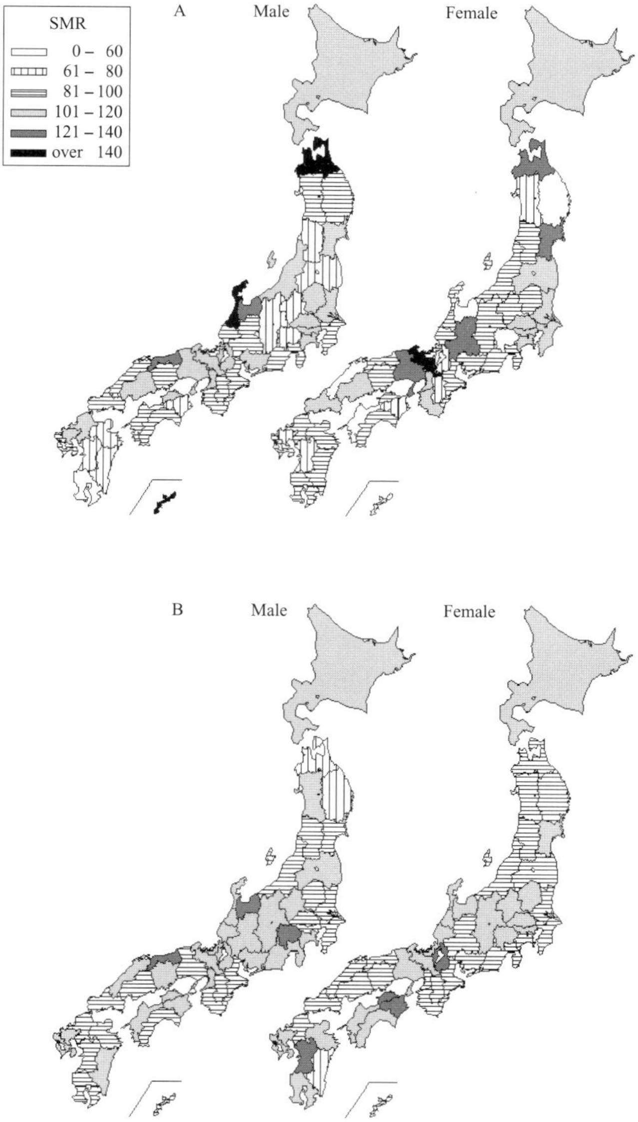

FIG. 4-10. Maps of the standardized mortality ratio (SMR) of cancer in Japan by prefecture (2000)
A: cancer of the kidney (ICD, 10th revision: C64, C65)
B: cancer of the lymphatic and hematopoietic systems other than leukemia (ICD, 10th revision: C81–C90, C96)

TABLE IV-11. Standardized Mortality Ratio (SMR) of Cancer in Japan by Prefecture (2000)

		A. Leukemia (ICD, 10th revision: C91–C95)	
		Male	Female
1	Hokkaido	112.0	93.9
2	Aomori	63.6	76.0
3	Iwate	89.8	141.9
4	Miyagi	94.7	93.7
5	Akita	99.2	98.9
6	Yamagata	66.4	97.6
7	Fukushima	83.8	82.1
8	Ibaraki	91.2	96.2
9	Tochigi	90.7	85.2
10	Gunma	77.4	92.2
11	Saitama	89.1	80.4
12	Chiba	85.2	84.8
13	Tokyo	83.3	85.2
14	Kanagawa	80.8	83.4
15	Niigata	114.5	76.5
16	Toyama	103.2	95.1
17	Ishikawa	105.4	108.0
18	Fukui	78.6	73.8
19	Yamanashi	124.4	85.8
20	Nagano	78.5	73.9
21	Gifu	106.7	88.6
22	Shizuoka	98.6	86.2
23	Aichi	89.2	90.3
24	Mie	100.8	88.0
25	Shiga	105.8	100.5
26	Kyoto	101.0	79.3
27	Osaka	101.8	101.2
28	Hyogo	90.0	97.0
29	Nara	104.2	95.3
30	Wakayama	103.3	54.9
31	Tottori	51.8	117.6
32	Shimane	103.8	111.0
33	Okayama	95.9	87.5
34	Hiroshima	87.1	83.6
35	Yamaguchi	96.5	98.1
36	Tokushima	83.1	111.7
37	Kagawa	93.0	96.9
38	Ehime	98.8	103.5
39	Kochi	77.6	88.2
40	Fukuoka	117.6	139.0
41	Saga	171.6	131.4
42	Nagasaki	197.3	175.9
43	Kumamoto	127.2	133.5
44	Oita	141.3	150.8
45	Miyazaki	193.3	186.4
46	Kagoshima	241.7	252.8
47	Okinawa	161.3	228.4

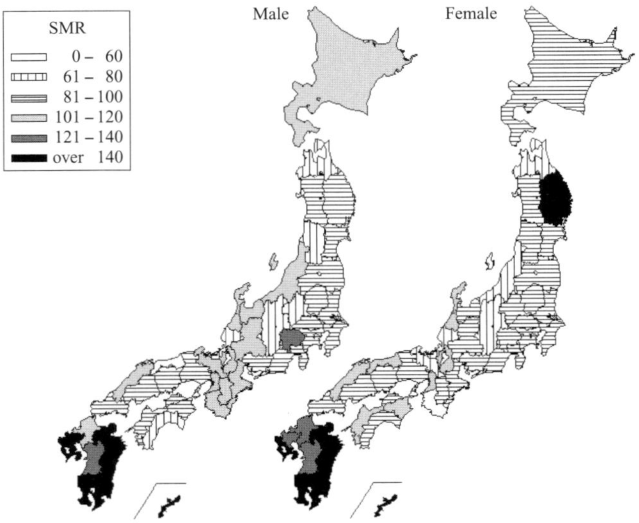

FIG. 4-11. Maps of the standardized mortality ratio (SMR) of cancer in Japan by prefecture (2000)
Leukemia (ICD, 10th revision: C91–C95)

CANCER INCIDENCE IN JAPAN

The Research Group for Population-based
Cancer Registration in Japan[*1,*2]

The Research Group for Population-based Cancer Registration in Japan has been conducting a cooperative study to estimate cancer incidence in Japan. Annual incidence has been estimated for 24 years, from 1975 to 1998. This report presents trends of the age-specific, age-standardized incidence rates, as well as the number of incident cases by sex and site during that period.

The Research Group for Population-based Cancer Registration in Japan has been operating since 1975 with a research grant from the Ministry of Health, Labour and Welfare of Japan. Since its inception, the Group has been conducting a cooperative estimation study on cancer incidence in Japan, the results of which have been reported annually in its report. Summaries of the results have been reported in scientific journals and in the Gann Monograph series (*1–5, 8–18*).

This report presents for outlines of the population-based cancer registration in Japan, estimated incidence and incidence rates in 1998, and trends in incidence and incidence rates during 1975–1998.

Population-based Cancer Registration in Japan

According to the 2002 survey of cancer registries by the Japanese Association of Cancer Registries (*6*), 33 population-based registries were operating and they covered about 64% of the Japanese population. Most registries are run by the prefectural governments in cooperation with the prefectural medical associations and the prefectural cancer centers or local universities/colleges.

Cancer registration in Japan has been carried out on a voluntary basis. Cancer records are collected actively in three registries (Miyagi, Hiroshima City, and Nagasaki), but only passively in 20 registries. Many cancer registries suffer from budgetary limitations and lack of trained personnel. Only a few large hospitals have medical record librarians. Under these circumstances, it is difficult to obtain high quality cancer data, *i.e.*, complete reporting of accurate cancer data from all these registries.

*1 This report was prepared by Hideaki Tsukuma, Wakiko Ajiki, and Akira Oshima, Osaka Cancer Registry, Department of Cancer Control and Statistics, Osaka Medical Center for Cancer and Cardiovascular Diseases, 3-3 Nakamichi 1-chome, Higashinari-ku, Osaka 537-8511, Japan.

*2 The chairpersons of the Research Group are Isaburo Fujimoto (1975-1980 and 1987–1992), Seigo Fukuma (1981–1986), Aya Hanai (1993-1995), Akira Oshima (1996–2001), and Hideaki Tsukuma (2002–). The study members of the Study Group as of 2003 include Takayoshi Tsubono, Daisuke Shibuya (Miyagi Cancer Registry), Toru Matsuda (Yamagata Cancer Registry), Kazuei Ogoshi (Niigata Cancer Registry), Haruo Mikami (Chiba Cancer Registry), Atsushi Miyamatsu, Naoyuki Okamoto (Kanagawa Cancer Registry), Manabu Fujita (Fukui Cancer Registry), Kazuo Tajima (Aichi Cancer Registry), Takumi Uehata (Shiga Cancer Registry), Wakiko Ajiki, Hideaki Tsukuma, Akira Oshima (Osaka Cancer Registry), Takuji Kishimoto (Tottori Cancer Registry), Kojiro Koyama (Hiroshima City Tumor Registry), Midori Sota (Nagasaki Cancer Registry), Mitsuo Shimoji (Okinawa Cancer Registry), and Tetsuo Kuroishi (Aichi Cancer Center).

According to the annual reports of cancer incidence in 1997 published by 27 of the existing 33 registries, the average proportion of death-certificate-only cases was 30%, ranging from 6% to 63% (*6*) . Cancer data from only six registries (Miyagi, Yamagata, Osaka, Hiroshima City, Saga, and Nagasaki) were accepted for publication in "*Cancer Incidence in Five Continents Volume VIII*" (*7*). Meanwhile, the Research Group for Population-based Cancer Registration in Japan has been making continuous efforts to estimate cancer statistics in Japan including incidence, survival, and clinical stage distribution at diagnosis from its inception. The Group is composed of 13–14 registries with active researchers and with data quality above the usual standard.

Estimated Incidence and Incidence Rates in Japan in 1998

National cancer incidence has been calculated annually in a cooperative study by the member registries of this Research Group. As details of the methodology have been described elsewhere (*9*) , only an outline is presented in the following.

The Research Group collects the most recent incidence data from all participating registries on an annual basis. Only registry data that fulfill the standard requirements for completeness are used in national incidence estimates. The present requirements are: 1) the proportion of death-certificate-only cases should be less than 25%, or the proportion of death certificate notification less than 30%, and 2) the ratio of incidence to death should be 1.5 or above. The most recent three-year incidence is calculated for each eligible registry. Cancer incidence rates in Japan, before correction, are estimated as the arithmetic mean of incidence rates of all eligible registries according to site, sex, and five-year age group. Since using data from only a limited number of registries may introduce some biases into estimating all-Japan incidence, correction coefficients are calculated as the ratio of actual cancer deaths in the country to those estimated from eligible registries' mortality data. Final estimates of the rates are obtained by multiplying the estimated incidence rates before correction by the correction coefficients.

Table I shows the characteristics of 13 regions of the cancer registries participating in the cooperative study estimating cancer incidence and incidence rates for 1998. The average of the proportion of death-certificate-only cases was 18.6%, the proportion of death certificate notification was 24.3%, and the ratio of incidence to deaths was 1.77. Twelve registries were selected for the estimation of incidence in 1998: Miyagi, Yamagata, Chiba (model area), Kanagawa (model area), Niigata, Fukui, Aichi (model area), Shiga, Osaka, Hiroshima City, Saga, and Nagasaki registries. These registries covered a population of 24,500,000, corresponding to 19.4% of the total population of Japan. The average of the proportion of death-certificate-only cases of the 12 registries was 17.3%, the proportion of death certificate notification was 23.4%, and the ratio of incidence to deaths was 1.77. The proportion of cases which had been histologically verified was 71.6%.

Table II shows the estimated incidence and incidence rate for cancer in 1998. Among males, the estimated incidence for all sites was 290,343. Stomach was the most common site (67,861), followed by lung (43,895), colon (33,008), and liver (25,931) in this order. Among females, the estimated cancer incidence for all sites (including carcinoma *in situ*) was 213,421, the most common site being breast (33,676), followed by stomach (33,518), colon (24,726), lung (17,723), and uterus

(17,686).

Trends in Cancer Incidence and Incidence Rates in Japan during 1975–1998

Before presenting data on the trends in cancer incidence and cancer incidence rates, some precautions should be mentioned. The first is that data from the same registries were not selected throughout the period and that the data quality might not be constant during the period observed. Table III shows the number and names of cancer registries selected in estimating cancer incidence, and data regarding the completeness and accuracy of diagnosis, *i.e.*, the proportion of death-certificate-only cases and the ratio of incidence to deaths, and the proportion of histologically verified cases. The second point to be mentioned is that a considerable number of delayed cancer reports were submitted to the relevant registries after the annual calculation of cancer incidence was conducted. For this reason, re-estimations were made for 1975–1979, 1980–1984, 1985–1989, and 1990–1994, but this has not yet been done for 1995–1998; therefore, estimates for 1995–1998 should be considered as tentative in a strict sense. According to the results of re-estimation for 1990–1994, the numbers on cancer incidence for all sites increased by 4–6% compared to the tentative figures before re-estimation.

Tables IV-1 and IV-2 and Figs. 1 and 2 show the trends of age-standardized cancer incidence rate in Japan by sex and primary site during 1975-1998. The standard population is the world population in Table IV-1 and Fig. 1, and the Japanese 1985 model population in Table IV-2 and Fig. 2, respectively. Among males, the age-standardized cancer incidence rate for all sites gradually increased until the early 1990s, while among females it increased only slightly until the early 1990s. When observed by site, the incidence rates have increased for colon, rectum, and lung in both sexes, prostate, and breast in females. On the other hand, incidence rates for stomach in both sexes and for uterus have decreased considerably during the period.

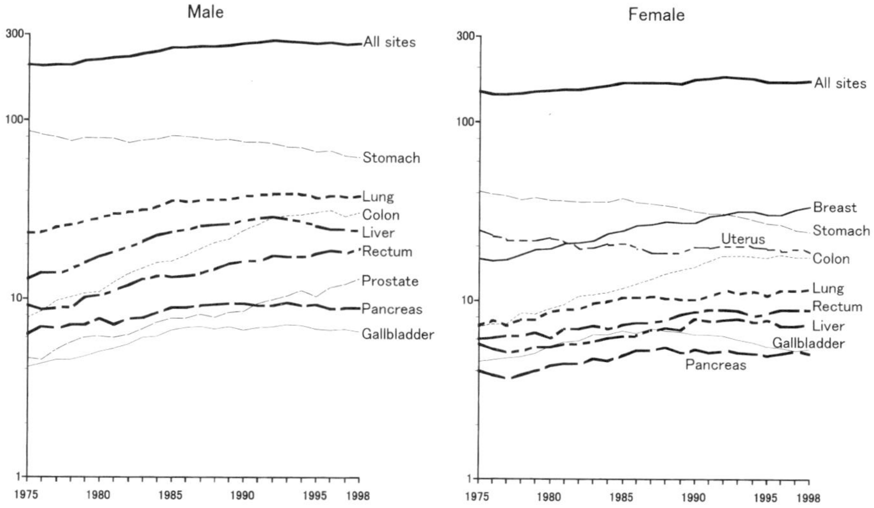

FIG. 1. Trends of age-standardized cancer incidence rates per 100,000 population for major sites in Japan during 1975–1998 (standard population: world population)

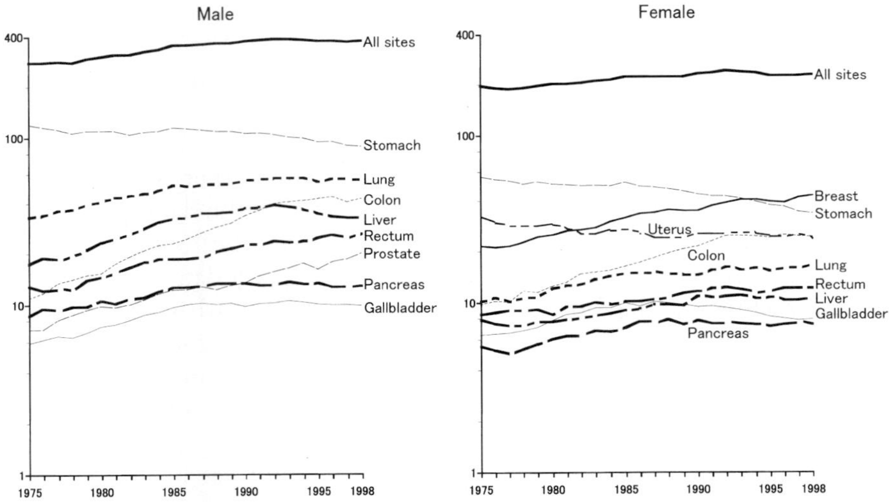

FIG. 2. Trends of age-standardized cancer incidence rates per 100,000 population for major sites in Japan during 1975–1998 (standard population: Japanese 1985 model population)

Incidence rates for liver increased especially in males until the early 1990s, but then began to decrease.

Table V shows the trends of the number of incident cases in Japan according to sex and primary site during 1975–1998. For most sites, the number of incident cases has increased due to the aging of the Japanese population.

Table VI shows the trends of age-specific incidence rates by sex and primary site during 1975–1998.

Estimated incidence rates in Japan by sex, site, five-year age groups, and calendar year during the period of 1975–1998 are now available on a Web site (http://www.mc.pref.osaka.jp/ocr/registry/) or through correspondence with Hideaki Tsukuma, Osaka Cancer Registry.

Acknowledgments

The authors would like to thank the following registries and all those who are associated with them: Miyagi Cancer Registry, Yamagata Cancer Registry, Chiba Cancer Registry, Kanagawa Cancer Registry, Niigata Cancer Registry, Fukui Cancer Registry, Aichi Cancer Registry, Shiga Cancer Registry, Osaka Cancer Registry, Tottori Cancer Registry, Hiroshima City Tumor Registry, Saga Cancer Registry, Nagasaki Cancer Registry, and Okinawa Cancer Registry. This study was supported in part by a grant-in-aid from the Ministry of Health, Labour and Welfare, Japan (14-2).

REFERENCES

1. Cancer incidence and incidence rates in Japan in 1994: estimates based on data from seven population-based cancer registries. *Jpn. J. Clin. Oncol.*, **29**, 361–364 (1999).
2. Cancer incidence and incidence rates in Japan in 1995: estimates based on data from nine population-based cancer registries. *Jpn. J. Clin. Oncol.*, **30**, 318–321 (2000).

3. Cancer incidence and incidence rates in Japan in 1996: estimates based on data from 10 population-based cancer registries. *Jpn. J. Clin. Oncol.*, **31**, 410–414 (2001).
4. Cancer incidence and incidence rates in Japan in 1997: estimates based on data from 12 population-based cancer registries. *Jpn. J. Clin. Oncol.*, **32**, 318–322 (2002).
5. Cancer incidence and incidence rates in Japan in 1998: estimates based on data from 12 population-based cancer registries. *Jpn. J. Clin. Oncol.*, **33**, 241–245 (2003).
6. Japanese Association of Cancer Registry. Annual Report 2002 (2003), Secretariat of JACR, Osaka (in Japanese).
7. Parkin, D. M., Whelan, S. L., Ferlay, J., Teppo, L., and Thomas, D. B. (eds.). "Cancer Incidence in Five Continents," vol. VIII, IARC Scientific Publications No. 155 (2002). IARC, Lyon.
8. Research Group for Population-based Cancer Registration in Japan. Cancer incidence in Japan, 1975. Cancer registry statistics. *In* "Cancer Mortality and Morbidity Statistics: Japan and the World," ed. M. Segi *et al.*, Gann Monograph on Cancer Research No. 26, pp. 92–116 (1981). Japan Sci. Soc. Press, Tokyo.
9. Research Group for Population-based Cancer Registration in Japan. Cancer incidence in Japan. *In* "Cancer Mortality and Morbidity Statistics: Japan and the World—1994," ed. S. Tominaga *et al.*, Gann Monograph on Cancer Research No. 41, pp. 107–158 (1994). Japan Sci. Soc. Press, Tokyo/CRC Press, Boca Raton.
10. Research Group for Population-based Cancer Registration in Japan. Cancer incidence in Japan. *In* "Cancer Mortality and Morbidity Statistics: Japan and the World—1999," ed. S. Tominaga *et al.*, Gann Monograph on Cancer Research No. 47, pp. 83–143 (1999). Japan Sci. Soc. Press, Tokyo/Karger, Basel.
11. Research Group for Population-based Cancer Registration in Japan. Cancer incidence and incidence rates in Japan in 1985: estimates based on data from seven cancer registries. *Jpn. J. Clin. Oncol.*, **20**, 212–218 (1990).
12. Research Group for Population-based Cancer Registration in Japan. Cancer incidence and incidence rates in Japan in 1986: estimates based on data from nine cancer registries. *Jpn. J. Clin. Oncol.*, **21**, 318–323 (1991).
13. Research Group for Population-based Cancer Registration in Japan. Cancer incidence and incidence rates in Japan in 1987: estimates based on data from nine cancer registries. *Jpn. J. Clin. Oncol.*, **22**, 437–442 (1992).
14. Research Group for Population-based Cancer Registration in Japan. Cancer incidence and incidence rates in Japan in 1988: estimates based on data from nine cancer registries. *Jpn. J. Clin. Oncol.*, **24**, 299–304 (1994).
15. Research Group for Population-based Cancer Registration in Japan. Cancer incidence in Japan, 1990. *Jpn. J. Clin. Oncol.*, **28**, 450–453 (1998).
16. Research Group for Population-based Cancer Registration in Japan. Cancer incidence in Japan, 1991. *Jpn. J. Clin. Oncol.*, **28**, 574–577 (1998).
17. Research Group for Population-based Cancer Registration in Japan. Cancer incidence in Japan, 1992-1993. *Jpn. J. Clin. Oncol.*, **28**, 641–647 (1998).
18. Research Group for Population-based Cancer Registration in Japan. Cancer incidence in Japan, 1985-89: re-estimation based on data from eight cancer registries. *Jpn. J. Clin. Oncol.*, **28**, 54–67 (1998).

TABLE I. Characteristics of 13 Regions Covered by the Research Group, 1998

Registry	Population	Number of incidence	Number of mortality	Completeness of registration			Accuracy of diagnosis	
				DCN/I (%)	DCO/I (%)	I/D	H/I (%)	H/R (%)
Miyagi	2,349,653	10,005	5,039	17.4	17.4	1.99	74.1	89.7*
Yamagata	1,244,891	6,146	3,475	21.4	15.7	1.77	75.2	89.3*
Chiba[a]	1,231,157	3,858	2,561	30.4	23.8	1.51	55.4	72.7*
Kanagawa[a]	1,694,361	6,268	3,743	23.4	23.4	1.68	59.8	78.0*
Niigata	2,478,877	11,663	6,489	25.8	25.8	1.80	68.3	92.0*
Fukui	827,955	3,806	1,983	15.2	8.5	1.92	76.5	83.6*
Aichi[a]	1,042,076	3,266	1,691	14.7	14.7	1.93	79.0	92.7*
Shiga	1,320,094	4,324	2,662	34.9	16.5	1.63	71.7	85.8*
Osaka	8,786,130	30,351	19,881	34.3	23.0	1.53	65.6	85.2*
Tottori	610,698	2,897	1,636	34.9	34.9	1.77	47.4	72.8
Hiroshima City	1,117,564	4,702	2,234	14.6	14.6	2.11	80.4	94.1*
Saga	879,630	3,728	2,408	35.6	11.0	1.55	73.2	82.2*
Nagasaki	1,522,771	7,743	4,088	12.9	12.9	1.89	80.6	92.5*
Total/Average	25,105,857	98,757	57,890	24.3	18.6	1.77	69.8	85.4
(Selected registries*)	24,495,159	95,860	56,254	23.4	17.3	1.77	71.6	86.5

All data in this table were annual average calculated by using data during the period of 1997–99.
DCN/I: proportion of cases notified by death certificate to incidence.
DCO/I: proportion of cases registered with death certificate only to incidence.
I/D: incidence to deaths.
H/I: proportion of cases verified histologically to incidence.
H/R: proportion of cases verified histologically to reported incident cases.
[a] Data of model area.
* Registry attaining a) DCN/I<30% or DCO/I<25% and b) I/D≧1.5.

TABLE II-1. Incidence, Completeness of Reporting, and Accuracy of Diagnosis in Japan according to Sex and Primary Site (1998), Male

Primary site	ICD-10th	Number of incidence	Crude rate[a]	Age-standardized rate[a]		Completeness of registration		Accuracy of diagnosis
				World population	Japanese 1985 model population	DCO/I (%)	I/D	H/I (%)
All sites	C00–C96	290,343	468.9	265.6	373.2	17.4	1.69	71.5
Oral & Pharynx	C00–C14	6,101	9.9	5.9	7.9	9.5	1.79	84.5
Esophagus	C15	11,742	19.0	10.7	14.9	14.5	1.42	78.3
Stomach	C16	67,861	109.6	62.0	87.1	13.2	2.07	82.0
Colon	C18	33,008	53.3	30.2	42.3	10.6	2.85	83.6
Rectum	C19–C21	20,144	32.5	18.9	25.9	9.3	2.65	84.7
Liver	C22	25,931	41.9	24.0	32.8	30.1	1.10	28.9
Gallbladder	C23, C24	7,672	12.4	6.5	9.8	29.2	1.15	44.4
Pancreas	C25	10,052	16.2	8.8	12.8	33.2	1.03	30.1
Larynx	C32	3,083	5.0	2.8	3.9	5.8	3.24	88.2
Lung	C33, C34	43,895	70.9	37.7	55.9	25.2	1.19	66.6
Skin	C43, C44	3,339	5.4	3.0	4.3	5.7	7.27	91.3
Prostate	C61	15,814	25.5	12.9	19.9	13.6	2.32	77.6
Bladder	C67	9,765	15.8	8.6	12.5	9.1	3.31	85.5
Kidney	C64–C66, C68	6,523	10.5	6.2	8.5	13.7	2.17	74.5
CNS	C70–C72	2,020	3.3	2.5	2.9	22.9	2.44	68.0
Thyroid	C73	1,411	2.3	1.5	1.9	7.0	3.62	86.2
Lymphoma	C81–C85, C96	6,530	10.5	6.6	8.7	17.5	1.51	80.9
Myeloma	C88–C90	1,690	2.7	1.5	2.2	34.1	1.07	65.0
Leukemias	C91–C95	4,565	7.4	5.4	6.4	27.4	1.21	72.6

ICD-10th: International Classification of Diseases, 10th Revision.
DCO/I: proportion of cases registered with death certificate only to incidence.
I/D: incidence to deaths.
H/I: proportion of cases verified histologically to incidence.
[a] per 100,000 population.

TABLE II-2. Incidence, Completeness of Reporting, and Accuracy of Diagnosis in Japan according to Sex and Primary Site (1998), Female

Primary site	ICD-10th	Number of incidence	Crude rate[a]	Age-standardized rate[a]		Completeness of registration		Accuracy of diagnosis
				World population	Japanese 1985 model population	DCO/I (%)	I/D	H/I (%)
All sites[b]	C00–C96, D05–D06	213,421	330.5	170.1	229.6	17.1	1.91	71.8
All sites	C00–C96	207,782	321.8	163.0	220.7	17.5	1.86	71.2
Oral & Pharynx	C00-C14	2,586	4.0	2.0	2.7	10.9	1.90	82.4
Esophagus	C15	2,111	3.3	1.4	2.0	21.0	1.44	70.6
Stomach	C16	33,518	51.9	24.2	33.7	17.0	1.88	77.6
Colon	C18	24,726	38.3	17.4	24.4	14.4	2.29	78.4
Rectum	C19–C21	11,693	18.1	8.8	12.1	11.5	2.52	82.5
Liver	C22	11,307	17.5	7.4	10.6	34.5	1.14	24.5
Gallbladder	C23, C24	9,177	14.2	5.3	7.9	31.5	1.12	36.9
Pancreas	C25	8,217	12.7	5.0	7.4	36.3	1.04	25.4
Larynx	C32	239	0.4	0.2	0.2	18.1	2.44	80.1
Lung	C33, C34	17,723	27.4	11.7	16.8	28.0	1.27	62.5
Skin	C43, C44	3,505	5.4	2.3	3.2	6.5	7.43	91.4
Breast[b]	C50, D05	33,676	52.2	33.8	43.6	5.2	3.92	89.3
Uterus[b]	C53–C55, D06	17,686	27.4	18.8	23.9	7.5	3.53	86.6
Uterus	C53–C55	12,885	20.0	12.4	16.1	9.9	2.57	83.2
Cervix uteri	C53	7,012	10.9	7.2	9.3	6.1	3.09	87.4
Corpus uteri	C54	4,763	7.4	4.5	5.8	5.8	4.54	88.6
Ovary	C56	6,742	10.4	6.5	8.3	17.6	1.62	72.4
Bladder	C67	3,243	5.0	2.0	2.9	16.4	2.41	75.2
Kidney	C64–C66, C68	3,204	5.0	2.3	3.2	16.9	2.10	69.0
CNS	C70–C72	1,842	2.9	2.0	2.3	26.1	2.78	64.5
Thyroid	C73	5,581	8.6	5.7	7.2	4.4	6.77	89.6
Lymphoma	C81–C85, C96	4,892	7.6	3.9	5.2	19.1	1.60	79.0
Myeloma	C88–C90	1,642	2.5	1.0	1.5	34.7	1.10	65.0
Leukemia	C91–C95	3,332	5.2	3.5	4.0	27.7	1.21	70.1

ICD-10th: International Classification of Diseases, 10th Revision.
DCO/I: proportion of cases registered with death certificate only to incidence.
I/D: incidence to deaths.
H/I: proportion of cases verified histologically to incidence.
[a] per 100,000 population.
[b] including carcinoma *in situ*.

TABLE III. Number and Names of Registries Selected in Estimating National Cancer Incidence, and Their Validity Indexes of Registration

Year	Number of registries	Name of registry	Completeness of reporting				Accuracy of diagnosis	
			DCO/I (%)		I/D		H/I (%)	
			Average	Range	Average	Range	Average	Range
1975	5	M,Y,O,H,NC	17.2	6.2–27.2	1.58	1.43–1.73	59.9	40.2–75.5
1976	5	M,Y,O,H,NC	16.6	6.7–25.0	1.56	1.42–1.71	61.9	45.1–75.3
1977	5	M,Y,O,H,NC	14.8	6.3–24.4	1.58	1.39–1.77	65.4	51.7–78.0
1978	5	M,Y,O,H,NC	13.4	5.2–23.2	1.60	1.44–1.81	67.6	55.4–80.9
1979	5	M,Y,O,H,NC	13.0	6.4–22.1	1.63	1.43–1.91	68.7	56.0–80.8
1980	7	M,Y,C,O,H,NC,S	15.5	7.1–35.2	1.58	1.43–1.97	63.2	47.2–80.8
1981	7	M,Y,C,O,H,NC,S	14.8	6.4–22.8	1.61	1.44–2.06	66.1	51.8–80.6
1982	7	M,Y,C,O,H,NC,S	13.8	7.0–22.9	1.63	1.41–2.06	67.7	51.5–82.3
1983	7	M,Y,C,O,H,NC,S	13.8	6.0–24.5	1.68	1.42–2.13	68.8	52.0–82.1
1984	7	M,Y,C,O,H,NC,S	15.9	6.0–26.3	1.70	1.39–2.13	68.9	52.2–81.3
1985	9	M,Y,K,F,O,T,H,NP,S	15.0	6.9–30.5	1.78	1.62–2.16	65.9	44.7–79.8
1986	9	M,Y,K,F,O,T,H,NP,S	14.7	4.7–27.9	1.80	1.57–2.15	66.8	50.3–79.3
1987	9	M,Y,K,F,O,T,H,NP,S	14.4	2.6–26.3	1.80	1.56–2.18	67.6	54.1–79.6
1988	9	M,Y,K,F,O,T,H,NP,S	15.4	2.0–24.8	1.80	1.58–2.22	67.6	53.6–81.1
1989	9	M,Y,K,F,O,T,H,NP,S	13.9	1.7–26.8	1.79	1.56–2.24	66.5	49.0–82.3
1990–94	10	M,Y,C[a],K[a],F,O,T,H,NP,Ok	16.6	3.6–28.3	1.87	1.64–2.31	71.2	54.5–84.8
1995	9	Y,C[a],K[a],Ni,F,O,H,Sa,NP	16.9	6.2–24.6	1.73	1.50–2.06	69.2	59.5–82.1
1996	10	M,Y,K[a],Ni,F,O,T,H,Sa,NP	18.2	7.4–28.3	1.74	1.51–2.00	69.7	49.6–79.0
1997	12	M,Y,C[a],K[a],Ni,F,A[a],Si,O,H, Sa,NP	17.4	8.6–25.7	1.76	1.50–2.00	71.3	57.8–79.5
1998	12	M,Y,C[a],K[a],Ni,F,A[a],Si,O,H, Sa,NP	17.3	8.5–25.7	1.77	1.51–2.11	71.6	55.4–80.6

M, Miyagi; Y, Yamagata; C, Chiba; K, Kanagawa; Ni, Niigata; F, Fukui; A, Aichi; Si, Shiga; O, Osaka; T, Tottori; H, Hiroshima City; S, Saga; NC, Nagasaki City; NP, Nagasaki Prefecture; Ok, Okinawa.
[a] Data of model area.

TABLE IV-1-1. Trends of Age-standardized Incidence Rates per 100,000 Population in Japan according to Sex, Primary Site, and Year —Standardized to World Population, Male—

Primary site	Year of diagnosis											
	1975	1980	1985	1990	1991	1992	1993	1994	1995	1996	1997	1998
All sites	202.0	216.9	252.4	268.2	271.4	276.7	273.7	270.7	265.8	268.9	262.6	265.6
Oral & Pharynx	3.1	3.9	4.6	5.5	5.6	5.4	5.2	5.3	6.0	5.4	5.6	5.9
Esophagus	8.3	8.3	9.2	9.5	9.8	10.0	10.2	9.9	10.0	10.3	10.8	10.7
Stomach	85.8	78.9	81.2	75.3	75.3	73.8	70.8	69.7	66.5	67.1	63.0	62.0
Colon	7.7	10.8	16.1	24.0	25.9	28.4	29.1	29.4	30.3	31.2	28.9	30.2
Rectum	9.1	10.4	13.2	16.3	16.2	17.3	17.1	17.2	17.7	18.6	17.9	18.9
Liver	12.8	17.0	23.6	27.6	28.1	28.6	28.0	26.8	25.5	24.4	24.0	24.0
Gallbladder	4.1	5.0	6.6	6.6	6.8	6.9	7.1	7.0	6.7	6.6	6.7	6.5
Pancreas	6.3	7.6	8.9	9.3	9.1	9.1	9.4	9.1	9.2	8.7	8.8	8.8
Larynx	2.4	3.4	3.6	3.6	3.4	3.4	3.1	3.1	2.9	2.9	2.9	2.8
Lung	23.2	28.1	35.4	37.7	38.2	38.9	38.8	38.3	36.6	37.9	37.3	37.7
Skin	1.8	3.0	3.0	3.1	2.6	3.5	3.3	2.5	2.5	2.5	2.8	3.0
Prostate	4.6	6.1	7.7	8.4	9.3	9.8	10.3	11.0	10.2	11.5	12.0	12.9
Bladder	5.0	7.9	7.6	8.4	8.3	8.2	7.9	8.0	8.2	8.5	8.5	8.6
Kidney	2.5	3.0	4.6	5.6	5.6	5.7	5.9	6.2	6.3	6.4	6.2	6.2
CNS	1.6	2.8	3.3	3.6	3.2	3.2	2.7	2.6	2.1	2.4	2.3	2.5
Thyroid	0.5	1.2	1.5	1.6	1.4	1.3	1.2	1.6	1.4	1.6	1.5	1.5
Lymphoma	4.5	4.6	5.7	6.5	6.4	6.7	6.4	6.8	6.8	6.4	6.3	6.6
Myeloma	0.9	1.6	1.7	1.8	1.7	1.6	1.5	1.5	1.4	1.4	1.4	1.5
Leukemia	5.2	5.6	5.5	5.2	5.0	5.3	5.0	4.9	4.8	4.8	5.4	5.4

TABLE IV-1-2. Trends of Age-standardized Incidence Rates per 100,000 Population in Japan according to Sex, Primary Site, and Year —Standardized to World Population, Female—

Primary site	Year of diagnosis											
	1975	1980	1985	1990	1991	1992	1993	1994	1995	1996	1997	1998
All sites*	146.1	149.9	165.9	173.0	175.6	179.8	176.8	174.7	167.3	167.5	168.8	170.1
All sites	142.7	146.1	160.5	166.8	168.7	172.4	169.3	167.2	160.6	160.9	161.7	163.0
Oral & Pharynx	1.2	2.1	2.2	1.8	1.9	1.9	2.0	1.7	2.0	1.9	2.0	2.0
Esophagus	1.9	1.9	1.6	1.3	1.5	1.6	1.6	1.6	1.3	1.4	1.4	1.4
Stomach	40.9	36.5	37.4	31.6	30.8	30.6	29.6	28.4	27.1	26.6	24.8	24.2
Colon	7.0	8.9	11.6	15.3	16.6	17.8	17.8	17.6	17.3	18.0	17.5	17.4
Rectum	6.0	6.1	7.3	8.6	8.9	8.9	8.7	8.2	8.5	8.8	8.8	8.8
Liver	5.6	5.4	6.3	7.9	7.6	7.8	7.9	7.5	7.7	7.2	7.2	7.4
Gallbladder	4.5	5.5	6.7	6.4	6.4	6.3	6.0	5.8	5.5	5.4	5.2	5.3
Pancreas	4.0	4.3	4.9	5.3	5.1	5.2	5.1	5.0	4.9	5.0	5.2	5.0
Larynx	0.2	0.3	0.3	0.2	0.2	0.2	0.1	0.2	0.2	0.3	0.2	0.2
Lung	7.2	8.6	10.3	10.1	10.7	11.3	10.9	11.2	10.7	11.3	11.3	11.7
Skin	1.2	2.9	1.9	2.6	3.0	3.0	2.9	2.2	2.4	2.2	1.9	2.3
Breast	17.0	19.6	24.8	27.6	29.6	30.6	32.0	31.8	30.8	30.4	32.8	33.8
Uterus[a]	24.7	22.3	20.9	19.9	19.8	20.3	20.3	20.1	19.4	19.1	19.6	18.8
Uterus	21.4	18.7	15.9	14.4	13.8	13.7	13.4	13.4	13.1	12.9	12.9	12.4
Cervix uteri	13.4	15.3	11.8	9.2	8.5	8.3	8.2	7.4	8.5	7.8	7.7	7.2
Corpus uteri	1.4	2.4	3.1	3.9	4.1	4.6	3.9	4.6	4.3	4.5	4.5	4.5
Ovary	3.6	4.0	5.7	6.3	6.1	6.2	6.0	6.5	6.4	6.3	6.6	6.5
Bladder	1.5	1.9	2.0	1.9	2.1	2.0	1.9	1.8	1.9	1.8	1.9	2.0
Kidney	0.8	1.3	1.4	2.0	2.0	2.3	2.3	2.2	2.1	2.3	2.2	2.3
CNS	1.1	2.3	2.5	2.8	2.4	2.4	2.0	2.4	1.7	1.7	2.1	2.0
Thyroid	2.1	3.0	4.8	7.3	6.8	7.8	6.1	6.9	5.6	5.7	5.8	5.7
Lymphoma	2.3	2.5	2.9	3.9	3.9	3.8	3.7	4.2	4.1	3.9	4.1	3.9
Myeloma	0.7	1.0	1.3	1.1	1.2	1.1	1.1	1.1	1.1	1.0	1.1	1.0
Leukemia	3.8	3.7	3.7	3.5	3.5	3.4	3.6	3.3	3.0	3.1	3.5	3.5

[a] including carcinoma *in situ*.

TABLE IV-2-1. Trends of Age-standardized Incidence Rates per 100,000 Population in Japan according to Sex, Primary Site, and Year —Standardized to Japanese 1985 Model Population, Male—

Primary site	Year of diagnosis											
	1975	1980	1985	1990	1991	1992	1993	1994	1995	1996	1997	1998
All sites	280.3	302.3	353.5	374.7	379.2	386.9	383.5	379.8	372.7	376.6	368.3	373.2
Oral & Pharynx	4.2	5.3	6.3	7.3	7.6	7.2	7.0	7.3	8.1	7.4	7.5	7.9
Esophagus	11.7	11.7	12.8	13.3	13.6	13.9	14.2	13.8	13.9	14.2	15.0	14.9
Stomach	119.3	109.5	113.7	105.3	105.5	103.4	99.5	97.8	93.4	93.9	88.4	87.1
Colon	10.9	15.3	23.0	33.4	36.1	39.6	40.5	41.2	42.3	43.4	40.3	42.3
Rectum	12.8	14.5	18.6	22.5	22.4	23.7	23.5	23.7	24.5	25.6	24.6	25.9
Liver	17.5	23.2	32.3	37.2	37.9	38.7	37.8	36.2	34.4	33.2	32.7	32.8
Gallbladder	5.9	7.4	9.6	9.7	10.1	10.2	10.5	10.3	10.0	9.9	9.9	9.8
Pancreas	8.6	10.6	12.7	13.3	13.0	13.1	13.6	13.1	13.3	12.6	12.7	12.8
Larynx	3.3	4.7	5.0	5.0	4.7	4.8	4.3	4.3	4.0	4.0	4.1	3.9
Lung	33.2	41.0	51.8	55.1	55.9	57.1	56.9	56.3	53.8	55.8	55.2	55.9
Skin	2.6	4.4	4.2	4.4	3.8	5.0	4.6	3.6	3.5	3.6	4.1	4.3
Prostate	7.1	9.8	12.2	13.4	14.7	15.6	16.4	17.5	16.1	17.8	18.5	19.9
Bladder	7.2	11.4	11.0	12.1	11.9	11.9	11.5	11.7	12.0	12.4	12.3	12.5
Kidney	3.3	4.0	6.3	7.6	7.7	7.8	8.2	8.5	8.7	8.9	8.5	8.5
CNS	1.8	3.1	3.7	4.2	3.8	3.7	3.2	3.1	2.4	2.9	2.7	2.9
Thyroid	0.7	1.6	2.0	2.1	1.8	1.7	1.6	2.0	1.8	2.0	1.9	1.9
Lymphoma	5.7	6.0	7.6	8.8	8.5	8.9	8.4	9.0	9.0	8.5	8.4	8.7
Myeloma	1.3	2.3	2.5	2.6	2.5	2.3	2.1	2.1	2.1	2.1	2.0	2.2
Leukemia	5.8	6.3	6.4	6.0	5.9	6.2	6.0	5.8	5.7	5.8	6.4	6.4

TABLE IV-2-2. Trends of Age-standardized Incidence Rates per 100,000 Population in Japan according to Sex, Primaryin Site, and Year —Standardized to Japanese 1985 Model Population, Female—

Primary site	Year of diagnosis											
	1975	1980	1985	1990	1991	1992	1993	1994	1995	1996	1997	1998
All sites[a]	196.5	202.2	224.8	233.2	236.9	242.6	238.8	235.9	225.7	226.2	227.6	229.6
All sites	192.3	197.4	218.0	225.4	228.3	233.4	229.4	226.6	217.5	218.1	218.9	220.7
Oral & Pharynx	1.6	2.8	2.9	2.4	2.5	2.7	2.7	2.3	2.7	2.5	2.6	2.7
Esophagus	2.7	2.7	2.4	2.0	2.1	2.3	2.3	2.2	1.9	1.9	2.0	2.0
Stomach	56.3	50.9	51.9	44.0	43.0	42.8	41.4	39.8	37.9	37.1	34.6	33.7
Colon	9.7	12.5	16.4	21.5	23.1	24.8	24.9	24.6	24.2	25.1	24.6	24.4
Rectum	8.4	8.5	10.1	11.7	12.2	12.3	12.0	11.4	11.7	12.1	12.1	12.1
Liver	7.9	7.7	8.9	10.9	10.7	10.9	11.0	10.6	10.8	10.3	10.3	10.6
Gallbladder	6.4	7.8	9.9	9.4	9.5	9.3	9.0	8.7	8.2	8.0	7.8	7.9
Pancreas	5.5	6.1	7.1	7.8	7.5	7.6	7.5	7.4	7.2	7.4	7.6	7.4
Larynx	0.3	0.4	0.4	0.3	0.3	0.3	0.1	0.2	0.2	0.4	0.2	0.2
Lung	10.2	12.1	14.9	14.6	15.5	16.2	15.6	16.0	15.3	16.1	16.1	16.8
Skin	1.6	4.1	2.6	3.7	4.3	4.4	4.1	3.2	3.5	3.2	2.7	3.2
Breast	21.7	25.2	31.9	35.5	38.1	39.4	41.4	41.1	39.8	39.2	42.3	43.6
Uterus[a]	32.4	29.2	27.3	25.8	25.5	26.1	26.0	25.8	24.8	24.3	25.0	23.9
Uterus	28.2	24.6	21.0	18.9	18.0	17.9	17.5	17.5	17.1	16.7	16.7	16.1
Cervix uteri	17.5	20.1	15.5	12.0	11.0	10.8	10.6	9.6	11.1	10.0	9.9	9.3
Corpus uteri	1.8	3.2	4.1	5.0	5.3	5.9	5.0	6.0	5.6	5.8	5.8	5.8
Ovary	4.5	4.9	7.2	7.9	7.8	7.9	7.6	8.2	8.0	7.9	8.4	8.3
Bladder	2.1	2.8	2.9	2.8	3.1	2.9	2.8	2.6	2.8	2.7	2.9	2.9
Kidney	1.1	1.7	1.9	2.7	2.8	3.1	3.2	3.0	3.0	3.2	3.1	3.2
CNS	1.1	2.5	2.8	3.1	2.7	2.7	2.3	2.7	1.9	2.0	2.3	2.3
Thyroid	2.7	3.8	6.1	9.3	8.6	9.8	7.8	8.8	7.0	7.2	7.3	7.2
Lymphoma	3.0	3.2	3.8	5.2	5.1	5.1	5.0	5.6	5.5	5.1	5.4	5.2
Myeloma	0.9	1.4	1.8	1.6	1.7	1.6	1.6	1.6	1.5	1.4	1.6	1.5
Leukemia	4.1	4.0	4.1	3.9	4.0	3.9	4.1	3.8	3.4	3.6	3.9	4.0

[a] including carcinoma *in situ*.

TABLE V-1. Trends of Number of Incident Cases in Japan according to Sex, Primary Site, and Year
—Male—

Primary site	Year of diagnosis											
	1975	1980	1985	1990	1991	1992	1993	1994	1995	1996	1997	1998
All sites	110,782	137,290	185,793	229,506	239,643	252,153	257,046	261,402	264,130	275,858	278,352	290,343
Oral & pharynx	1,717	2,478	3,382	4,571	4,867	4,784	4,759	5,017	5,720	5,354	5,659	6,101
Esophagus	4,449	5,166	6,698	8,220	8,701	9,178	9,679	9,640	9,992	10,600	11,493	11,742
Stomach	47,254	50,035	60,130	64,763	66,893	67,614	66,901	67,609	66,440	68,931	66,928	67,861
Colon	4,310	6,913	12,047	20,628	23,004	26,016	27,365	28,548	30,201	32,019	30,590	33,008
Rectum	4,995	6,582	9,805	13,920	14,287	15,659	15,967	16,453	17,466	18,806	18,655	20,144
Liver	6,979	10,712	17,404	23,497	24,659	25,877	25,983	25,487	25,000	24,795	25,198	25,931
Gallbladder	2,222	3,230	4,881	5,798	6,285	6,544	6,963	7,068	7,071	7,213	7,550	7,672
Pancreas	3,393	4,826	6,569	8,088	8,196	8,519	9,125	9,018	9,440	9,282	9,627	10,052
Larynx	1,268	2,135	2,610	3,081	3,038	3,166	2,943	2,998	2,876	2,950	3,122	3,083
Lung	12,701	17,998	26,527	33,217	34,864	36,816	37,849	38,545	38,052	40,976	41,953	43,895
Skin	997	1,908	2,176	2,685	2,348	3,218	3,079	2,473	2,481	2,606	3,050	3,339
Prostate	2,412	3,944	5,960	7,840	8,927	9,855	10,704	11,807	11,304	13,086	14,170	15,814
Bladder	2,674	4,959	5,627	7,305	7,463	7,654	7,656	8,036	8,471	9,085	9,341	9,765
Kidney	1,354	1,834	3,331	4,701	4,897	5,072	5,481	5,870	6,107	6,443	6,344	6,523
CNS	862	1,662	2,124	2,575	2,328	2,345	2,080	2,019	1,615	1,976	1,811	2,020
Thyroid	288	821	1,108	1,291	1,128	1,133	1,067	1,353	1,213	1,409	1,339	1,411
Lymphoma	2,492	2,889	4,084	5,382	5,338	5,753	5,570	6,063	6,269	6,062	6,172	6,530
Myeloma	506	1,036	1,266	1,557	1,559	1,490	1,406	1,461	1,500	1,512	1,540	1,690
Leukemia	2,779	3,240	3,534	3,664	3,609	3,916	3,822	3,793	3,775	3,931	4,514	4,565

TABLE V-2. Trends of Number of Incident Cases in Japan according to Sex, Primary Site, and Year
—Female—

Primary site	Year of diagnosis											
	1975	1980	1985	1990	1991	1992	1993	1994	1995	1996	1997	1998
All sites[a]	98,149	116,536	149,918	177,383	184,782	193,870	195,563	197,767	194,579	200,501	206,434	213,421
All sites	95,920	113,751	145,692	172,435	179,305	188,092	189,684	191,992	189,434	195,459	200,930	207,782
Oral & pharynx	780	1,581	1,919	1,873	1,972	2,166	2,295	2,040	2,398	2,272	2,433	2,586
Esophagus	1,312	1,553	1,651	1,640	1,839	2,059	2,083	2,120	1,808	1,915	2,003	2,111
Stomach	27,879	29,370	34,948	34,493	34,757	35,608	35,380	34,916	34,402	34,625	33,384	33,518
Colon	4,752	7,223	11,153	17,083	18,852	20,801	21,563	21,993	22,266	23,830	24,039	24,726
Rectum	4,115	4,875	6,816	9,101	9,757	10,126	10,155	9,874	10,381	10,971	11,341	11,693
Liver	3,856	4,425	6,143	8,830	8,928	9,420	9,817	9,701	10,288	10,191	10,598	11,307
Gallbladder	3,118	4,507	6,850	7,972	8,396	8,524	8,551	8,554	8,368	8,634	8,702	9,177
Pancreas	2,682	3,536	4,928	6,495	6,460	6,788	7,010	7,131	7,170	7,751	8,122	8,217
Larynx	150	210	268	219	212	226	125	213	220	348	244	239
Lung	4,971	6,979	10,246	11,913	13,080	14,090	14,068	14,863	14,689	15,954	16,464	17,723
Skin	808	2,372	1,820	3,050	3,668	3,928	3,806	3,017	3,478	3,339	2,850	3,505
Breast[a]	11,123	14,447	20,296	24,697	26,866	28,186	30,107	30,326	29,818	29,699	32,347	33,676
Uterus[a]	16,397	16,777	17,623	17,872	17,871	18,408	18,277	18,289	17,735	17,596	18,190	17,686
Uterus	14,176	14,142	13,685	13,541	13,112	13,034	13,034	13,203	13,001	12,946	13,157	12,885
Cervix uteri	8,832	11,552	10,071	8,477	7,873	7,735	7,735	7,057	8,099	7,424	7,419	7,012
Corpus uteri	892	1,826	2,636	3,574	3,837	3,776	3,776	4,550	4,367	4,567	4,609	4,763
Ovary	2,295	2,842	4,638	5,624	5,589	5,704	5,704	6,250	6,144	6,256	6,705	6,742
Bladder	998	1,618	2,065	2,358	2,688	2,630	2,630	2,599	2,826	2,810	3,119	3,243
Kidney	542	975	1,292	2,175	2,297	2,718	2,718	2,662	2,706	3,007	2,970	3,204
CNS	619	1,444	1,793	2,178	1,962	1,705	1,705	2,090	1,461	1,607	1,883	1,842
Thyroid	1,403	2,175	3,893	6,394	6,055	5,615	5,615	6,414	5,243	5,481	5,625	5,581
Lymphoma	1,521	1,852	2,551	3,915	4,047	4,155	4,155	4,723	4,724	4,554	5,026	4,892
Myeloma	460	784	1,267	1,339	1,441	1,426	1,426	1,511	1,494	1,470	1,632	1,642
Leukemia	2,234	2,343	2,617	2,786	2,855	3,043	3,043	2,910	2,662	2,907	3,196	3,332

[a] including carcinoma *in situ*.

TABLE V-3. Trends of Number of Incident Cases in Japan according to Sex, Primary Site, and Year
—Both Sexes—

Primary site	Year of diagnosis											
	1975	1980	1985	1990	1991	1992	1993	1994	1995	1996	1997	1998
All sites[a]	208,931	253,826	335,711	406,889	424,425	446,023	452,609	459,169	458,710	476,360	484,787	503,764
All sites	206,702	251,041	331,485	401,941	418,948	440,245	446,730	453,394	453,564	471,317	479,282	498,125
Oral & pharynx	2,497	4,059	5,301	6,444	6,839	6,950	7,054	7,057	8,118	7,626	8,092	8,687
Esophagus	5,761	6,719	8,349	9,860	10,540	11,237	11,762	11,760	11,800	12,515	13,496	13,853
Stomach	75,133	79,405	95,078	99,256	101,650	103,222	102,281	102,525	100,842	103,556	100,312	101,379
Colon	9,062	14,136	23,200	37,711	41,856	46,817	48,928	50,541	52,467	55,849	54,629	57,734
Rectum	9,110	11,457	16,621	23,021	24,044	25,785	26,122	26,327	27,847	29,777	29,996	31,837
Liver	10,835	15,137	23,547	32,327	33,587	35,297	35,800	35,188	35,288	34,986	35,796	37,238
Gallbladder	5,340	7,737	11,731	13,770	14,681	15,068	15,514	15,622	15,439	15,847	16,252	16,849
Pancreas	6,075	8,362	11,497	14,583	14,656	15,307	16,135	16,149	16,610	17,033	17,749	18,269
Larynx	1,418	2,345	2,878	3,300	3,250	3,392	3,068	3,211	3,096	3,298	3,366	3,322
Lung	17,672	24,977	36,773	45,130	47,944	50,906	51,917	53,408	52,741	56,930	58,417	61,618
Skin	1,805	4,280	3,996	5,735	6,016	7,146	6,885	5,490	5,959	5,945	5,900	6,844
Breast[a]	11,123	14,447	20,296	24,697	26,866	28,186	30,107	30,326	29,818	29,699	32,347	33,676
Uterus[a]	16,397	16,777	17,623	17,872	17,871	18,408	18,277	18,289	17,735	17,596	18,190	17,686
Uterus	14,176	14,142	13,685	13,541	13,112	13,034	13,034	13,203	13,001	12,946	13,157	12,885
Cervix uteri	8,832	11,552	10,071	8,477	7,873	7,735	7,735	7,057	8,099	7,424	7,419	7,012
Corpus uteri	892	1,826	2,636	3,574	3,837	3,776	3,776	4,550	4,367	4,567	4,609	4,763
Ovary	2,295	2,842	4,638	5,624	5,589	5,704	5,704	6,250	6,144	6,256	6,705	6,742
Prostate	2,412	3,944	5,960	7,840	8,927	9,855	10,704	11,807	11,304	13,086	14,170	15,814
Bladder	3,672	6,577	7,692	9,663	10,151	10,284	10,286	10,635	11,297	11,895	12,460	13,008
Kidney	1,896	2,809	4,623	6,876	7,194	7,790	8,199	8,532	8,813	9,450	9,314	9,727
CNS	1,481	3,106	3,917	4,753	4,290	4,050	3,785	4,109	3,076	3,583	3,694	3,862
Thyroid	1,691	2,996	5,001	7,685	7,183	6,748	6,682	7,767	6,456	6,890	6,964	6,992
Lymphoma	4,013	4,741	6,635	9,297	9,385	9,908	9,725	10,786	10,993	10,616	11,198	11,422
Myeloma	966	1,820	2,533	2,896	3,000	2,916	2,832	2,972	2,994	2,982	3,172	3,332
Leukemia	5,013	5,583	6,151	6,450	6,464	6,959	6,865	6,703	6,437	6,838	7,710	7,897

[a] including carcinoma *in situ*.

TABLE VI-1. Trends of Age-specific Incidence Rates per 100,000 Population in Japan according to Sex, Primary Site, and Year
—All Sites (including carcinoma *in situ*), Female—

Age	Year of diagnosis											
	1975	1980	1985	1990	1991	1992	1993	1994	1995	1996	1997	1998
All age	173.4	192.3	254.5	281.9	292.7	306.0	307.8	310.4	304.0	312.4	320.7	330.5
0–4	11.8	12.8	14.1	13.9	14.3	14.4	14.1	13.2	15.1	12.9	12.5	10.9
5–9	7.7	6.9	6.8	7.6	7.2	7.6	7.5	5.9	5.6	4.7	6.1	5.8
10–14	7.7	5.5	7.7	8.8	8.5	7.7	8.3	8.3	8.3	6.8	6.9	7.1
15–19	7.3	7.2	8.5	9.5	9.4	9.8	9.5	9.3	8.5	7.6	7.4	7.8
20–24	15.0	15.3	14.8	16.0	16.5	16.9	15.7	16.5	15.6	16.6	16.1	15.8
25–29	30.2	24.9	29.0	37.4	38.8	38.7	38.4	38.2	35.5	36.6	33.9	34.7
30–34	54.0	60.4	74.4	76.9	78.3	80.5	82.1	83.7	80.5	80.4	78.8	78.2
35–39	98.7	113.5	129.0	140.4	138.5	143.9	135.8	131.1	131.1	127.4	131.5	130.2
40–44	166.2	167.5	197.4	222.6	236.0	249.0	235.1	228.1	205.1	200.5	201.3	199.9
45–49	231.4	228.7	254.3	277.5	273.0	278.4	276.7	285.4	280.9	300.3	313.8	311.1
50–54	291.6	297.3	320.6	324.9	334.0	352.5	352.1	347.9	325.1	311.7	310.7	320.0
55–59	370.1	382.9	412.6	417.8	423.2	430.7	430.7	430.0	402.1	403.2	411.3	417.5
60–64	507.6	518.7	542.3	561.4	568.3	575.9	562.4	543.5	514.9	522.9	531.5	544.4
65–69	663.1	662.9	697.9	731.1	740.4	746.8	740.2	726.4	692.2	695.9	703.9	709.2
70–74	836.6	870.3	945.2	924.9	944.8	957.0	932.5	923.8	912.6	908.3	896.8	905.8
75–79	1,040.0	1,035.9	1,149.9	1,138.9	1,154.7	1,188.2	1,180.6	1,162.0	1,109.2	1,114.2	1085.1	1,099.1
80–84	992.5	1,094.2	1,370.6	1,378.1	1,414.1	1,445.0	1,427.7	1,399.4	1,338.9	1,347.3	1,352.7	1,357.4
85–	841.8	1,009.2	1,375.2	1,497.4	1,500.1	1,519.1	1,511.9	1,522.7	1,539.2	1,569.2	1,589.8	1,615.6

TABLE VI-2-1. Trends of Age-specific Incidence Rates per 100,000 Population in Japan according to Sex, Primary Site, and Year
—All Sites, Male—

Age	Year of diagnosis											
	1975	1980	1985	1990	1991	1992	1993	1994	1995	1996	1997	1998
All age	203.9	234.4	329.0	378.1	393.5	412.7	419.8	426.2	429.0	447.2	450.4	468.9
0–4	14.7	15.2	17.7	17.3	16.7	15.4	13.8	14.8	17.1	15.0	16.3	15.0
5–9	8.3	7.3	8.5	8.9	9.8	9.8	9.0	8.5	8.0	7.5	8.1	8.7
10–14	8.1	7.5	8.9	7.5	7.2	7.1	7.5	8.1	7.8	8.0	7.5	7.9
15–19	10.4	10.0	12.2	10.1	11.3	11.8	12.4	11.3	10.3	9.7	9.6	10.3
20–24	11.7	9.3	11.9	12.2	13.4	14.0	13.1	12.5	13.6	12.8	13.2	13.1
25–29	20.0	18.0	21.0	19.6	18.0	20.1	20.3	20.1	18.9	19.0	17.0	18.1
30–34	33.6	34.1	35.8	37.0	34.5	35.6	33.6	34.5	30.8	30.2	29.4	29.3
35–39	56.7	61.0	68.7	70.4	68.0	64.3	62.6	62.7	58.7	60.1	57.8	58.7
40–44	103.4	102.3	111.2	126.4	134.4	137.0	129.0	120.6	114.7	115.5	109.3	111.2
45–49	202.8	208.4	203.3	215.2	208.2	203.5	198.7	201.1	207.7	228.9	228.3	223.1
50–54	319.1	369.3	411.9	390.5	383.0	392.8	381.4	384.0	377.2	360.5	337.9	343.1
55–59	511.5	554.5	695.3	718.4	719.6	728.2	711.7	674.7	658.7	640.1	613.7	627.0
60–64	805.0	841.3	992.9	1,128.3	1,162.3	1,191.0	1,168.4	1,127.9	1,088.1	1,096.2	1,045.2	1,027.6
65–69	1,150.2	1,232.5	1,374.9	1,553.5	1,600.2	1,647.4	1,650.3	1,645.6	1,583.5	1,643.6	1,605.3	1,628.5
70–74	1,595.4	1,710.0	1,962.9	1,991.6	2,007.6	2,034.5	2,034.3	2,053.0	2,079.8	2,149.7	2,170.7	2,226.8
75–79	1,844.7	2,027.5	2,422.6	2,504.7	2,555.3	2,637.8	2,635.6	2,618.0	2,560.9	2,485.3	2,396.6	2,467.5
80–84	1,959.5	2,157.6	2,699.3	2,870.7	2,914.8	2,972.8	3,003.6	3,026.3	2,924.0	2,979.9	3,030.4	3,069.9
85–	1,624.5	1,950.0	2,687.6	2,979.1	2,955.5	3,041.5	3,082.2	3,113.7	3,183.3	3,315.1	3,285.6	3,336.3

TABLE VI-2-2. Trends of Age-specific Incidence Rates per 100,000 Population in Japan according to Sex, Primary Site, and Year
—All Sites, Female—

Age	Year of diagnosis											
	1975	1980	1985	1990	1991	1992	1993	1994	1995	1996	1997	1998
All age	169.5	187.7	247.7	274.1	284.0	296.9	298.5	301.4	296.0	304.6	312.2	321.8
0–4	11.8	12.8	14.1	13.9	14.3	14.4	14.1	13.2	15.1	12.9	12.5	10.9
5–9	7.7	6.9	6.8	7.6	7.2	7.6	7.5	5.9	5.6	4.7	6.1	5.8
10–14	7.7	5.5	7.7	8.8	8.5	7.7	8.3	8.3	8.3	6.8	6.9	7.1
15–19	7.3	7.2	8.5	9.4	9.4	9.8	9.5	9.3	8.4	7.5	7.3	7.7
20–24	14.7	15.0	14.3	15.1	15.3	16.0	14.6	15.4	14.5	15.5	14.8	14.2
25–29	29.1	23.7	26.1	32.5	32.6	31.9	31.2	31.5	28.5	29.0	26.4	26.8
30–34	50.3	53.8	64.1	61.8	62.1	60.8	60.4	60.6	60.3	59.4	58.2	57.3
35–39	87.1	101.4	111.8	122.4	118.2	121.5	113.3	109.7	109.7	107.0	107.9	107.2
40–44	153.2	152.8	178.7	199.9	211.1	222.3	209.3	203.8	186.1	182.7	181.7	180.3
45–49	219.1	219.2	238.2	262.3	256.5	261.6	259.2	266.8	263.1	281.7	293.5	291.0
50–54	284.7	287.7	310.8	315.2	323.3	341.2	340.4	336.3	315.0	303.7	301.8	310.7
55–59	366.7	376.8	404.7	410.9	415.7	423.6	423.4	423.1	395.0	396.4	403.1	409.3
60–64	502.2	513.5	534.8	552.8	559.4	567.4	554.5	535.7	509.4	517.0	525.9	537.3
65–69	661.6	658.9	692.2	723.6	733.1	739.8	732.5	719.1	687.0	691.3	698.7	703.8
70–74	833.6	868.4	941.2	920.2	938.7	950.8	926.3	918.6	909.0	904.7	892.0	900.1
75–79	1,039.8	1,035.0	1,147.4	1,134.0	1,148.9	1,183.0	1,176.6	1,157.6	1,105.7	1,110.7	1,081.3	1,094.9
80–84	992.5	1,094.1	1,368.4	1,377.0	1,412.9	1,443.8	1,425.9	1,397.1	1,336.7	1,345.6	1,350.3	1,354.0
85–	841.8	1,009.0	1,373.9	1,494.6	1,496.7	1,516.2	1,509.4	1,520.8	1,537.3	1,567.7	1,588.4	1,613.9

TABLE VI-3-1. Trends of Age-specific Incidence Rates per 100,000 Population in Japan according to Sex, Primary Site, and Year
—Oral & pharynx, Male—

Age	Year of diagnosis											
	1975	1980	1985	1990	1991	1992	1993	1994	1995	1996	1997	1998
All age	2.8	4.2	5.8	7.5	8.0	7.8	7.8	8.2	9.3	8.7	9.2	9.9
0–4	0.2	0.0	0.1	0.2	0.1	0.0	0.0	0.0	0.0	0.0	0.0	0.0
5–9	0.2	0.0	0.0	0.0	0.0	0.0	0.0	0.0	0.1	0.1	0.0	0.0
10–14	0.4	0.3	0.0	0.1	0.1	0.1	0.0	0.1	0.0	0.1	0.1	0.1
15–19	0.3	0.3	0.1	0.5	0.3	0.3	0.3	0.3	0.2	0.2	0.1	0.4
20–24	0.3	0.5	0.6	0.5	0.5	0.5	0.5	0.5	0.5	0.5	0.8	0.9
25–29	0.5	0.2	0.3	0.8	0.6	0.4	0.5	0.6	1.0	0.8	0.9	1.3
30–34	1.3	0.9	1.1	0.6	0.7	0.8	0.8	1.2	1.0	0.8	0.7	0.9
35–39	1.3	1.5	2.6	2.1	1.8	1.7	1.6	1.7	2.0	2.0	1.8	1.9
40–44	2.9	2.7	3.4	3.4	3.6	3.7	3.8	4.1	4.4	3.5	3.1	3.2
45–49	3.4	4.8	5.9	5.8	6.1	5.6	5.7	6.3	6.9	7.7	7.8	7.4
50–54	5.7	8.6	9.6	11.7	11.9	11.2	10.8	12.6	14.9	12.4	11.9	11.6
55–59	9.2	12.2	13.3	18.9	18.0	16.7	15.5	15.9	20.2	17.8	19.4	18.4
60–64	12.3	15.0	17.6	24.6	27.3	25.5	24.8	24.1	27.4	23.5	24.1	24.8
65–69	13.1	20.1	25.7	33.1	31.8	32.4	29.5	28.7	29.4	26.7	27.8	32.1
70–74	19.0	28.8	27.2	30.3	36.7	34.2	32.4	30.4	34.2	34.9	36.5	40.2
75–79	21.5	24.0	35.4	35.2	37.5	37.2	37.6	41.9	40.9	36.5	34.6	36.7
80–84	25.7	33.6	32.7	29.2	28.8	28.6	31.5	32.1	35.7	35.5	36.3	38.8
85–	32.8	12.6	36.2	28.8	31.7	27.4	31.1	31.5	33.2	29.7	39.8	44.9

TABLE VI-3-2. Trends of Age-specific Incidence Rates per 100,000 Population in Japan according to Sex, Primary Site, and Year
—Oral & pharynx, Female—

Age	Year of diagnosis											
	1975	1980	1985	1990	1991	1992	1993	1994	1995	1996	1997	1998
All age	1.1	2.5	3.2	3.0	3.1	3.4	3.6	3.2	3.7	3.5	3.8	4.0
0–4	0.1	0.0	0.1	0.0	0.0	0.0	0.0	0.0	0.0	0.0	0.0	0.0
5–9	0.1	0.1	0.0	0.0	0.1	0.1	0.1	0.0	0.0	0.1	0.1	0.1
10–14	0.2	0.0	0.3	0.1	0.1	0.1	0.3	0.2	0.3	0.2	0.2	0.2
15–19	0.2	0.2	0.3	0.2	0.2	0.1	0.1	0.1	0.1	0.2	0.1	0.1
20–24	0.4	0.7	0.3	0.2	0.2	0.4	0.4	0.4	0.4	0.3	0.4	0.2
25–29	0.2	0.2	0.3	0.9	0.9	0.6	0.6	0.4	0.1	0.9	1.1	1.2
30–34	0.5	0.8	1.6	0.8	1.1	0.9	0.9	0.7	1.2	1.1	0.8	0.6
35–39	0.7	1.6	1.4	1.1	1.0	1.2	1.2	1.2	1.2	1.0	0.9	1.3
40–44	0.8	1.1	1.3	2.1	1.9	2.2	1.6	1.4	1.3	1.5	2.2	2.3
45–49	1.6	4.3	3.6	1.7	1.4	1.8	2.3	2.4	2.5	2.4	2.3	2.7
50–54	1.8	3.4	5.4	3.9	4.1	3.8	3.6	2.7	4.4	3.8	3.6	3.1
55–59	3.0	5.9	5.9	4.8	4.8	4.7	5.2	4.4	5.4	4.1	4.9	4.9
60–64	5.5	9.3	8.2	5.6	6.8	7.2	7.7	6.3	6.5	6.5	6.8	7.3
65–69	3.6	7.3	8.5	8.3	8.4	9.6	8.8	7.8	8.7	8.1	8.7	9.4
70–74	6.2	8.5	10.1	9.5	8.9	9.3	11.0	8.8	11.7	9.6	9.1	9.3
75–79	8.6	17.0	13.6	12.9	13.0	13.9	14.4	13.0	15.7	13.9	15.2	13.8
80–84	10.6	12.0	13.6	16.1	17.5	19.2	19.1	16.6	16.2	14.8	15.9	18.4
85–	8.0	19.1	18.0	16.4	15.9	18.7	21.7	20.1	21.0	21.3	20.5	22.6

TABLE VI-4-1. Trends of Age-specific Incidence Rates per 100,000 Population in Japan according to Sex, Primary Site, and Year
—Esophagus, Male—

Age	Year of diagnosis											
	1975	1980	1985	1990	1991	1992	1993	1994	1995	1996	1997	1998
All age	7.9	8.8	11.7	13.5	14.3	15.0	15.8	15.7	16.2	17.2	18.6	19.0
0–4	0.2	0.0	0.0	0.0	0.0	0.0	0.0	0.0	0.1	0.1	0.0	0.0
5–9	0.2	0.0	0.0	0.0	0.0	0.0	0.0	0.0	0.0	0.0	0.0	0.0
10–14	0.2	0.0	0.0	0.0	0.0	0.0	0.0	0.0	0.0	0.0	0.0	0.0
15–19	0.3	0.0	0.2	0.0	0.0	0.0	0.0	0.0	0.0	0.0	0.0	0.0
20–24	0.3	0.0	0.0	0.0	0.0	0.0	0.0	0.0	0.0	0.0	0.0	0.0
25–29	0.2	0.0	0.0	0.0	0.0	0.1	0.0	0.0	0.0	0.0	0.0	0.0
30–34	0.2	0.0	0.0	0.1	0.1	0.0	0.2	0.1	0.0	0.0	0.1	0.1
35–39	1.0	0.5	0.6	0.7	0.6	0.6	0.5	0.3	0.2	0.1	0.4	0.3
40–44	1.3	1.8	1.6	1.6	2.6	2.6	3.0	1.9	1.8	1.7	2.5	2.6
45–49	5.2	5.4	7.4	6.8	7.1	6.4	6.3	6.4	7.6	8.7	8.0	7.3
50–54	10.1	13.4	16.1	17.1	17.6	19.2	19.0	19.6	19.2	18.7	17.3	16.6
55–59	20.1	23.3	26.6	29.6	29.9	30.4	32.2	31.7	33.1	33.8	37.5	39.7
60–64	37.0	35.0	45.9	49.3	52.1	53.0	51.0	46.4	48.1	49.8	52.3	51.6
65–69	56.5	49.2	58.3	59.2	62.6	67.9	71.0	69.1	66.3	72.3	75.4	76.1
70–74	74.2	75.0	75.4	78.3	77.2	73.0	78.6	76.6	78.7	80.6	87.7	84.9
75–79	79.4	88.5	80.5	85.5	82.0	82.6	83.6	84.9	81.1	79.2	81.2	81.4
80–84	89.2	77.2	86.6	82.0	86.2	88.6	92.5	88.0	83.7	80.5	90.4	82.8
85–	111.1	108.3	73.7	72.7	68.9	72.1	69.9	72.8	80.3	82.2	82.1	85.9

TABLE VI-4-2. Trends of Age-specific Incidence Rates per 100,000 Population in Japan according to Sex, Primary Site, and Year
—Esophagus, Female—

Age	Year of diagnosis											
	1975	1980	1985	1990	1991	1992	1993	1994	1995	1996	1997	1998
All age	2.0	2.5	2.8	2.6	2.9	3.2	3.3	3.3	2.8	3.0	3.1	3.3
0–4	0.1	0.0	0.0	0.0	0.0	0.0	0.0	0.0	0.0	0.0	0.0	0.0
5–9	0.2	0.0	0.0	0.0	0.0	0.0	0.0	0.0	0.0	0.0	0.0	0.0
10–14	0.2	0.0	0.0	0.0	0.0	0.0	0.0	0.0	0.0	0.0	0.0	0.0
15–19	0.2	0.0	0.0	0.0	0.0	0.0	0.0	0.0	0.0	0.0	0.0	0.0
20–24	0.2	0.0	0.0	0.0	0.0	0.0	0.0	0.0	0.0	0.0	0.0	0.0
25–29	0.1	0.0	0.0	0.0	0.0	0.0	0.0	0.0	0.0	0.0	0.0	0.0
30–34	0.1	0.0	0.1	0.1	0.0	0.0	0.0	0.0	0.0	0.1	0.1	0.1
35–39	0.4	0.0	0.0	0.1	0.2	0.1	0.0	0.0	0.2	0.2	0.2	0.3
40–44	0.6	0.8	0.6	0.5	0.7	0.6	0.6	0.6	0.7	0.5	0.4	0.4
45–49	0.9	1.0	0.8	0.7	0.8	0.9	1.5	1.4	1.1	1.1	0.9	1.0
50–54	3.1	1.6	2.2	2.1	2.7	2.5	3.0	2.6	2.4	2.6	2.4	3.1
55–59	3.4	4.5	3.0	2.5	3.5	4.6	4.7	4.6	4.4	4.4	4.2	4.0
60–64	7.5	9.3	5.1	4.0	4.1	4.3	5.2	5.2	5.5	5.6	6.2	6.4
65–69	9.8	10.6	9.3	7.8	9.7	10.3	8.9	7.9	6.1	6.4	7.3	6.9
70–74	13.5	15.8	13.7	12.1	11.1	12.3	11.1	12.6	9.6	10.5	10.0	10.2
75–79	25.7	26.7	22.2	17.0	16.4	17.3	16.0	16.9	11.0	11.6	12.1	12.3
80–84	23.3	18.1	27.3	19.0	22.2	23.8	23.0	21.4	17.9	18.9	16.8	16.3
85–	31.8	28.4	29.4	28.1	28.4	31.3	29.4	27.9	23.3	21.0	23.6	24.5

TABLE VI-5-1. Trends of Age-specific Incidence Rates per 100,000 Population in Japan according to Sex, Primary Site, and Year
—Stomach, Male—

Age	Year of diagnosis											
	1975	1980	1985	1990	1991	1992	1993	1994	1995	1996	1997	1998
All age	88.5	86.6	107.7	106.7	109.8	110.7	109.3	110.2	107.9	111.7	108.3	109.6
0–4	0.2	0.0	0.0	0.0	0.0	0.0	0.0	0.2	0.3	0.2	0.0	0.0
5–9	0.2	0.1	0.0	0.0	0.0	0.0	0.0	0.1	0.0	0.0	0.0	0.0
10–14	0.2	0.1	0.0	0.0	0.0	0.0	0.0	0.0	0.0	0.0	0.0	0.0
15–19	0.7	0.3	0.7	0.3	0.3	0.2	0.2	0.1	0.3	0.3	0.2	0.1
20–24	2.8	1.3	0.5	1.6	1.5	1.3	0.8	0.7	0.6	0.7	0.6	0.7
25–29	5.4	6.2	5.5	2.4	2.0	2.3	2.7	2.6	2.9	2.3	1.9	1.9
30–34	12.6	12.2	12.0	10.4	8.6	9.3	7.7	7.9	5.8	4.8	4.8	4.4
35–39	25.7	24.5	26.2	24.4	23.5	20.8	19.3	18.6	16.6	16.9	16.9	16.1
40–44	48.9	43.3	47.7	43.7	46.6	46.8	41.7	38.4	34.0	35.4	30.7	29.8
45–49	97.4	86.4	75.9	71.6	66.8	60.9	58.4	59.9	59.2	63.8	64.9	63.6
50–54	151.1	145.7	148.2	130.8	125.8	122.8	112.7	112.2	105.9	102.4	90.1	89.5
55–59	231.5	219.0	242.1	210.2	211.2	204.8	198.2	188.8	180.2	180.3	163.1	162.2
60–64	356.4	324.3	330.4	319.9	322.7	322.7	306.4	304.8	291.3	293.3	263.6	255.5
65–69	512.2	456.1	443.3	443.4	451.6	446.0	431.5	425.7	395.4	409.2	387.9	378.3
70–74	673.4	621.7	617.4	554.4	552.5	541.3	522.2	513.5	515.3	530.1	516.7	516.1
75–79	735.4	674.4	717.9	666.9	663.0	658.3	633.5	625.0	603.4	584.2	542.6	539.0
80–84	762.1	641.2	773.9	719.1	750.2	725.4	743.1	729.8	682.1	652.1	657.0	651.9
85–	565.3	625.4	782.7	705.3	727.8	718.2	732.0	726.1	695.4	705.5	688.5	683.7

TABLE VI-5-2. Trends of Age-specific Incidence Rates per 100,000 Population in Japan according to Sex, Primary Site, and Year
—Stomach, Female—

Age	Year of diagnosis											
	1975	1980	1985	1990	1991	1992	1993	1994	1995	1996	1997	1998
All age	49.9	49.1	60.4	54.8	55.0	56.2	55.7	54.8	53.8	54.0	51.9	51.9
0–4	0.2	0.1	0.0	0.1	0.0	0.0	0.1	0.1	0.0	0.1	0.0	0.0
5–9	0.2	0.0	0.0	0.0	0.0	0.1	0.1	0.1	0.0	0.0	0.0	0.0
10–14	0.3	0.0	0.0	0.0	0.0	0.0	0.0	0.0	0.0	0.0	0.0	0.0
15–19	0.6	0.0	0.2	0.2	0.3	0.3	0.5	0.3	0.4	0.1	0.2	0.2
20–24	3.0	2.2	2.0	1.1	1.3	1.6	1.4	1.0	0.7	0.6	0.9	0.8
25–29	8.1	5.5	6.5	4.3	3.5	3.3	3.9	3.9	3.5	2.4	2.3	2.3
30–34	16.6	14.2	14.5	9.4	9.9	9.9	10.2	10.2	8.5	7.8	5.7	5.8
35–39	24.4	22.7	26.8	22.8	20.9	21.2	17.7	17.5	16.0	16.6	13.5	13.0
40–44	38.9	33.6	37.0	33.3	33.1	35.7	33.8	32.0	27.1	27.0	24.7	23.9
45–49	47.9	46.4	50.5	38.5	35.1	36.8	36.4	34.5	34.1	37.3	37.3	35.3
50–54	73.0	62.5	65.9	54.4	51.3	53.4	51.7	47.5	44.2	43.2	38.9	37.8
55–59	98.3	89.5	89.9	77.5	77.1	73.3	70.8	69.6	66.9	65.0	60.2	57.5
60–64	161.6	125.8	128.0	113.0	110.8	104.4	99.4	93.3	89.7	91.5	87.8	88.6
65–69	206.5	189.9	174.7	155.7	147.1	143.5	139.5	136.6	131.3	126.9	120.1	116.0
70–74	272.3	248.9	256.4	202.4	207.9	203.4	197.4	192.7	192.4	181.6	166.6	159.8
75–79	336.0	312.5	297.4	256.5	250.3	253.4	248.3	240.7	232.5	225.7	208.0	204.8
80–84	328.9	367.5	353.3	329.6	328.4	331.9	322.2	304.6	276.1	268.5	247.9	248.1
85–	304.0	294.7	370.9	326.0	324.6	328.7	317.0	309.7	318.9	309.9	310.5	306.3

Table VI-6-1. Trends of Age-specific Incidence Rates per 100,000 Population in Japan according to Sex, Primary Site, and Year
—Colon, Male—

Age	Year of diagnosis											
	1975	1980	1985	1990	1991	1992	1993	1994	1995	1996	1997	1998
All age	7.4	11.6	21.0	34.0	37.8	42.6	44.7	46.5	49.0	51.9	49.5	53.3
0–4	0.2	0.0	0.0	0.0	0.0	0.0	0.0	0.0	0.0	0.0	0.0	0.0
5–9	0.2	0.0	0.0	0.0	0.0	0.0	0.0	0.0	0.0	0.0	0.0	0.0
10–14	0.2	0.0	0.1	0.1	0.0	0.0	0.0	0.0	0.0	0.0	0.0	0.0
15–19	0.4	0.2	0.2	0.1	0.2	0.2	0.2	0.0	0.1	0.1	0.1	0.2
20–24	0.6	0.5	0.9	0.4	0.5	0.6	0.5	0.6	0.6	0.8	0.7	0.6
25–29	1.1	0.8	0.8	1.8	1.4	1.9	1.1	1.0	1.1	1.0	0.9	0.7
30–34	1.9	2.4	2.3	2.0	2.4	2.5	3.1	3.1	2.5	2.5	2.5	2.9
35–39	3.0	4.1	5.8	5.4	6.2	5.8	6.0	5.8	5.5	7.0	5.7	6.5
40–44	5.6	6.1	6.8	11.8	13.2	13.8	13.8	12.5	14.1	13.3	12.9	14.0
45–49	8.0	11.1	13.0	22.8	21.5	22.5	23.5	23.2	26.6	28.9	27.7	26.4
50–54	13.2	18.4	27.8	44.4	47.2	50.0	49.1	47.7	48.4	44.7	41.2	43.9
55–59	13.5	24.7	44.5	67.3	75.9	87.8	87.2	84.2	88.4	85.9	78.3	79.3
60–64	32.4	40.1	59.6	109.7	119.9	131.1	131.4	131.2	136.1	146.2	131.1	130.6
65–69	36.7	56.4	84.0	140.1	153.8	173.0	182.2	193.5	190.1	199.2	181.3	192.1
70–74	62.8	81.1	130.9	158.6	179.0	199.8	212.1	219.3	225.2	241.7	232.0	247.7
75–79	84.1	113.7	166.9	215.3	228.8	243.2	251.8	262.5	280.5	272.2	240.3	270.2
80–84	80.5	133.9	181.5	236.8	241.1	268.9	273.3	289.1	267.5	272.9	272.0	290.7
85–	58.5	114.0	205.1	244.3	257.4	266.3	266.1	267.2	296.6	310.2	308.9	321.3

TABLE VI-6-2. Trends of Age-specific Incidence Rates per 100,000 Population in Japan according to Sex, Primary Site, and Year
—Colon, Female—

Age	Year of diagnosis											
	1975	1980	1985	1990	1991	1992	1993	1994	1995	1996	1997	1998
All age	8.0	11.9	19.2	27.2	29.9	32.8	33.9	34.5	34.8	37.1	37.4	38.3
0–4	0.2	0.0	0.0	0.0	0.0	0.0	0.0	0.0	0.0	0.0	0.0	0.0
5–9	0.4	0.0	0.0	0.0	0.0	0.0	0.0	0.0	0.0	0.0	0.0	0.0
10–14	0.3	0.0	0.0	0.0	0.1	0.1	0.1	0.1	0.0	0.0	0.0	0.0
15–19	0.5	0.2	0.0	0.2	0.2	0.2	0.2	0.3	0.3	0.5	0.3	0.2
20–24	0.4	0.6	0.3	0.8	0.6	0.9	0.3	0.6	0.5	0.6	0.3	0.2
25–29	0.8	0.4	0.5	0.7	1.2	1.4	1.5	1.0	0.9	0.5	0.6	0.5
30–34	1.5	1.7	1.8	1.9	1.9	2.2	2.3	2.0	2.4	2.7	3.2	2.6
35–39	3.1	2.7	4.2	5.4	6.6	7.5	6.4	5.1	4.4	5.2	4.7	4.5
40–44	4.2	5.4	7.8	10.8	12.0	11.7	10.6	10.5	9.6	11.2	10.0	9.1
45–49	10.2	8.2	12.3	18.2	19.8	19.9	20.0	19.4	20.1	20.1	21.2	19.4
50–54	11.9	18.0	24.2	28.9	32.4	34.2	32.7	33.3	34.3	33.5	30.9	28.9
55–59	19.1	22.8	29.1	41.3	43.0	48.6	52.1	53.0	47.8	48.1	49.4	49.4
60–64	23.4	36.7	45.1	59.9	67.4	69.9	71.9	68.6	68.9	71.7	69.0	69.5
65–69	36.0	50.5	58.1	81.4	84.3	92.0	93.9	91.2	89.4	96.6	96.0	98.1
70–74	51.2	64.0	82.7	100.2	113.8	128.0	124.3	123.0	125.7	131.4	126.1	126.7
75–79	60.5	93.5	104.6	134.1	137.4	146.6	153.7	157.7	149.6	155.0	151.1	151.9
80–84	62.1	77.2	134.0	165.9	174.1	180.7	183.1	181.3	177.1	184.3	184.6	186.2
85–	63.3	74.8	138.1	179.4	179.6	186.1	183.8	190.7	194.7	201.2	197.4	204.9

TABLE VI-7-1. Trends of Age-specific Incidence Rates per 100,000 Population in Japan according to Sex, Primary Site, and Year
—Rectum, Male—

Age	Year of diagnosis											
	1975	1980	1985	1990	1991	1992	1993	1994	1995	1996	1997	1998
All age	8.8	11.1	17.4	22.9	23.5	25.6	26.1	26.8	28.4	30.5	30.2	32.5
0–4	0.2	0.0	0.2	0.0	0.0	0.0	0.0	0.0	0.0	0.0	0.0	0.0
5–9	0.2	0.0	0.0	0.0	0.0	0.0	0.0	0.0	0.0	0.0	0.0	0.0
10–14	0.2	0.0	0.0	0.0	0.0	0.0	0.0	0.0	0.0	0.0	0.0	0.0
15–19	0.4	0.1	0.3	0.1	0.0	0.0	0.0	0.0	0.0	0.0	0.0	0.1
20–24	0.3	0.1	0.4	0.2	0.3	0.3	0.3	0.2	0.2	0.3	0.3	0.2
25–29	0.8	0.4	0.4	0.6	0.5	0.7	0.4	0.3	0.4	0.7	0.5	0.7
30–34	2.1	2.2	1.6	1.4	1.3	1.6	2.0	2.0	1.9	1.7	1.7	1.4
35–39	3.2	4.9	2.7	3.1	3.3	3.2	3.8	4.2	4.5	4.1	4.1	4.5
40–44	4.6	7.3	5.3	9.0	9.5	9.4	9.1	9.0	9.6	10.1	9.2	9.6
45–49	9.9	10.9	14.3	17.9	17.4	17.9	17.9	17.0	17.9	21.5	21.6	22.8
50–54	14.0	15.6	25.5	30.4	29.1	30.2	30.0	31.7	33.9	34.6	31.8	33.3
55–59	22.6	27.3	42.2	50.9	51.4	56.5	58.5	58.0	57.6	57.2	56.5	60.2
60–64	31.9	44.2	53.3	72.9	77.7	84.9	84.5	81.0	77.7	82.9	80.5	85.1
65–69	52.1	61.7	74.2	96.8	95.1	101.9	102.7	102.9	106.3	108.8	110.2	115.3
70–74	70.7	74.0	87.0	116.7	109.4	116.0	108.9	112.2	122.9	136.5	129.8	141.9
75–79	89.7	82.8	121.6	122.3	122.4	133.7	128.5	134.6	131.4	133.8	122.8	124.8
80–84	94.2	108.2	143.0	130.6	132.8	134.3	131.4	138.8	158.2	155.1	141.3	144.4
85–	93.4	99.6	138.8	157.5	145.6	139.1	134.2	132.1	146.4	158.7	152.0	150.4

TABLE VI-7-2. Trends of Age-specific Incidence Rates per 100,000 Population in Japan according to Sex, Primary Site, and Year
—Rectum, Female—

Age	Year of diagnosis											
	1975	1980	1985	1990	1991	1992	1993	1994	1995	1996	1997	1998
All age	7.1	8.1	11.7	14.5	15.5	16.0	16.0	15.5	16.2	17.1	17.6	18.1
0–4	0.2	0.0	0.0	0.0	0.0	0.0	0.0	0.0	0.0	0.0	0.0	0.0
5–9	0.2	0.0	0.0	0.0	0.0	0.0	0.0	0.0	0.0	0.0	0.0	0.0
10–14	0.2	0.0	0.0	0.1	0.1	0.0	0.0	0.0	0.0	0.0	0.0	0.0
15–19	0.3	0.0	0.0	0.0	0.0	0.0	0.0	0.1	0.1	0.1	0.1	0.1
20–24	0.4	0.1	0.2	0.1	0.2	0.3	0.3	0.3	0.3	0.2	0.1	0.2
25–29	0.9	0.3	0.4	0.3	0.3	0.1	0.3	0.4	0.6	0.7	0.7	0.6
30–34	1.9	1.4	1.6	1.4	1.2	1.4	1.2	1.1	0.4	1.1	1.1	1.3
35–39	3.4	3.8	2.0	3.5	3.3	3.8	3.5	3.5	3.4	3.5	2.5	2.7
40–44	4.4	4.7	7.9	7.2	6.7	6.5	6.3	6.3	6.9	6.7	7.1	6.5
45–49	5.3	7.9	11.3	12.6	12.5	12.4	10.2	9.7	9.9	13.2	13.6	13.4
50–54	12.4	11.8	14.3	17.9	19.5	19.4	18.7	16.7	20.0	19.2	18.7	17.6
55–59	17.5	17.2	19.1	27.3	28.6	28.3	28.9	28.2	28.7	27.8	26.9	26.5
60–64	20.0	24.0	27.1	33.8	36.1	36.3	37.0	34.5	35.6	35.3	37.8	37.0
65–69	25.5	31.6	35.6	45.1	44.5	43.5	42.8	41.2	42.5	44.4	43.7	43.6
70–74	40.2	35.1	49.0	56.3	59.6	58.0	55.6	52.1	54.0	54.1	53.9	56.3
75–79	57.0	47.5	54.9	53.2	58.0	64.4	65.0	60.6	58.3	62.1	62.0	64.4
80–84	73.9	65.4	73.6	64.3	72.4	74.9	73.4	72.5	68.0	67.5	67.9	70.8
85–	46.9	59.7	71.7	79.6	80.6	81.4	75.6	68.3	72.6	78.0	83.3	84.6

TABLE VI-8-1. Trends of Age-specific Incidence Rates per 100,000 Population in Japan according to Sex, Primary Site, and Year
—Liver, Male—

Age	Year of diagnosis											
	1975	1980	1985	1990	1991	1992	1993	1994	1995	1996	1997	1998
All age	12.6	18.1	30.0	38.7	40.5	42.4	42.4	41.6	40.6	40.2	40.8	41.9
0–4	0.7	0.4	0.2	0.3	0.3	0.3	0.7	1.0	0.9	0.5	0.7	0.8
5–9	0.2	0.1	0.1	0.0	0.1	0.2	0.2	0.1	0.2	0.3	0.4	0.5
10–14	0.3	0.0	0.1	0.2	0.1	0.1	0.1	0.1	0.0	0.0	0.0	0.0
15–19	0.3	0.0	0.2	0.1	0.2	0.3	0.5	0.2	0.3	0.2	0.0	0.0
20–24	0.3	0.1	0.4	0.1	0.2	0.4	0.3	0.3	0.2	0.4	0.3	0.3
25–29	0.5	0.1	0.7	0.3	0.3	0.2	0.1	0.3	0.3	0.6	0.4	0.4
30–34	1.8	1.2	1.0	1.9	1.6	1.4	0.9	0.7	0.5	0.9	0.6	0.7
35–39	2.2	2.6	5.1	4.2	4.1	4.2	4.1	4.1	2.1	2.3	1.8	2.2
40–44	7.8	8.7	8.9	13.0	12.2	11.6	9.2	9.4	7.6	7.4	6.3	5.9
45–49	18.1	27.4	22.6	24.3	23.7	23.9	22.1	21.8	21.2	20.8	20.0	19.8
50–54	26.5	43.8	61.4	49.0	46.4	44.0	41.5	38.3	37.4	35.4	33.7	34.2
55–59	42.7	57.4	98.8	125.8	123.7	115.7	101.7	88.8	76.7	67.7	60.7	63.2
60–64	51.6	76.3	112.6	156.5	164.3	173.9	173.7	160.6	153.6	137.4	136.2	124.6
65–69	62.8	84.0	122.3	157.7	165.3	176.3	182.2	184.7	181.6	180.1	180.6	185.8
70–74	88.3	105.5	145.9	155.8	160.1	162.1	168.3	174.7	179.4	181.4	186.3	187.2
75–79	105.2	109.8	151.6	154.5	171.2	180.0	181.1	171.2	164.3	168.7	168.9	174.2
80–84	97.9	136.2	173.7	178.4	174.2	183.7	181.7	178.8	160.9	171.1	172.0	181.8
85–	91.7	111.4	145.1	163.7	178.3	196.2	199.7	178.9	171.6	161.6	174.2	175.8

TABLE VI-8-2. Trends of Age-specific Incidence Rates per 100,000 Population in Japan according to Sex, Primary Site, and Year
—Liver, Female—

Age	Year of diagnosis											
	1975	1980	1985	1990	1991	1992	1993	1994	1995	1996	1997	1998
All age	6.6	7.3	10.6	14.0	14.1	14.9	15.5	15.2	16.1	15.9	16.5	17.5
0–4	0.7	0.2	0.2	0.3	0.7	0.6	0.7	0.3	0.3	0.1	0.4	0.1
5–9	0.2	0.0	0.0	0.1	0.1	0.1	0.0	0.0	0.2	0.2	0.2	0.1
10–14	0.4	0.0	0.0	0.0	0.0	0.1	0.1	0.1	0.0	0.0	0.0	0.0
15–19	0.3	0.1	0.1	0.1	0.0	0.0	0.0	0.0	0.1	0.1	0.1	0.1
20–24	0.4	0.1	0.0	1.0	0.6	0.4	0.2	0.1	0.1	0.0	0.0	0.1
25–29	0.4	0.3	0.1	0.4	0.5	0.4	0.3	0.4	0.3	0.1	0.0	0.2
30–34	0.9	0.3	0.3	0.7	0.5	0.3	0.2	0.3	0.1	0.2	0.3	0.4
35–39	1.0	0.8	0.9	1.1	0.9	0.9	1.0	0.8	1.1	0.4	0.4	0.4
40–44	2.0	1.6	1.5	2.4	2.4	2.8	2.0	1.8	1.4	1.4	1.7	1.8
45–49	5.3	4.1	4.0	4.6	4.2	4.2	3.7	3.0	3.6	3.0	3.3	3.3
50–54	6.9	6.8	8.2	9.8	9.8	9.3	9.2	7.9	7.3	6.7	6.3	6.4
55–59	14.0	13.9	18.2	20.9	18.6	20.2	17.9	16.8	16.2	14.3	13.2	14.1
60–64	18.2	22.1	26.1	36.9	34.0	34.8	37.4	37.3	36.2	33.5	33.0	32.5
65–69	33.7	33.7	41.1	50.5	51.9	56.4	59.8	58.0	58.8	55.7	55.9	57.8
70–74	47.1	44.7	47.2	65.2	64.8	64.1	65.8	65.4	68.7	70.2	68.6	73.4
75–79	61.6	52.1	65.2	65.6	64.3	69.4	71.1	71.9	74.1	71.9	69.2	74.5
80–84	65.1	75.9	79.8	80.9	85.0	83.9	82.2	73.7	80.6	81.4	90.6	91.8
85–	57.3	65.3	78.6	96.9	94.8	84.2	87.1	80.3	89.1	84.9	91.7	91.9

TABLE VI-9-1. Trends of Age-specific Incidence Rates per 100,000 Population in Japan according to Sex, Primary Site, and Year
—Gallbladder, Male—

Age	Year of diagnosis											
	1975	1980	1985	1990	1991	1992	1993	1994	1995	1996	1997	1998
All age	3.9	5.6	8.9	9.6	10.3	10.7	11.4	11.5	11.5	11.7	12.2	12.4
0–4	0.1	0.0	0.0	0.0	0.0	0.0	0.0	0.0	0.2	0.0	0.0	0.0
5–9	0.2	0.0	0.0	0.0	0.0	0.0	0.0	0.0	0.0	0.0	0.0	0.0
10–14	0.2	0.0	0.0	0.0	0.0	0.0	0.0	0.0	0.0	0.0	0.0	0.0
15–19	0.3	0.0	0.1	0.0	0.0	0.0	0.0	0.0	0.0	0.0	0.0	0.0
20–24	0.2	0.0	0.1	0.0	0.0	0.0	0.0	0.0	0.0	0.0	0.0	0.0
25–29	0.2	0.1	0.0	0.0	0.0	0.0	0.0	0.0	0.1	0.1	0.1	0.1
30–34	0.3	0.1	0.3	0.1	0.1	0.2	0.2	0.4	0.4	0.4	0.2	0.2
35–39	0.6	0.7	0.6	0.8	0.6	0.6	0.5	0.5	1.0	1.2	0.8	0.6
40–44	1.1	0.9	2.5	1.7	2.0	2.5	2.5	2.1	1.9	1.4	1.5	1.6
45–49	2.4	3.1	4.3	3.0	2.8	3.2	3.1	3.2	2.9	4.0	3.4	3.2
50–54	6.4	5.8	6.3	6.3	6.1	6.6	6.2	6.9	6.0	5.0	5.8	5.6
55–59	8.6	12.2	12.0	13.9	14.0	13.9	15.3	14.5	12.5	11.4	12.5	11.7
60–64	16.9	19.8	22.3	21.9	23.4	22.0	22.6	22.9	21.5	21.5	22.3	22.1
65–69	24.7	29.0	45.0	40.6	42.4	42.6	45.4	43.6	38.5	36.2	38.3	36.1
70–74	37.1	51.7	59.5	62.0	64.3	64.5	68.6	66.8	61.6	58.7	58.0	60.0
75–79	37.1	69.2	80.7	84.3	96.2	99.4	95.1	89.6	88.9	92.7	85.1	83.0
80–84	68.6	64.9	98.8	101.1	102.0	100.5	110.0	114.2	126.3	120.8	129.1	124.5
85–	36.8	48.5	114.9	132.2	134.3	133.1	131.3	131.9	150.6	161.7	162.7	165.5

TABLE VI-9-2. Trends of Age-specific Incidence Rates per 100,000 Population in Japan according to Sex, Primary Site, and Year
—Gallbladder, Female—

Age	Year of diagnosis											
	1975	1980	1985	1990	1991	1992	1993	1994	1995	1996	1997	1998
All age	5.2	7.6	12.0	12.7	13.3	13.5	13.5	13.4	13.1	13.5	13.5	14.2
0–4	0.2	0.0	0.0	0.0	0.0	0.0	0.0	0.0	0.0	0.0	0.0	0.0
5–9	0.5	0.1	0.0	0.0	0.0	0.0	0.0	0.0	0.0	0.0	0.0	0.0
10–14	0.2	0.0	0.0	0.0	0.0	0.0	0.0	0.0	0.0	0.0	0.0	0.0
15–19	0.3	0.0	0.0	0.0	0.0	0.0	0.0	0.0	0.0	0.0	0.0	0.0
20–24	0.2	0.1	0.3	0.1	0.1	0.1	0.0	0.0	0.0	0.0	0.0	0.0
25–29	0.2	0.5	0.1	0.1	0.2	0.2	0.2	0.2	0.5	0.4	0.2	0.0
30–34	0.5	0.1	0.6	0.3	0.2	0.2	0.3	0.2	0.2	0.1	0.1	0.1
35–39	0.7	0.5	0.6	0.9	0.8	0.8	0.7	0.7	1.0	0.5	0.5	0.6
40–44	1.7	1.6	2.8	1.8	1.5	1.9	1.7	1.5	1.3	1.4	0.9	1.0
45–49	4.2	4.1	3.9	3.3	4.0	3.6	3.9	3.4	3.2	2.7	3.1	2.8
50–54	6.8	5.7	7.7	6.6	6.1	6.1	5.5	6.3	5.6	5.3	4.4	4.4
55–59	9.7	16.2	15.3	12.5	12.0	12.2	11.5	10.6	10.0	9.7	8.9	9.3
60–64	14.8	23.8	24.7	21.5	19.6	18.4	17.4	17.4	16.5	18.3	17.7	18.8
65–69	27.9	29.3	37.9	38.8	40.5	38.0	37.0	33.6	31.5	31.7	28.9	28.0
70–74	43.1	54.6	57.6	55.5	54.8	57.4	54.6	54.3	46.8	43.3	42.4	43.9
75–79	50.3	64.1	92.0	84.2	85.6	82.9	77.8	73.9	71.2	68.9	70.1	71.6
80–84	50.4	57.4	103.4	105.6	115.1	111.9	111.8	105.9	100.4	104.3	102.9	106.4
85–	32.2	48.3	94.5	131.6	136.8	131.7	134.1	136.2	135.8	137.8	135.5	135.8

TABLE VI-10-1. Trends of Age-specific Incidence Rates per 100,000 Population in Japan according to Sex, Primary Site, and Year
—Pancreas, Male—

Age	Year of diagnosis											
	1975	1980	1985	1990	1991	1992	1993	1994	1995	1996	1997	1998
All age	6.0	8.3	11.8	13.3	13.5	13.9	14.9	14.7	15.3	15.0	15.6	16.2
0–4	0.2	0.0	0.0	0.0	0.0	0.0	0.0	0.0	0.3	0.1	0.1	0.0
5–9	0.2	0.2	0.0	0.1	0.1	0.0	0.0	0.0	0.1	0.1	0.1	0.0
10–14	0.2	0.0	0.0	0.0	0.0	0.0	0.0	0.0	0.0	0.0	0.1	0.1
15–19	0.3	0.1	0.0	0.0	0.0	0.0	0.1	0.1	0.1	0.0	0.0	0.1
20–24	0.3	0.0	0.0	0.0	0.0	0.1	0.1	0.1	0.0	0.0	0.0	0.0
25–29	0.2	0.2	0.1	0.0	0.1	0.1	0.2	0.3	0.1	0.3	0.1	0.1
30–34	0.7	0.8	0.6	0.3	0.2	0.0	0.0	0.4	0.3	0.4	0.3	0.2
35–39	1.8	2.0	1.6	1.4	1.5	1.2	1.0	0.8	0.8	0.9	0.9	0.7
40–44	2.9	2.1	3.8	3.3	3.8	4.0	4.1	3.26	3.5	2.7	2.7	2.4
45–49	6.0	7.1	6.5	6.8	6.9	7.1	7.9	8.0	6.8	7.5	6.7	6.6
50–54	8.9	11.9	11.0	10.8	10.3	12.1	12.3	13.1	13.6	12.6	12.0	13.2
55–59	17.7	19.6	21.3	22.0	20.9	19.8	21.2	20.5	23.5	20.7	20.8	21.2
60–64	24.5	31.0	37.2	37.6	36.9	39.0	38.7	36.7	32.5	32.5	33.6	32.2
65–69	42.0	50.0	56.0	61.3	58.5	55.0	56.6	52.6	53.1	53.8	53.3	53.3
70–74	45.7	65.6	72.3	77.3	75.6	73.5	75.7	73.8	78.8	70.5	72.1	75.5
75–79	60.4	81.9	101.1	99.7	95.5	98.5	107.4	101.4	104.9	93.7	93.5	95.8
80–84	38.7	65.1	106.3	122.7	126.2	126.1	132.9	126.8	138.4	130.8	134.4	137.0
85–	71.1	41.8	109.9	124.7	126.4	132.3	132.6	126.5	121.6	128.1	133.6	132.8

TABLE VI-10-2. Trends of Age-specific Incidence Rates per 100,000 Population in Japan according to Sex, Primary Site, and Year
— Pancreas, Female —

Age	Year of diagnosis											
	1975	1980	1985	1990	1991	1992	1993	1994	1995	1996	1997	1998
All age	4.5	6.0	8.7	10.3	10.2	10.7	11.0	11.2	11.2	12.1	12.6	12.7
0–4	0.2	0.0	0.0	0.0	0.0	0.0	0.0	0.0	0.0	0.0	0.0	0.0
5–9	0.2	0.0	0.0	0.0	0.0	0.0	0.0	0.0	0.0	0.0	0.0	0.0
10–14	0.2	0.0	0.0	0.0	0.0	0.0	0.0	0.0	0.0	0.0	0.0	0.0
15–19	0.4	0.0	0.0	0.0	0.0	0.0	0.0	0.0	0.1	0.1	0.1	0.0
20–24	0.3	0.0	0.0	0.2	0.2	0.0	0.2	0.2	0.2	0.0	0.1	0.0
25–29	0.3	0.2	0.1	0.1	0.1	0.1	0.1	0.1	0.2	0.1	0.1	0.2
30–34	0.4	0.6	0.1	0.1	0.2	0.2	0.3	0.3	0.2	0.4	0.1	0.2
35–39	1.1	0.8	0.3	1.5	1.1	0.5	0.7	0.6	0.5	0.4	0.5	0.5
40–44	2.4	1.1	1.5	1.5	1.6	1.5	1.5	1.2	1.8	0.9	1.2	1.5
45–49	4.1	2.6	3.1	4.1	3.0	2.8	2.7	3.3	3.4	3.8	3.5	3.0
50–54	6.5	5.4	6.5	6.9	6.3	6.5	6.4	6.1	5.8	5.3	5.4	6.0
55–59	11.5	11.9	10.1	11.0	10.5	11.8	10.1	10.2	8.7	11.7	12.6	12.6
60–64	17.6	17.1	20.6	18.5	19.0	19.4	19.4	17.9	16.6	17.6	18.8	17.3
65–69	23.5	26.9	27.3	30.4	29.1	29.3	28.8	29.0	27.1	26.7	28.4	28.0
70–74	24.4	40.6	43.9	46.1	44.1	44.9	44.2	41.0	41.1	42.1	43.2	39.8
75–79	39.7	44.8	57.8	69.2	69.8	70.1	67.9	65.3	64.1	65.0	63.0	61.8
80–84	24.4	52.1	72.3	80.1	73.9	78.2	77.8	81.5	80.4	87.7	82.4	80.6
85–	34.4	35.5	75.5	87.0	83.0	80.9	96.3	98.9	97.0	102.0	105.1	107.7

TABLE VI-11-1. Trends of Age-specific Incidence Rates per 100,000 Population in Japan according to Sex, Primary Site, and Year
—Larynx, Male—

Age	Year of diagnosis											
	1975	1980	1985	1990	1991	1992	1993	1994	1995	1996	1997	1998
All age	1.9	3.6	4.6	5.1	5.0	5.2	4.8	4.9	4.7	4.8	5.1	5.0
0–4	0.1	0.0	0.0	0.0	0.0	0.0	0.0	0.1	0.2	0.1	0.0	0.0
5–9	0.1	0.0	0.0	0.0	0.0	0.0	0.0	0.0	0.0	0.0	0.0	0.0
10–14	0.2	0.0	0.0	0.0	0.0	0.0	0.0	0.0	0.0	0.0	0.0	0.0
15–19	0.2	0.0	0.0	0.0	0.0	0.0	0.0	0.0	0.0	0.0	0.0	0.0
20–24	0.2	0.0	0.0	0.0	0.0	0.0	0.0	0.0	0.0	0.0	0.0	0.0
25–29	0.1	0.0	0.0	0.0	0.0	0.0	0.0	0.0	0.0	0.0	0.0	0.0
30–34	0.2	0.0	0.1	0.0	0.0	0.1	0.1	0.1	0.1	0.1	0.0	0.1
35–39	0.2	0.5	0.2	0.2	0.3	0.3	0.3	0.2	0.2	0.3	0.1	0.1
40–44	0.6	0.6	0.8	1.1	1.3	1.1	0.7	0.3	0.3	0.4	0.7	0.8
45–49	0.8	2.5	2.9	2.6	2.0	2.1	1.8	2.3	1.8	2.2	2.2	2.1
50–54	3.0	6.7	7.0	4.4	3.8	4.8	4.9	5.0	5.5	5.0	5.0	4.6
55–59	7.3	11.2	10.2	11.3	11.6	11.6	10.5	9.1	9.0	8.9	9.4	9.2
60–64	11.1	16.0	18.5	18.5	18.2	17.1	14.8	14.6	12.7	13.3	13.3	13.3
65–69	12.5	27.3	23.2	28.6	25.3	25.8	21.3	21.6	20.7	20.5	20.0	17.4
70–74	20.2	20.3	28.4	24.7	23.4	22.9	24.8	25.4	27.1	25.0	25.8	24.2
75–79	19.0	36.6	30.9	32.0	31.8	33.4	27.1	27.9	20.6	22.1	21.9	22.3
80–84	33.9	21.6	28.3	28.4	27.2	27.8	28.2	27.1	22.4	20.7	26.7	27.4
85–	29.5	9.3	25.8	23.2	25.4	24.8	24.6	23.6	22.5	22.4	22.5	24.3

TABLE VI-11-2. Trends of Age-specific Incidence Rates per 100,000 Population in Japan according to Sex, Primary Site, and Year
—Larynx, Female—

Age	Year of diagnosis											
	1975	1980	1985	1990	1991	1992	1993	1994	1995	1996	1997	1998
All age	0.1	0.3	0.4	0.3	0.3	0.4	0.2	0.3	0.3	0.5	0.4	0.4
0–4	0.1	0.0	0.0	0.0	0.0	0.0	0.0	0.0	0.0	0.0	0.0	0.0
5–9	0.1	0.0	0.0	0.0	0.0	0.0	0.0	0.0	0.0	0.0	0.0	0.0
10–14	0.1	0.0	0.0	0.0	0.0	0.0	0.0	0.0	0.0	0.0	0.0	0.0
15–19	0.1	0.0	0.0	0.0	0.0	0.0	0.0	0.0	0.0	0.0	0.0	0.0
20–24	0.1	0.0	0.0	0.0	0.0	0.0	0.0	0.0	0.0	0.0	0.0	0.0
25–29	0.1	0.0	0.1	0.0	0.0	0.0	0.0	0.0	0.1	0.0	0.1	0.0
30–34	0.1	0.0	0.1	0.1	0.0	0.0	0.1	0.1	0.1	0.0	0.0	0.0
35–39	0.1	0.1	0.1	0.1	0.1	0.1	0.0	0.0	0.1	0.3	0.1	0.0
40–44	0.1	0.1	0.2	0.0	0.0	0.0	0.0	0.0	0.0	0.0	0.0	0.0
45–49	0.1	0.1	0.2	0.2	0.1	0.0	0.0	0.1	0.1	0.0	0.0	0.2
50–54	0.4	0.9	0.2	0.5	0.3	0.3	0.1	0.2	0.3	0.3	0.2	0.2
55–59	0.3	0.5	0.9	0.6	0.7	0.5	0.2	0.3	0.2	0.8	0.6	0.7
60–64	0.8	0.4	1.0	0.8	0.4	0.5	0.3	0.6	0.8	1.5	0.7	0.6
65–69	1.2	1.5	2.3	0.8	1.5	1.5	0.8	1.0	0.9	0.9	1.0	1.0
70–74	1.3	2.3	1.6	1.4	1.4	1.1	0.7	1.0	1.1	2.2	1.1	1.5
75–79	1.1	2.9	1.8	1.8	1.5	2.6	1.5	2.5	1.7	2.4	1.7	1.4
80–84	3.0	2.8	3.0	2.1	1.8	1.8	0.9	2.0	2.1	4.3	2.7	1.5
85–	2.4	4.5	4.6	2.6	2.0	2.1	1.5	2.4	2.3	1.5	1.8	2.0

TABLE VI-12-1. Trends of Age-specific Incidence Rates per 100,000 Population in Japan according to Sex, Primary Site, and Year
— Lung, Male —

Age	Year of diagnosis											
	1975	1980	1985	1990	1991	1992	1993	1994	1995	1996	1997	1998
All age	22.7	30.7	47.5	54.7	57.2	60.3	61.8	62.9	61.8	66.4	67.9	70.9
0–4	0.1	0.0	0.0	0.0	0.0	0.0	0.0	0.0	0.5	0.0	0.0	0.0
5–9	0.2	0.2	0.0	0.0	0.0	0.0	0.0	0.0	0.0	0.0	0.0	0.0
10–14	0.2	0.0	0.0	0.0	0.0	0.0	0.0	0.1	0.0	0.1	0.0	0.0
15–19	0.5	0.1	0.0	0.0	0.0	0.0	0.0	0.1	0.1	0.3	0.1	0.1
20–24	0.4	0.1	0.2	0.2	0.3	0.3	0.3	0.3	0.5	0.3	0.4	0.1
25–29	0.6	0.4	0.3	0.3	0.7	0.7	0.7	0.5	0.5	0.6	0.3	0.2
30–34	0.8	1.0	1.5	1.8	1.5	1.6	1.2	1.6	1.4	1.4	0.7	0.9
35–39	2.6	3.3	4.7	4.7	4.9	4.7	4.5	4.3	5.2	5.2	4.3	4.1
40–44	6.0	4.5	6.9	9.5	10.4	10.6	10.4	10.7	11.3	10.5	9.9	9.8
45–49	17.6	13.8	13.2	16.6	16.9	17.0	15.8	15.9	16.0	18.9	19.9	20.4
50–54	26.0	35.6	34.8	30.4	30.1	34.1	35.5	35.7	33.9	33.9	34.7	34.8
55–59	46.5	62.2	82.2	74.1	72.0	73.8	70.2	66.4	62.5	64.2	62.9	67.4
60–64	94.3	104.4	141.1	150.2	152.8	156.3	155.7	147.0	131.4	131.5	122.2	120.9
65–69	158.5	193.6	229.3	257.4	267.6	268.1	264.0	257.0	242.3	257.8	246.7	246.1
70–74	239.5	282.4	361.4	363.4	364.5	369.2	370.3	377.7	365.2	383.7	394.1	397.2
75–79	270.3	353.7	455.0	478.4	497.8	516.6	525.7	512.2	489.9	478.1	481.4	491.0
80–84	240.9	391.7	482.1	550.1	555.2	561.0	557.0	559.6	536.7	594.9	601.7	611.5
85–	212.2	243.9	409.0	526.9	497.6	503.0	519.5	552.6	567.0	596.0	586.8	601.0

TABLE VI-12-2. Trends of Age-specific Incidence Rates per 100,000 Population in Japan according to Sex, Primary Site, and Year
— Lung, Female —

Age	Year of diagnosis											
	1975	1980	1985	1990	1991	1992	1993	1994	1995	1996	1997	1998
All age	8.4	11.3	17.6	18.9	20.7	22.2	22.1	23.3	23.0	24.9	25.6	27.4
0–4	0.3	0.0	0.0	0.0	0.0	0.0	0.0	0.0	0.4	0.2	0.0	0.0
5–9	0.2	0.0	0.0	0.0	0.0	0.0	0.0	0.0	0.0	0.0	0.1	0.1
10–14	0.2	0.0	0.0	0.1	0.0	0.0	0.0	0.0	0.0	0.1	0.1	0.1
15–19	0.3	0.0	0.0	0.1	0.0	0.0	0.1	0.1	0.1	0.0	0.2	0.1
20–24	0.4	0.0	0.0	0.1	0.2	0.3	0.2	0.1	0.1	0.1	0.0	0.1
25–29	0.3	0.9	0.4	0.7	0.7	0.7	0.5	0.6	0.3	0.9	0.5	0.6
30–34	0.8	0.8	1.5	1.2	1.2	1.3	0.8	1.0	0.6	0.6	1.2	1.2
35–39	2.5	1.7	2.6	2.1	2.2	2.2	2.0	2.1	2.3	3.0	2.2	2.7
40–44	4.5	4.5	6.4	4.5	4.8	6.0	5.5	5.8	6.8	7.2	6.2	5.1
45–49	6.1	8.8	9.3	9.3	8.3	8.4	8.1	10.3	10.5	11.4	11.9	11.4
50–54	11.0	10.1	13.0	14.0	15.3	17.2	17.6	18.2	15.5	15.6	16.3	18.4
55–59	17.7	18.6	22.8	22.6	23.1	23.5	23.5	24.3	24.3	26.2	29.6	32.9
60–64	27.5	36.9	35.8	34.5	40.0	45.2	42.1	42.1	37.4	39.7	37.9	40.5
65–69	41.0	53.5	60.3	57.8	61.9	63.0	59.9	60.7	55.7	59.9	61.5	64.5
70–74	58.8	78.1	94.1	86.9	90.5	92.9	90.4	91.0	88.9	90.5	88.2	88.3
75–79	79.0	79.1	116.4	115.9	122.2	124.7	123.5	125.1	116.4	119.7	115.5	121.9
80–84	81.7	92.3	135.4	140.6	146.5	143.9	134.6	135.8	130.1	141.6	150.8	156.5
85–	45.5	88.8	114.8	131.3	146.2	156.8	159.9	166.8	175.7	179.7	170.7	177.9

TABLE VI-13-1. Trends of Age-specific Incidence Rates per 100,000 Population in Japan according to Sex, Primary Site, and Year
— Skin, Male —

Age	Year of diagnosis											
	1975	1980	1985	1990	1991	1992	1993	1994	1995	1996	1997	1998
All age	1.5	3.2	3.9	4.4	3.9	5.3	5.0	4.0	4.0	4.2	4.9	5.4
0–4	0.1	0.0	0.0	0.1	0.0	0.0	0.0	0.0	0.0	0.0	0.1	0.1
5–9	0.2	0.0	0.1	0.2	0.2	0.2	0.1	0.1	0.0	0.0	0.1	0.1
10–14	0.2	0.0	0.3	0.1	0.1	0.1	0.1	0.1	0.2	0.2	0.1	0.2
15–19	0.2	0.0	0.3	0.2	0.2	0.3	0.3	0.3	0.4	0.2	0.2	0.0
20–24	0.4	0.1	0.0	0.2	0.2	0.2	0.2	0.2	0.5	0.3	0.2	0.2
25–29	0.5	0.3	0.5	0.4	0.3	0.6	0.6	0.5	0.4	0.3	0.2	0.1
30–34	0.3	0.2	0.5	0.7	0.4	0.2	0.6	0.8	0.8	0.6	0.9	0.9
35–39	0.7	1.1	0.5	1.2	1.0	1.0	0.7	0.6	0.5	0.5	0.7	0.7
40–44	0.9	1.8	1.6	1.7	1.4	2.2	2.1	1.4	0.7	0.9	1.7	1.9
45–49	1.2	2.0	2.3	2.3	1.8	2.3	1.9	1.6	1.6	2.2	2.1	2.7
50–54	1.7	4.4	5.0	3.3	3.4	4.8	4.1	2.8	2.4	2.4	2.6	2.9
55–59	4.5	5.6	6.3	6.4	5.5	7.2	7.1	5.0	5.4	5.3	5.9	6.7
60–64	5.5	12.8	9.7	10.7	8.7	10.6	11.2	8.0	7.7	7.7	8.2	9.4
65–69	9.0	13.2	15.4	14.3	13.7	18.0	16.3	11.4	13.0	12.7	14.6	14.4
70–74	11.8	20.7	23.0	21.9	16.6	23.9	21.7	18.0	18.1	17.9	23.8	23.2
75–79	23.7	39.9	27.2	36.3	30.4	37.8	35.2	28.8	24.7	23.7	24.7	29.9
80–84	22.4	50.0	41.3	48.2	36.1	48.9	43.0	40.5	33.7	38.6	45.7	45.5
85–	31.6	50.9	53.4	59.9	60.7	87.2	78.8	61.5	66.8	67.5	69.4	72.4

TABLE VI-13-2. Trends of Age-specific Incidence Rates per 100,000 Population in Japan according to Sex, Primary Site, and Year
— Skin, Female —

Age	Year of diagnosis											
	1975	1980	1985	1990	1991	1992	1993	1994	1995	1996	1997	1998
All age	1.2	3.8	3.1	4.8	5.8	6.2	6.0	4.7	5.4	5.2	4.4	5.4
0–4	0.3	0.0	0.0	0.0	0.0	0.0	0.0	0.0	0.1	0.1	0.2	0.1
5–9	0.2	0.2	0.1	0.1	0.1	0.2	0.1	0.1	0.0	0.0	0.0	0.0
10–14	0.2	0.0	0.0	0.2	0.1	0.1	0.1	0.1	0.2	0.2	0.0	0.1
15–19	0.3	0.5	0.3	0.2	0.1	0.2	0.5	0.4	0.2	0.1	0.1	0.0
20–24	0.2	0.3	0.1	0.1	0.4	0.4	0.5	0.3	0.2	0.1	0.3	0.4
25–29	0.3	0.7	0.5	0.6	0.5	0.3	0.5	0.7	0.4	0.7	0.5	0.8
30–34	0.3	1.2	0.5	0.6	1.1	1.2	1.1	0.6	0.7	0.6	0.7	0.8
35–39	0.7	1.0	1.0	1.0	1.3	1.6	1.3	0.9	1.1	1.1	1.0	0.9
40–44	0.4	2.7	1.8	2.1	2.0	2.5	1.9	1.9	2.1	1.2	1.3	1.5
45–49	0.6	2.8	1.5	2.3	2.4	2.4	2.0	1.5	2.1	1.9	1.9	2.4
50–54	1.5	3.8	2.5	3.9	5.4	4.0	4.9	3.0	3.2	2.7	2.1	2.8
55–59	2.0	5.4	4.0	4.8	4.9	5.9	5.2	4.7	4.3	4.7	3.5	4.6
60–64	3.7	8.3	5.8	6.2	7.1	7.5	6.7	4.6	5.9	5.3	5.9	6.7
65–69	4.8	11.2	6.9	10.6	13.6	13.4	12.1	8.1	9.2	8.9	7.6	8.4
70–74	8.9	19.0	11.1	17.5	20.9	19.2	20.0	15.5	18.0	15.1	12.2	14.0
75–79	12.1	30.3	15.4	27.1	28.8	31.8	27.4	22.4	24.5	24.0	16.8	22.7
80–84	14.3	37.9	28.2	35.4	46.7	54.0	50.8	39.3	43.1	40.1	29.7	34.4
85–	25.7	71.5	51.3	70.1	75.3	73.2	68.8	53.1	60.3	57.4	49.7	56.0

TABLE VI-14. Trends of Age-specific Incidence Rates per 100,000 Population in Japan according to Sex, Primary Site, and Year
—Breast (including carcinoma *in situ*), Female—

Age	Year of diagnosis											
	1975	1980	1985	1990	1991	1992	1993	1994	1995	1996	1997	1998
All age	19.1	23.7	33.1	39.3	42.6	44.5	47.4	47.6	46.6	46.3	50.3	52.2
0–4	0.2	0.0	0.0	0.0	0.0	0.0	0.0	0.0	0.0	0.0	0.0	0.1
5–9	0.2	0.0	0.2	0.0	0.0	0.0	0.0	0.0	0.0	0.0	0.0	0.0
10–14	0.3	0.1	0.0	0.0	0.0	0.0	0.0	0.0	0.0	0.0	0.1	0.1
15–19	0.3	0.0	0.2	0.0	0.1	0.0	0.1	0.0	0.0	0.0	0.0	0.1
20–24	1.2	1.1	0.8	0.7	0.5	0.5	0.5	0.9	0.9	0.9	0.7	0.5
25–29	5.4	3.5	4.5	6.5	6.4	6.8	6.0	5.2	3.6	4.3	3.9	4.4
30–34	10.7	12.1	17.4	16.6	18.1	16.7	17.2	15.7	14.4	14.5	15.3	16.5
35–39	19.2	28.5	36.0	38.0	39.8	40.2	40.2	37.7	39.9	36.9	42.1	40.8
40–44	36.1	46.9	56.8	70.8	83.2	86.3	86.4	81.8	76.0	73.6	75.4	77.1
45–49	55.3	56.9	75.6	86.4	89.4	93.2	99.3	101.8	105.0	110.6	122.0	123.7
50–54	46.3	59.8	70.4	72.9	78.6	87.7	92.4	94.8	86.0	82.9	88.1	92.2
55–59	37.6	56.3	65.6	69.8	73.7	73.3	82.9	84.7	80.9	81.8	89.2	90.6
60–64	50.1	55.7	69.6	78.0	79.7	81.2	83.9	82.7	80.6	76.4	85.0	92.2
65–69	53.2	43.5	66.5	76.6	80.7	81.4	88.5	88.3	86.6	81.9	88.2	88.0
70–74	41.5	47.5	63.4	68.4	71.1	71.8	76.4	79.7	80.6	80.0	84.7	92.2
75–79	36.1	41.0	53.7	62.2	71.4	75.3	82.4	76.6	76.2	71.0	76.1	77.0
80–84	46.4	35.3	48.8	49.9	54.6	63.4	72.5	73.9	67.9	63.1	66.3	71.5
85–	42.8	50.7	40.7	51.8	56.1	55.4	54.6	54.4	51.4	52.5	61.0	66.2

TABLE VI-15. Trends of Age-specific Incidence Rates per 100,000 Population in Japan according to Sex, Primary Site, and Year
—Uterus (including carcinoma *in situ*), Female—

Age	Year of diagnosis											
	1975	1980	1985	1990	1991	1992	1993	1994	1995	1996	1997	1998
All age	28.1	27.4	29.0	28.4	28.3	29.1	28.8	28.7	27.7	27.4	28.3	27.4
0–4	0.2	0.0	0.0	0.0	0.0	0.0	0.0	0.0	0.2	0.0	0.0	0.0
5–9	0.2	0.0	0.0	0.0	0.0	0.0	0.0	0.0	0.0	0.0	0.0	0.0
10–14	0.3	0.0	0.1	0.0	0.0	0.0	0.0	0.0	0.0	0.0	0.0	0.0
15–19	0.5	0.0	0.1	0.1	0.2	0.1	0.2	0.2	0.2	0.2	0.3	0.3
20–24	1.7	1.3	0.8	1.5	1.8	1.5	2.0	2.1	2.0	2.2	2.2	2.4
25–29	5.0	4.0	5.9	10.0	12.0	13.3	14.2	13.3	13.1	13.4	12.8	12.1
30–34	10.0	14.8	19.9	26.7	27.0	30.5	34.2	36.4	36.6	36.2	37.4	34.3
35–39	29.7	31.3	34.2	37.1	36.4	38.3	38.3	38.6	40.4	40.1	43.1	41.7
40–44	49.3	40.0	44.5	47.8	47.7	50.4	49.4	48.4	43.9	40.5	41.8	39.1
45–49	57.6	49.0	44.2	44.5	44.6	42.5	43.4	44.0	46.0	48.0	47.5	44.5
50–54	64.5	62.8	49.1	40.0	40.3	43.6	44.4	43.5	39.8	38.1	41.2	40.2
55–59	78.0	64.2	61.8	45.8	45.3	45.0	44.4	43.6	43.3	42.1	40.8	39.8
60–64	78.0	74.4	60.5	51.1	48.1	48.9	45.5	43.7	36.5	37.6	37.8	39.4
65–69	80.8	68.9	60.4	51.1	50.9	48.9	46.0	44.4	39.8	38.4	41.0	39.7
70–74	90.1	77.3	65.2	51.4	46.5	45.0	40.6	40.3	38.1	36.3	39.9	38.4
75–79	106.2	76.8	66.8	58.4	55.8	52.2	48.6	48.5	45.6	42.3	39.3	37.2
80–84	65.4	82.8	71.8	57.6	53.5	57.1	53.9	54.7	50.5	43.8	42.0	40.3
85–	35.0	48.0	59.4	67.5	68.6	65.1	54.1	51.4	53.6	58.8	61.0	57.9

TABLE VI-16. Trends of Age-specific Incidence Rates per 100,000 Population in Japan according to Sex, Primary Site, and Year
—Uterus (only invasive), Female—

Age	Year of diagnosis											
	1975	1980	1985	1990	1991	1992	1993	1994	1995	1996	1997	1998
All age	24.2	23.0	22.7	21.5	20.8	21.0	20.5	20.7	20.3	20.2	20.4	20.0
0–4	0.2	0.0	0.0	0.0	0.0	0.0	0.0	0.0	0.2	0.0	0.0	0.0
5–9	0.2	0.0	0.0	0.0	0.0	0.0	0.0	0.0	0.0	0.0	0.0	0.0
10–14	0.3	0.0	0.1	0.0	0.0	0.0	0.0	0.0	0.0	0.0	0.0	0.0
15–19	0.5	0.0	0.1	0.1	0.2	0.1	0.2	0.2	0.2	0.1	0.2	0.2
20–24	1.4	1.0	0.4	0.7	0.7	0.6	0.9	1.0	0.9	1.0	0.8	0.8
25–29	3.8	2.8	3.1	5.4	6.1	6.7	7.1	6.6	6.0	5.8	5.0	4.2
30–34	6.2	8.4	9.8	12.0	11.2	11.2	13.0	13.8	15.9	14.5	15.7	13.6
35–39	18.1	19.9	17.6	20.1	17.4	17.2	16.8	18.3	19.2	19.6	19.4	19.5
40–44	36.2	26.4	26.5	26.9	25.6	26.2	25.6	26.1	26.0	23.8	23.4	21.7
45–49	45.0	40.0	29.6	31.9	30.8	28.5	28.4	27.9	29.8	31.4	29.9	28.5
50–54	57.9	53.6	40.3	32.3	31.6	33.8	34.5	34.4	31.3	31.2	33.2	33.2
55–59	74.5	58.7	54.6	40.0	39.1	39.1	38.3	38.1	36.9	36.2	34.0	33.3
60–64	72.8	69.2	53.6	43.9	40.6	41.9	39.1	38.1	32.5	33.1	33.7	35.0
65–69	79.7	65.0	55.4	46.1	45.8	43.9	40.0	38.8	35.8	35.0	37.4	36.2
70–74	87.1	75.4	62.2	47.4	41.8	40.4	36.2	36.5	35.6	34.2	37.0	34.9
75–79	106.0	75.9	65.3	55.9	52.7	48.6	46.2	46.0	43.8	40.4	36.9	34.7
80–84	65.4	82.6	70.6	56.8	52.6	56.3	52.9	53.2	50.0	43.1	41.5	39.1
85–	35.0	47.7	59.0	65.9	67.4	64.2	53.2	50.3	52.2	58.0	60.1	57.2

TABLE VI-17. Trends of Age-specific Incidence Rates per 100,000 Population in Japan according to Sex, Primary Site, and Year
—Cervix Uteri, Female—

Age	Year of diagnosis											
	1975	1980	1985	1990	1991	1992	1993	1994	1995	1996	1997	1998
All age	14.7	18.7	16.6	13.5	12.5	12.4	12.2	11.1	12.7	11.6	11.5	10.9
0–4	0.2	0.0	0.0	0.0	0.0	0.0	0.0	0.0	0.0	0.0	0.0	0.0
5–9	0.2	0.0	0.0	0.0	0.0	0.0	0.0	0.0	0.0	0.0	0.0	0.0
10–14	0.2	0.0	0.0	0.0	0.0	0.0	0.0	0.0	0.0	0.0	0.0	0.0
15–19	0.3	0.0	0.0	0.0	0.1	0.1	0.1	0.1	0.1	0.0	0.0	0.0
20–24	0.7	0.2	0.4	0.6	0.7	0.4	0.6	0.5	0.6	0.6	0.5	0.5
25–29	1.7	2.4	2.6	4.1	4.8	5.1	5.4	4.8	5.6	5.4	4.4	3.5
30–34	3.9	8.5	8.0	10.0	9.1	9.1	11.1	10.9	14.6	12.3	13.2	11.4
35–39	13.3	18.3	15.3	16.0	13.5	13.4	13.2	12.8	16.8	15.9	16.4	15.7
40–44	26.0	24.2	21.3	20.0	18.6	18.9	18.2	17.3	20.2	18.0	17.6	16.5
45–49	29.8	34.5	22.4	20.7	18.6	17.2	17.3	15.9	19.3	18.7	17.6	16.7
50–54	36.2	41.5	27.7	16.5	15.6	16.6	17.6	15.3	16.2	13.8	14.4	14.5
55–59	44.5	45.9	37.0	19.4	18.3	18.7	18.4	16.2	17.4	16.1	15.0	14.0
60–64	46.7	58.5	39.3	25.4	23.5	22.9	20.2	17.1	16.7	16.2	15.4	15.5
65–69	49.7	52.1	44.4	30.0	28.9	26.3	23.3	19.4	21.0	20.1	19.1	17.0
70–74	48.6	60.7	46.4	30.4	25.5	23.6	22.5	20.7	22.3	18.8	21.1	19.2
75–79	59.8	55.5	44.6	37.2	32.8	30.6	28.0	24.4	26.2	21.5	21.2	19.1
80–84	26.6	56.7	45.8	30.8	26.3	30.4	30.3	29.5	29.9	23.5	20.8	19.8
85–	14.7	22.2	30.2	32.1	29.2	27.5	23.4	19.9	26.1	24.8	28.2	25.3

TABLE VI-18. Trends of Age-specific Incidence Rates per 100,000 Population in Japan according to Sex, Primary Site, and Year
— Corpus Uteri, Female —

Age	Year of diagnosis											
	1975	1980	1985	1990	1991	1992	1993	1994	1995	1996	1997	1998
All age	1.3	2.9	4.4	5.7	6.1	6.9	5.9	7.1	6.8	7.1	7.2	7.4
0–4	0.1	0.0	0.0	0.0	0.0	0.0	0.0	0.0	0.0	0.0	0.0	0.0
5–9	0.1	0.0	0.0	0.0	0.0	0.0	0.0	0.0	0.0	0.0	0.0	0.0
10–14	0.2	0.0	0.1	0.0	0.0	0.0	0.0	0.0	0.0	0.0	0.0	0.0
15–19	0.2	0.0	0.0	0.0	0.0	0.0	0.1	0.1	0.0	0.1	0.1	0.1
20–24	0.2	0.0	0.0	0.0	0.0	0.0	0.1	0.1	0.3	0.5	0.2	0.2
25–29	0.2	0.3	0.2	0.6	0.7	1.0	1.1	1.1	0.5	0.2	0.5	0.7
30–34	0.4	0.3	1.1	1.0	0.9	0.9	0.9	1.2	1.7	2.0	2.1	1.9
35–39	0.4	2.4	1.9	2.9	2.6	2.8	2.5	3.7	2.7	3.3	2.5	3.1
40–44	1.5	2.6	4.4	5.1	5.3	6.4	6.0	6.7	5.9	5.4	5.3	4.6
45–49	1.8	5.4	6.3	9.2	10.3	10.4	8.9	9.8	10.6	11.9	10.8	10.8
50–54	4.8	11.4	11.9	13.8	14.8	17.2	14.0	16.9	15.2	16.1	17.1	16.9
55–59	8.1	10.4	16.8	18.7	19.3	20.3	17.0	20.2	20.1	19.6	17.7	17.3
60–64	4.8	8.0	11.3	14.8	14.3	17.2	15.2	18.0	15.4	15.5	16.7	17.7
65–69	3.4	7.6	7.0	12.1	13.5	15.4	12.9	15.6	13.8	12.8	16.2	17.1
70–74	4.2	5.4	9.6	10.6	10.1	11.7	8.5	10.6	11.2	13.1	13.2	13.3
75–79	4.3	10.3	8.6	7.7	9.8	10.1	9.3	11.7	11.4	11.4	9.6	11.0
80–84	7.4	4.4	6.7	7.8	9.0	9.5	7.6	8.8	8.4	8.3	8.3	8.7
85–	3.5	2.3	6.9	6.2	9.8	10.5	7.8	8.0	9.1	11.3	8.0	8.1

TABLE VI-19. Trends of Age-specific Incidence Rates per 100,000 Population in Japan according to Sex, Primary Site, and Year
— Ovary, Female —

Age	Year of diagnosis											
	1975	1980	1985	1990	1991	1992	1993	1994	1995	1996	1997	1998
All age	3.7	4.3	7.7	8.9	8.9	9.2	9.0	9.8	9.6	9.7	10.4	10.4
0–4	0.7	0.3	0.0	0.2	0.1	0.0	0.0	0.0	0.3	0.1	0.1	0.0
5–9	0.2	0.6	0.3	0.5	0.5	0.4	0.4	0.3	0.4	0.3	0.3	0.1
10–14	1.0	0.8	0.7	0.9	0.7	0.3	0.6	1.0	1.1	0.9	0.8	0.6
15–19	1.2	1.4	1.5	1.6	1.4	2.1	2.2	2.2	2.0	1.4	1.3	0.9
20–24	1.9	1.7	2.8	1.9	2.1	1.8	1.9	2.2	2.3	2.5	2.3	2.5
25–29	1.1	1.9	1.8	3.5	3.3	2.7	2.6	2.6	3.2	2.9	2.8	3.3
30–34	1.4	2.7	4.0	3.0	2.5	2.4	3.1	3.6	4.3	4.7	4.3	4.1
35–39	2.5	3.3	4.9	5.6	5.9	6.1	6.1	5.5	6.7	5.9	6.4	5.0
40–44	5.6	5.9	8.9	10.7	10.7	10.7	10.9	10.9	10.3	8.5	9.8	9.5
45–49	8.6	7.3	12.8	15.7	14.6	15.3	13.8	15.9	14.3	15.5	16.1	15.4
50–54	9.7	10.1	15.3	16.6	16.7	16.6	17.1	18.9	17.8	17.5	17.1	19.4
55–59	9.5	9.6	15.6	16.9	15.8	16.5	15.1	17.4	15.5	16.1	18.5	18.8
60–64	10.6	11.3	16.2	16.4	16.1	17.1	15.3	15.7	15.4	16.6	17.9	18.0
65–69	9.6	11.6	14.3	17.4	17.8	18.8	17.0	18.1	17.3	17.2	18.9	18.8
70–74	9.9	15.9	18.0	18.1	18.2	18.1	17.9	18.1	17.8	17.8	20.7	19.1
75–79	9.7	12.0	19.0	20.6	19.4	18.4	17.8	17.8	18.6	19.5	18.7	18.1
80–84	10.1	9.8	21.1	20.1	22.2	21.9	22.3	25.2	25.0	24.4	27.0	25.2
85–	12.8	8.6	20.2	22.3	19.5	23.2	22.7	26.8	21.8	25.4	24.8	25.5

TABLE VI-20. Trends of Age-specific Incidence Rates per 100,000 Population in Japan according to Sex, Primary Site, and Year
— Prostate, Male —

Age	Year of diagnosis											
	1975	1980	1985	1990	1991	1992	1993	1994	1995	1996	1997	1998
All age	4.0	6.5	10.7	12.9	14.7	16.1	17.5	19.3	18.4	21.2	22.9	25.5
0–4	0.1	0.0	0.0	0.0	0.0	0.0	0.1	0.1	0.0	0.0	0.0	0.0
5–9	0.2	0.0	0.0	0.0	0.0	0.0	0.0	0.0	0.0	0.0	0.0	0.0
10–14	0.2	0.1	0.0	0.0	0.0	0.0	0.0	0.0	0.0	0.0	0.0	0.0
15–19	0.3	0.0	0.1	0.1	0.0	0.0	0.0	0.0	0.0	0.0	0.1	0.1
20–24	0.2	0.1	0.0	0.0	0.0	0.0	0.0	0.0	0.0	0.0	0.0	0.0
25–29	0.1	0.0	0.0	0.0	0.1	0.1	0.1	0.0	0.1	0.1	0.0	0.0
30–34	0.2	0.0	0.0	0.2	0.3	0.3	0.0	0.1	0.0	0.0	0.0	0.1
35–39	0.2	0.0	0.0	0.1	0.1	0.0	0.0	0.2	0.1	0.1	0.1	0.0
40–44	0.2	0.6	0.3	0.1	0.2	0.1	0.1	0.1	0.1	0.1	0.1	0.1
45–49	0.7	0.1	0.2	0.3	0.5	0.5	0.7	0.7	0.9	0.7	0.9	0.7
50–54	1.2	1.8	2.8	2.0	2.1	1.9	1.7	2.1	2.1	2.4	2.6	3.0
55–59	3.5	4.9	6.1	6.4	7.8	8.2	8.6	8.3	8.6	10.0	11.5	12.4
60–64	12.7	8.2	15.4	24.5	26.7	24.8	24.2	23.8	24.6	28.9	34.8	35.1
65–69	22.0	34.4	34.4	40.8	47.6	54.1	61.2	68.3	60.5	74.3	77.1	85.5
70–74	48.1	70.2	96.1	89.8	98.6	101.8	105.9	113.4	109.4	124.0	136.1	151.5
75–79	75.8	122.4	147.8	154.2	170.3	188.8	202.8	216.0	190.1	181.3	178.0	193.8
80–84	120.0	159.4	197.5	232.6	247.4	265.4	270.7	285.3	253.3	282.0	282.6	294.2
85–	138.1	194.3	238.8	264.6	277.1	298.1	308.2	332.5	313.0	358.1	346.5	359.1

TABLE VI-21-1. Trends of Age-specific Incidence Rates per 100,000 Population in Japan according to Sex, Primary Site, and Year
—Bladder, Male—

Age	Year of diagnosis											
	1975	1980	1985	1990	1991	1992	1993	1994	1995	1996	1997	1998
All age	4.4	8.1	9.8	12.0	12.3	12.5	12.5	13.1	13.8	14.7	15.1	15.8
0–4	0.1	0.0	0.0	0.0	0.0	0.0	0.0	0.0	0.0	0.0	0.1	0.1
5–9	0.1	0.3	0.0	0.0	0.1	0.1	0.1	0.0	0.0	0.0	0.0	0.0
10–14	0.2	0.0	0.0	0.0	0.0	0.0	0.0	0.0	0.0	0.0	0.0	0.0
15–19	0.2	0.3	0.1	0.0	0.0	0.0	0.0	0.0	0.0	0.1	0.1	0.1
20–24	0.2	0.6	0.0	0.1	0.1	0.0	0.0	0.1	0.1	0.3	0.2	0.1
25–29	0.5	0.5	0.3	0.6	0.6	0.4	0.3	0.4	0.7	0.5	0.4	0.3
30–34	0.4	1.1	1.0	1.2	1.2	1.3	1.1	1.0	0.9	0.9	0.9	0.8
35–39	0.3	2.6	2.0	2.1	1.3	1.3	1.3	1.4	1.4	1.2	1.5	1.7
40–44	1.8	2.3	1.9	3.5	3.8	3.6	3.4	2.6	3.0	2.9	2.9	2.8
45–49	3.2	3.7	4.8	5.1	5.1	4.7	5.4	4.5	5.6	5.7	5.8	5.2
50–54	6.4	10.6	7.2	8.8	8.1	8.9	8.7	9.4	9.6	10.3	10.4	10.3
55–59	10.7	16.2	17.9	18.0	17.3	16.1	15.8	15.7	16.5	15.2	14.5	14.8
60–64	23.2	31.8	31.3	31.8	32.4	30.5	29.7	28.5	29.1	31.0	27.6	28.7
65–69	21.8	41.8	42.2	46.5	49.2	48.2	48.7	49.7	47.3	49.4	51.4	53.9
70–74	43.4	70.4	64.5	73.7	70.3	69.6	64.7	67.3	74.1	81.0	78.6	80.6
75–79	47.5	81.7	88.5	95.5	99.0	100.2	95.1	98.3	95.1	90.9	97.0	94.7
80–84	89.0	118.1	108.5	113.3	111.2	118.6	115.2	126.8	120.6	131.0	130.8	132.2
85–	88.3	131.3	123.7	155.3	137.0	144.7	136.0	141.8	153.8	160.6	157.1	158.7

TABLE VI-21-2. Trends of Age-specific Incidence Rates per 100,000 Population in Japan according to Sex, Primary Site, and Year
—Bladder, Female—

Age	Year of diagnosis											
	1975	1980	1985	1990	1991	1992	1993	1994	1995	1996	1997	1998
All age	1.5	2.6	3.5	3.7	4.3	4.2	4.1	4.1	4.4	4.4	4.8	5.0
0–4	0.1	0.0	0.1	0.0	0.0	0.1	0.1	0.2	0.1	0.1	0.0	0.0
5–9	0.2	0.0	0.0	0.0	0.0	0.0	0.0	0.0	0.1	0.1	0.1	0.0
10–14	0.2	0.0	0.0	0.0	0.0	0.0	0.0	0.0	0.0	0.0	0.0	0.0
15–19	0.2	0.0	0.1	0.0	0.0	0.0	0.0	0.0	0.0	0.0	0.0	0.0
20–24	0.2	0.0	0.3	0.2	0.1	0.1	0.0	0.1	0.1	0.2	0.1	0.2
25–29	0.1	0.1	0.0	0.0	0.0	0.1	0.2	0.1	0.1	0.1	0.1	0.1
30–34	0.1	0.3	0.5	0.4	0.3	0.2	0.1	0.1	0.4	0.3	0.3	0.2
35–39	0.3	0.7	0.3	0.3	0.4	0.2	0.4	0.3	0.3	0.2	0.7	0.7
40–44	0.4	0.5	0.4	0.7	0.9	0.8	0.6	0.4	0.4	0.8	0.7	0.7
45–49	0.6	0.6	0.8	1.3	1.3	1.1	0.9	1.1	1.1	1.0	0.6	1.0
50–54	1.9	2.4	2.8	1.8	1.6	1.6	1.7	1.6	2.4	2.2	2.4	2.4
55–59	3.1	1.8	2.6	4.3	4.8	4.3	4.1	3.7	3.4	3.4	4.5	4.3
60–64	4.2	6.5	6.9	6.9	7.8	7.4	6.2	5.1	5.4	5.7	5.7	5.6
65–69	8.3	12.8	10.0	9.9	10.3	10.1	10.3	10.1	9.6	9.1	9.8	10.2
70–74	12.3	22.7	16.7	18.4	20.3	18.9	16.0	14.2	15.1	14.2	14.2	15.4
75–79	18.4	24.6	28.5	21.9	26.0	25.8	24.1	22.9	22.9	22.1	24.5	24.3
80–84	16.6	23.1	34.7	30.7	31.5	29.0	35.4	37.4	36.7	33.7	35.7	34.1
85–	24.3	26.1	41.9	36.8	42.6	41.5	39.9	37.7	45.7	43.3	47.0	45.9

TABLE VI-22-1. Trends of Age-specific Incidence Rates per 100,000 Population in Japan according to Sex, Primary Site, and Year
—Kidney, Male—

Age	Year of diagnosis											
	1975	1980	1985	1990	1991	1992	1993	1994	1995	1996	1997	1998
All age	2.1	3.1	5.8	7.7	8.0	8.3	9.0	9.6	9.9	10.4	10.3	10.5
0–4	1.6	1.4	1.7	0.7	0.6	0.5	0.6	0.7	0.9	1.0	0.8	0.7
5–9	0.4	0.2	0.1	0.1	0.1	0.1	0.2	0.2	0.2	0.1	0.2	0.2
10–14	0.3	0.0	0.0	0.0	0.0	0.0	0.0	0.0	0.2	0.2	0.2	0.2
15–19	0.3	0.0	0.0	0.0	0.0	0.1	0.1	0.1	0.1	0.1	0.0	0.0
20–24	0.4	0.0	0.0	0.0	0.2	0.4	0.4	0.2	0.1	0.0	0.2	0.2
25–29	0.3	0.2	0.3	0.3	0.1	0.3	0.2	0.3	0.0	0.2	0.4	0.3
30–34	0.4	0.3	0.5	0.6	0.8	0.9	1.0	1.0	1.1	1.2	1.1	1.1
35–39	0.5	1.1	1.5	1.6	2.0	2.1	1.9	1.9	1.8	1.8	1.7	2.0
40–44	0.8	1.7	1.1	2.5	3.6	4.2	5.0	4.5	4.7	5.0	4.3	4.5
45–49	2.3	2.1	3.6	5.8	5.8	4.8	4.9	5.6	7.0	8.0	8.2	7.6
50–54	3.8	3.5	8.2	9.5	9.9	9.7	9.9	10.8	12.2	11.4	10.1	11.2
55–59	9.9	8.2	11.0	15.3	15.3	16.4	18.0	16.4	16.2	14.2	14.1	13.4
60–64	9.2	13.3	18.8	24.4	23.6	24.1	23.8	25.2	19.6	23.7	22.7	24.6
65–69	13.8	18.9	28.0	35.0	33.5	33.5	34.2	36.2	35.0	37.0	35.0	33.4
70–74	13.1	23.6	34.3	40.9	38.2	39.6	43.1	47.7	48.4	45.8	47.4	46.3
75–79	16.2	23.9	41.5	45.5	47.1	41.5	48.2	50.0	56.7	51.5	45.8	49.0
80–84	18.0	20.0	45.8	46.6	53.1	49.2	48.4	52.9	57.4	66.3	62.6	61.5
85–	11.8	10.9	43.3	39.4	39.0	47.6	50.4	55.1	62.1	67.6	61.3	59.0

TABLE VI-22-2. Trends of Age-specific Incidence Rates per 100,000 Population in Japan according to Sex, Primary Site, and Year
—Kidney, Female—

Age	Year of diagnosis											
	1975	1980	1985	1990	1991	1992	1993	1994	1995	1996	1997	1998
All age	0.7	1.6	2.2	3.5	3.6	4.2	4.3	4.2	4.2	4.7	4.6	5.0
0–4	0.4	1.2	0.5	0.9	0.6	0.6	0.5	0.5	0.5	0.7	0.5	0.5
5–9	0.1	0.2	0.1	0.2	0.2	0.0	0.0	0.0	0.0	0.1	0.1	0.1
10–14	0.2	0.0	0.0	0.1	0.1	0.3	0.3	0.2	0.0	0.0	0.0	0.1
15–19	0.2	0.0	0.0	0.1	0.1	0.1	0.1	0.0	0.0	0.0	0.1	0.1
20–24	0.3	0.1	0.5	0.1	0.1	0.1	0.1	0.2	0.1	0.2	0.1	0.2
25–29	0.2	0.0	0.3	0.3	0.2	0.1	0.1	0.0	0.0	0.3	0.4	0.4
30–34	0.2	0.3	0.3	0.3	0.3	0.3	0.2	0.3	0.2	0.4	0.2	0.3
35–39	0.2	0.2	0.3	0.6	0.4	0.4	0.4	1.0	0.7	0.9	0.6	0.8
40–44	0.2	0.5	0.7	1.0	1.2	1.8	1.8	1.7	1.3	1.7	1.7	1.7
45–49	0.8	1.1	1.4	1.6	1.1	1.2	1.7	2.3	2.8	3.5	3.0	2.9
50–54	1.3	1.2	1.7	2.7	3.0	3.5	3.8	3.5	3.5	3.3	2.9	3.6
55–59	1.9	3.4	4.3	6.0	7.2	7.8	7.8	6.2	6.2	5.2	4.7	5.0
60–64	3.8	5.6	6.3	8.4	8.0	8.6	8.7	8.4	7.6	8.0	8.3	7.9
65–69	3.5	6.1	7.3	9.0	10.0	11.7	11.9	10.7	11.0	11.6	11.8	12.1
70–74	4.6	13.4	9.0	14.3	14.6	15.6	15.5	15.1	15.3	15.4	16.1	17.1
75–79	5.5	9.0	12.6	15.6	16.9	20.7	19.7	20.0	20.6	26.0	21.4	21.2
80–84	7.4	6.1	11.4	25.6	23.4	23.4	23.4	19.9	23.0	23.6	24.4	24.6
85–	9.9	3.3	11.4	19.3	19.5	22.1	21.1	22.2	17.8	18.7	19.4	24.5

TABLE VI-23-1. Trends of Age-specific Incidence Rates per 100,000 Population in Japan according to Sex, Primary Site, and Year
—CNS, Male—

Age	Year of diagnosis											
	1975	1980	1985	1990	1991	1992	1993	1994	1995	1996	1997	1998
All age	1.3	2.9	3.7	4.2	3.8	3.8	3.4	3.3	2.6	3.2	2.9	3.3
0–4	1.3	3.0	2.5	2.8	2.3	1.7	1.8	1.3	1.1	1.2	1.8	1.9
5–9	1.3	1.5	2.9	2.1	2.5	2.8	1.8	1.6	1.6	1.5	1.4	1.3
10–14	1.3	1.7	2.5	2.0	1.6	1.2	1.2	1.5	1.6	1.6	1.1	1.3
15–19	1.2	1.5	2.2	1.9	1.5	1.3	1.1	1.2	1.4	1.3	1.3	1.2
20–24	0.9	0.5	0.8	1.1	1.1	1.7	1.3	1.1	0.8	0.8	0.8	0.7
25–29	0.8	0.8	1.3	1.6	1.4	1.6	1.2	0.8	1.3	1.5	1.2	1.5
30–34	1.3	2.8	1.8	2.3	2.0	1.8	1.3	1.3	1.0	1.2	1.1	1.2
35–39	1.6	2.7	3.0	2.9	2.8	2.5	2.2	2.1	1.2	2.0	1.7	2.1
40–44	1.3	2.5	2.9	2.3	2.5	2.7	2.3	2.0	1.6	2.6	2.2	2.8
45–49	1.3	4.9	3.5	3.6	3.3	3.0	3.1	2.9	2.4	2.6	2.6	2.9
50–54	2.4	2.8	3.7	5.3	4.3	3.2	3.1	3.3	2.6	2.3	2.2	2.6
55–59	2.8	3.3	7.4	6.3	5.0	5.6	5.2	4.5	3.2	4.5	4.1	4.6
60–64	1.9	7.4	8.7	8.5	7.5	7.7	6.8	6.9	4.3	5.6	4.8	5.4
65–69	4.9	8.6	7.7	10.6	9.7	11.0	10.0	8.6	6.6	7.1	6.2	7.1
70–74	2.7	7.1	9.1	14.6	13.3	13.7	9.8	8.4	6.9	7.9	6.8	7.9
75–79	3.9	10.6	10.3	16.0	13.8	13.7	12.0	13.3	11.3	14.6	11.1	11.5
80–84	5.3	3.8	12.4	20.3	17.4	14.8	15.2	17.8	10.1	17.7	15.6	16.3
85–	9.7	5.0	9.8	19.9	18.4	14.9	13.7	14.4	13.5	15.6	17.3	13.9

TABLE VI-23-2. Trends of Age-specific Incidence Rates per 100,000 Population in Japan according to Sex, Primary Site, and Year
—CNS, Female—

Age	Year of diagnosis											
	1975	1980	1985	1990	1991	1992	1993	1994	1995	1996	1997	1998
All age	0.9	2.4	3.0	3.5	3.1	3.2	2.7	3.3	2.3	2.5	2.9	2.9
0–4	1.5	2.6	2.9	2.5	2.2	1.5	1.3	1.8	1.4	1.4	1.7	1.6
5–9	0.8	1.3	1.1	2.0	1.7	2.5	2.2	2.2	1.3	0.9	1.8	1.7
10–14	0.7	1.4	1.5	1.9	1.6	1.5	1.3	1.5	2.0	1.2	1.1	1.0
15–19	0.6	0.7	1.0	1.0	1.1	0.9	0.8	0.6	0.5	0.5	0.6	0.8
20–24	0.4	1.4	1.6	1.3	1.0	0.8	0.4	0.6	0.9	1.1	1.5	1.2
25–29	0.6	1.0	0.7	1.3	0.7	0.7	0.7	1.5	0.8	0.7	1.0	1.2
30–34	1.0	1.5	1.9	1.3	1.2	1.2	0.9	1.1	0.6	0.8	0.9	0.9
35–39	0.5	1.9	2.7	1.8	1.9	1.8	1.4	1.2	0.9	1.1	1.2	1.4
40–44	1.6	2.4	1.6	2.3	2.1	2.3	1.4	1.8	1.4	1.3	1.5	1.2
45–49	0.9	2.7	2.1	3.1	3.0	2.9	2.3	3.1	2.2	2.1	2.9	2.4
50–54	2.1	3.5	3.1	4.1	3.8	3.5	2.8	2.9	2.2	2.3	2.5	2.8
55–59	1.7	3.6	4.3	4.3	3.6	3.7	3.3	4.2	2.2	2.9	3.3	3.6
60–64	1.5	6.3	6.7	5.6	5.2	5.5	4.6	5.4	4.4	4.7	4.3	4.1
65–69	2.3	7.6	7.1	8.5	7.0	5.9	5.6	6.9	4.8	5.6	5.7	5.5
70–74	1.1	5.2	8.1	10.6	9.4	9.2	8.6	9.2	6.0	5.8	7.4	6.6
75–79	1.8	3.5	8.8	8.3	8.1	8.7	8.4	10.5	6.0	7.0	7.1	7.3
80–84	1.9	1.0	8.3	11.7	10.6	13.4	9.2	10.3	5.4	8.0	9.8	8.9
85–	3.3	0.7	3.7	10.7	8.4	9.1	7.8	13.0	7.2	8.6	11.0	10.4

TABLE VI-24-1. Trends of Age-specific Incidence Rates per 100,000 Population in Japan according to Sex, Primary Site, and Year
—Thyroid, Male—

Age	Year of diagnosis											
	1975	1980	1985	1990	1991	1992	1993	1994	1995	1996	1997	1998
All age	0.3	1.4	1.9	2.1	1.9	1.9	1.7	2.2	2.0	2.3	2.2	2.3
0–4	0.1	0.0	0.0	0.0	0.0	0.0	0.0	0.0	0.2	0.0	0.0	0.0
5–9	0.1	0.0	0.1	0.1	0.0	0.1	0.1	0.1	0.0	0.0	0.0	0.0
10–14	0.1	0.1	0.1	0.0	0.0	0.1	0.2	0.2	0.2	0.0	0.1	0.2
15–19	0.2	0.0	0.0	0.2	0.3	0.2	0.3	0.3	0.3	0.2	0.2	0.3
20–24	0.2	0.0	0.4	0.5	0.5	0.5	0.5	0.5	0.7	0.8	0.6	0.5
25–29	0.2	0.6	1.0	0.7	0.7	0.6	0.7	1.1	0.8	0.8	0.8	1.0
30–34	0.2	1.3	1.4	1.2	0.9	0.8	0.7	0.7	0.5	1.2	0.9	1.1
35–39	0.3	1.5	1.1	1.6	1.1	1.2	1.3	2.0	1.6	1.8	1.3	1.4
40–44	0.6	2.1	1.6	2.6	1.7	1.6	1.4	1.8	1.6	2.2	2.2	2.2
45–49	0.8	2.6	2.9	3.0	2.1	2.3	1.9	3.1	2.3	3.1	2.5	2.0
50–54	0.6	1.8	3.3	2.9	2.5	2.5	2.6	3.0	3.3	2.7	2.7	2.3
55–59	1.0	2.7	3.3	3.6	3.0	3.8	3.4	4.4	2.8	3.9	3.0	3.6
60–64	1.1	3.3	5.3	6.0	5.0	4.8	4.4	5.4	3.9	4.2	4.6	4.5
65–69	2.2	4.6	4.1	5.8	6.2	5.7	4.4	4.4	4.4	5.4	6.4	6.4
70–74	3.5	5.6	7.6	6.9	6.2	4.7	3.9	5.7	5.9	7.7	6.2	7.8
75–79	3.9	6.0	11.0	6.9	6.8	5.9	6.1	6.5	7.1	6.0	7.1	6.8
80–84	4.6	10.7	6.7	5.3	7.2	7.8	6.8	6.2	6.2	6.6	5.4	6.4
85–	5.5	4.3	7.0	6.8	8.0	5.5	8.1	10.0	10.8	10.3	7.3	7.2

TABLE VI-24-2. Trends of Age-specific Incidence Rates per 100,000 Population in Japan according to Sex, Primary Site, and Year
—Thyroid, Female—

Age	Year of diagnosis											
	1975	1980	1985	1990	1991	1992	1993	1994	1995	1996	1997	1998
All age	2.2	3.6	6.4	10.2	9.6	11.0	8.8	10.1	8.2	8.5	8.7	8.6
0–4	0.1	0.2	0.0	0.0	0.0	0.0	0.0	0.0	0.0	0.0	0.0	0.0
5–9	0.1	0.0	0.0	0.1	0.1	0.0	0.0	0.0	0.1	0.0	0.1	0.0
10–14	0.3	0.2	0.1	0.2	0.2	0.3	0.3	0.3	0.1	0.2	0.3	0.4
15–19	0.2	0.9	0.9	1.2	1.2	1.8	0.8	0.9	0.6	0.6	0.7	0.8
20–24	0.9	1.8	1.5	2.6	2.7	3.3	2.3	2.9	2.4	3.0	2.4	2.1
25–29	2.0	1.3	3.5	3.9	3.8	3.7	3.1	3.4	3.5	3.7	3.2	3.0
30–34	1.6	3.2	3.6	6.8	5.9	6.5	5.0	5.7	5.8	5.1	4.3	4.6
35–39	1.5	2.7	6.2	10.5	8.6	9.6	8.0	9.0	7.4	7.4	7.9	7.7
40–44	2.4	4.6	9.3	15.5	14.7	16.0	11.1	13.1	9.8	10.7	10.4	9.8
45–49	3.1	5.9	7.9	16.8	15.1	17.6	13.7	17.2	13.1	13.5	14.6	14.5
50–54	4.0	6.2	12.4	18.4	17.5	20.0	17.7	20.2	14.0	13.6	14.3	14.7
55–59	5.1	5.9	12.4	19.0	18.4	21.1	17.3	17.9	13.9	14.5	15.2	14.1
60–64	5.8	8.0	11.5	20.5	19.8	22.4	17.0	17.6	14.0	13.7	15.5	15.8
65–69	7.7	9.4	14.0	17.7	17.1	19.3	16.4	18.4	15.2	16.9	15.8	16.1
70–74	8.4	13.1	17.6	18.3	17.0	19.6	14.0	16.9	14.7	16.4	15.4	15.6
75–79	12.5	8.6	14.6	16.7	15.1	16.4	14.0	15.3	13.8	14.7	14.5	12.7
80–84	12.9	11.0	12.5	14.4	13.6	17.2	15.7	15.5	12.7	13.0	14.6	13.6
85–	12.8	13.5	15.4	14.9	12.5	12.2	12.5	13.8	15.1	13.1	13.0	13.0

TABLE VI-25-1. Trends of Age-specific Incidence Rates per 100,000 Population in Japan according to Sex, Primary Site, and Year
— Lymphoma, Male —

Age	Year of diagnosis											
	1975	1980	1985	1990	1991	1992	1993	1994	1995	1996	1997	1998
All age	4.2	5.1	7.2	8.9	8.8	9.4	9.1	9.9	10.2	9.8	10.0	10.5
0–4	0.6	0.9	1.1	0.9	1.2	1.1	1.0	0.8	1.3	1.2	1.4	1.3
5–9	0.8	0.6	1.3	1.2	1.1	1.2	0.9	1.3	1.5	1.4	1.2	0.9
10–14	1.2	1.2	1.5	1.1	1.2	1.5	1.1	1.3	1.1	1.4	1.0	1.0
15–19	1.4	1.2	1.2	0.6	1.2	1.6	1.8	1.4	1.3	1.0	1.6	2.1
20–24	1.3	0.6	1.5	1.3	1.5	1.7	2.1	2.1	2.6	1.4	1.6	1.6
25–29	1.9	1.0	1.1	1.7	1.2	2.0	2.1	2.3	1.0	1.5	1.3	1.5
30–34	2.2	1.6	2.2	2.8	2.7	2.7	2.1	1.9	1.7	1.3	1.5	2.2
35–39	2.8	1.8	2.7	2.9	3.2	3.6	3.9	4.1	3.1	2.8	3.0	3.4
40–44	3.7	3.6	3.4	4.8	4.4	4.8	4.2	4.6	3.8	4.3	4.3	5.0
45–49	5.1	5.9	5.8	5.6	5.3	6.3	6.5	7.5	8.0	7.7	6.9	6.5
50–54	7.4	11.2	9.2	9.5	9.4	10.0	9.4	10.4	9.6	8.3	8.2	8.3
55–59	12.2	11.0	14.5	14.1	12.7	14.6	15.0	16.1	15.6	12.9	12.6	13.0
60–64	16.6	14.3	18.8	24.3	24.3	24.6	22.2	23.1	23.8	22.0	21.8	20.4
65–69	21.2	21.8	24.2	32.4	33.6	30.8	27.8	29.4	29.7	30.3	30.6	33.3
70–74	20.8	25.1	37.4	37.5	34.4	37.6	36.3	40.8	40.8	38.5	41.7	44.8
75–79	19.5	28.8	42.7	54.6	52.1	51.3	48.1	47.1	52.4	47.3	46.1	46.0
80–84	28.5	27.6	46.6	66.3	59.6	60.2	56.8	59.9	66.4	64.2	62.1	59.1
85–	22.8	39.9	45.6	65.4	54.2	60.5	55.0	61.4	68.0	74.4	65.8	70.7

TABLE VI-25-2. Trends of Age-specific Incidence Rates per 100,000 Population in Japan according to Sex, Primary Site, and Year
— Lymphoma, Female —

Age	Year of diagnosis											
	1975	1980	1985	1990	1991	1992	1993	1994	1995	1996	1997	1998
All age	2.4	3.1	4.4	6.2	6.4	6.5	6.5	7.4	7.4	7.1	7.8	7.6
0–4	0.4	0.5	0.9	0.9	1.1	1.1	0.4	0.5	1.1	1.3	0.8	0.5
5–9	0.4	0.4	0.7	0.6	0.5	0.3	0.5	0.5	0.8	0.6	0.4	0.4
10–14	0.6	0.1	0.4	0.7	0.7	0.5	0.3	0.3	0.5	0.5	0.8	0.7
15–19	0.7	0.6	0.6	0.7	0.7	0.6	0.6	0.6	0.8	1.0	0.7	0.6
20–24	0.9	0.6	0.5	0.9	0.7	1.1	1.1	1.2	0.9	1.1	1.4	1.7
25–29	1.0	0.7	0.5	1.4	1.1	1.1	1.0	1.3	1.4	1.5	1.1	0.7
30–34	0.7	0.3	0.9	1.8	1.6	1.5	1.4	1.9	1.9	1.8	1.5	1.4
35–39	1.6	2.1	0.9	3.0	2.1	2.6	2.3	2.6	2.5	1.7	2.3	2.6
40–44	1.3	1.6	2.1	2.8	3.2	3.7	3.7	3.3	3.0	2.5	3.0	3.2
45–49	3.5	3.8	3.5	4.3	4.4	4.6	4.4	4.9	4.6	5.0	5.6	5.2
50–54	3.8	5.1	3.7	6.1	5.2	6.1	6.5	8.1	7.6	5.5	6.3	6.2
55–59	5.4	7.2	7.4	8.3	9.2	9.0	9.6	10.8	9.8	9.0	8.4	8.4
60–64	6.8	8.8	9.5	12.7	13.2	13.4	12.6	13.2	12.7	11.4	12.3	11.2
65–69	12.5	11.6	14.4	18.0	17.6	15.1	15.2	16.7	15.3	14.5	18.1	17.7
70–74	12.3	12.6	19.7	22.1	21.9	19.0	20.8	23.8	25.0	24.1	26.3	24.8
75–79	14.3	13.6	22.4	29.1	30.4	30.2	29.1	30.7	30.8	27.6	30.4	27.9
80–84	10.5	12.9	22.3	34.9	36.6	37.7	34.1	37.6	36.5	35.3	37.8	34.0
85–	13.2	12.4	16.5	23.1	25.1	28.7	28.0	32.7	32.2	35.2	33.6	33.1

TABLE VI-26-1. Trends of Age-specific Incidence Rates per 100,000 Population in Japan according to Sex, Primary Site, and Year
—Myeloma, Male—

Age	Year of diagnosis											
	1975	1980	1985	1990	1991	1992	1993	1994	1995	1996	1997	1998
All age	0.7	1.7	2.3	2.6	2.6	2.4	2.3	2.4	2.4	2.5	2.5	2.7
0–4	0.1	0.0	0.0	0.0	0.0	0.0	0.0	0.0	0.0	0.0	0.0	0.0
5–9	0.1	0.0	0.0	0.2	0.2	0.0	0.0	0.0	0.0	0.0	0.0	0.0
10–14	0.2	0.1	0.0	0.0	0.0	0.0	0.0	0.0	0.0	0.0	0.0	0.0
15–19	0.2	0.0	0.0	0.0	0.0	0.0	0.0	0.0	0.0	0.0	0.0	0.0
20–24	0.2	0.0	0.0	0.0	0.0	0.0	0.0	0.0	0.0	0.0	0.0	0.0
25–29	0.1	0.0	0.0	0.0	0.0	0.0	0.0	0.0	0.0	0.0	0.0	0.0
30–34	0.1	0.0	0.2	0.1	0.0	0.1	0.1	0.2	0.0	0.1	0.1	0.1
35–39	0.2	0.4	0.1	0.1	0.0	0.1	0.2	0.2	0.4	0.3	0.2	0.2
40–44	0.4	0.8	0.4	0.6	0.6	0.4	0.5	0.4	0.3	0.5	0.4	0.6
45–49	1.2	0.8	1.4	1.3	0.9	1.0	0.8	1.0	0.8	1.1	1.4	1.5
50–54	1.0	3.4	2.5	2.1	2.1	2.1	1.8	1.7	1.0	1.2	1.3	1.6
55–59	3.7	4.4	4.2	4.7	4.1	3.4	2.4	2.7	2.1	2.4	2.1	2.6
60–64	3.0	3.4	6.6	7.4	6.7	5.4	5.4	4.8	6.4	5.6	5.3	5.2
65–69	4.2	9.7	8.8	8.7	9.9	9.7	9.5	9.7	9.6	8.8	7.2	7.7
70–74	4.6	13.9	16.6	15.6	16.6	14.2	11.6	11.5	12.6	12.2	13.2	14.0
75–79	8.2	22.0	18.2	21.1	22.7	20.5	19.3	17.5	16.6	16.9	16.2	17.4
80–84	12.6	21.5	23.2	20.6	17.8	22.1	19.2	22.4	23.2	21.7	25.0	22.0
85–	9.0	13.8	25.6	31.4	27.7	26.7	29.5	30.1	28.4	25.7	24.3	29.9

TABLE VI-26-2. Trends of Age-specific Incidence Rates per 100,000 Population in Japan according to Sex, Primary Site, and Year
—Myeloma, Female—

Age	Year of diagnosis											
	1975	1980	1985	1990	1991	1992	1993	1994	1995	1996	1997	1998
All age	0.6	1.3	2.2	2.1	2.3	2.2	2.2	2.4	2.3	2.3	2.5	2.5
0–4	0.1	0.0	0.0	0.0	0.0	0.0	0.0	0.0	0.2	0.2	0.0	0.0
5–9	0.1	0.0	0.0	0.0	0.0	0.0	0.0	0.0	0.0	0.0	0.0	0.0
10–14	0.1	0.0	0.0	0.0	0.0	0.0	0.0	0.0	0.0	0.0	0.0	0.0
15–19	0.2	0.0	0.0	0.0	0.0	0.0	0.0	0.0	0.0	0.0	0.0	0.0
20–24	0.1	0.0	0.0	0.0	0.0	0.0	0.0	0.0	0.0	0.0	0.0	0.0
25–29	0.1	0.0	0.0	0.0	0.0	0.0	0.0	0.0	0.0	0.0	0.0	0.0
30–34	0.1	0.0	0.0	0.0	0.0	0.0	0.0	0.0	0.0	0.0	0.0	0.0
35–39	0.3	0.1	0.2	0.1	0.1	0.2	0.2	0.2	0.1	0.2	0.2	0.1
40–44	0.2	0.1	0.6	0.3	0.4	0.5	0.2	0.3	0.2	0.1	0.1	0.2
45–49	0.8	0.7	0.7	0.4	0.7	0.6	0.6	0.4	0.4	0.7	0.9	0.9
50–54	1.4	2.0	2.4	1.3	1.4	1.4	1.1	1.0	1.6	1.3	1.3	1.3
55–59	1.0	2.3	4.3	2.6	2.2	2.3	2.6	2.9	2.7	2.0	2.0	1.8
60–64	2.9	4.5	5.2	4.8	4.8	4.8	4.4	4.7	4.2	4.1	4.9	3.9
65–69	4.9	7.6	6.9	7.4	8.7	7.7	7.0	6.8	6.0	6.0	6.6	6.7
70–74	5.8	7.1	11.3	9.4	10.6	9.7	9.7	8.5	8.5	7.2	8.9	10.4
75–79	2.7	11.9	9.1	12.9	13.6	12.7	13.4	14.0	12.9	12.6	13.3	13.5
80–84	3.4	7.5	17.8	17.4	15.3	13.3	15.0	18.8	18.2	17.1	16.6	13.4
85–	5.8	1.9	18.8	13.7	13.3	13.9	13.7	13.9	13.2	14.8	14.6	14.8

TABLE VI-27-1. Trends of Age-specific Incidence Rates per 100,000 Population in Japan according to Sex, Primary Site, and Year
—Leukemia, Male—

Age	Year of diagnosis											
	1975	1980	1985	1990	1991	1992	1993	1994	1995	1996	1997	1998
All age	4.7	5.5	6.1	6.0	5.9	6.4	6.2	6.2	6.1	6.4	7.3	7.4
0–4	5.2	5.8	5.4	5.6	5.5	5.7	4.3	3.8	4.3	3.6	4.6	4.1
5–9	3.8	3.4	2.7	2.7	2.8	2.9	3.2	3.0	3.4	2.9	3.0	3.2
10–14	2.7	3.1	2.3	2.3	2.1	2.1	2.2	2.3	2.7	2.5	2.4	2.4
15–19	2.5	3.1	2.6	2.5	2.5	2.6	2.4	2.3	2.3	2.4	2.4	2.5
20–24	1.4	1.9	1.5	2.2	1.7	1.8	1.3	1.7	2.2	2.0	2.1	2.1
25–29	3.6	2.5	3.1	1.8	2.1	2.4	2.6	2.1	1.8	1.9	2.1	2.1
30–34	3.4	3.0	2.4	2.5	2.2	2.4	2.7	2.6	2.3	2.2	2.7	2.3
35–39	3.7	3.0	3.4	3.8	3.0	2.8	2.4	2.3	2.9	2.4	2.5	2.5
40–44	3.4	5.6	4.2	4.5	4.1	4.4	3.8	3.6	3.0	3.0	3.1	3.2
45–49	5.0	4.5	5.0	4.3	4.9	5.2	3.7	3.7	3.5	4.2	5.9	5.8
50–54	8.4	6.9	8.2	5.2	5.5	5.8	5.6	5.5	4.4	5.1	5.8	5.7
55–59	10.3	11.5	8.4	9.9	9.2	9.8	10.0	9.9	7.6	8.6	9.2	9.0
60–64	10.7	14.6	12.5	12.0	11.1	12.0	10.8	10.1	11.0	10.4	13.7	13.1
65–69	9.7	14.7	19.7	13.9	13.8	15.3	14.8	15.6	16.4	18.2	19.4	19.8
70–74	15.5	22.1	25.8	20.9	21.3	23.1	21.1	21.9	20.9	21.8	24.6	23.9
75–79	18.4	15.2	25.3	26.5	24.3	27.3	30.9	30.0	29.2	27.1	27.5	28.1
80–84	28.4	18.9	24.6	30.1	34.3	33.8	37.2	30.4	31.5	33.9	39.1	37.5
85–	31.9	33.6	22.4	38.4	33.7	36.7	40.3	42.2	36.5	37.1	38.4	42.0

TABLE VI-27-2. Trends of Age-specific Incidence Rates per 100,000 Population in Japan according to Sex, Primary Site, and Year
—Leukemia, Female—

Age	Year of diagnosis											
	1975	1980	1985	1990	1991	1992	1993	1994	1995	1996	1997	1998
All age	3.5	3.9	4.4	4.4	4.5	4.5	4.8	4.6	4.2	4.5	5.0	5.2
0–4	4.6	5.3	4.4	4.3	4.0	3.7	4.5	4.3	3.9	3.3	3.8	3.8
5–9	4.0	3.0	2.7	2.2	1.9	1.9	2.2	1.8	1.7	1.6	2.0	2.0
10–14	2.5	2.2	2.5	2.3	2.4	2.0	2.6	2.2	1.9	1.6	2.0	2.0
15–19	2.6	1.5	1.3	1.8	1.7	1.4	1.4	1.3	1.3	1.3	1.4	1.5
20–24	1.5	1.8	1.0	1.5	1.5	1.3	1.7	1.6	1.8	1.6	1.5	1.2
25–29	2.5	2.6	1.8	1.0	1.1	1.0	1.1	1.5	1.4	1.7	1.6	1.5
30–34	2.5	2.1	2.5	2.4	2.4	2.5	1.5	1.3	1.5	1.9	2.4	2.2
35–39	2.3	3.3	2.7	2.3	2.5	2.6	2.2	1.6	1.7	1.5	1.8	1.7
40–44	3.2	4.2	3.2	2.2	2.5	2.8	3.2	2.6	2.8	2.7	3.0	3.0
45–49	3.9	4.5	4.1	2.9	2.9	2.9	3.4	3.6	2.6	3.6	3.7	3.5
50–54	5.0	2.7	4.5	5.1	5.6	5.6	5.5	4.4	4.4	4.2	4.1	4.1
55–59	5.8	5.2	6.2	5.5	5.3	5.1	5.0	5.0	3.4	4.9	5.1	6.2
60–64	4.9	7.2	7.6	6.9	6.8	7.0	7.2	6.5	6.6	6.5	7.4	8.1
65–69	10.0	8.3	8.7	7.8	8.8	9.3	10.6	9.0	8.1	8.8	10.3	10.6
70–74	11.8	7.8	10.9	14.0	13.3	13.2	12.7	13.0	10.1	12.1	11.7	12.2
75–79	9.4	13.7	14.3	15.6	14.4	13.1	15.6	15.8	11.2	13.6	13.6	15.9
80–84	11.0	6.8	14.7	19.5	20.7	17.5	17.6	16.6	19.4	16.2	18.7	16.9
85–	8.6	12.5	14.7	14.8	14.7	15.3	16.9	18.5	16.1	18.9	20.8	19.8

ESTIMATION OF SURVIVAL OF CANCER PATIENTS IN JAPAN (preliminary report)

Akira OSHIMA, Wakiko AJIKI, and Hideaki TSUKUMA for the Research Group for Population-based Cancer Registration in Japan

Department of Cancer Control and Statistics, Osaka Medical Center for Cancer and Cardiovascular Diseases

Survival of cancer patients diagnosed in Japan was estimated based on 80,607 cases from 12 registries as one of the collaborative studies of the Research Group for Population-based Cancer Registration in Japan. The survivals from this collaborative study were moderately higher than those reported from the Osaka Cancer Registry. It should be taken into consideration that passive follow-up methods were conducted in 8 registries and that some of the participating registries did not have as complete records as did the Osaka Cancer Registry. The Group is going to continue the collaborative study in order to establish methods of estimating survival for cancer patients throughout Japan, and to monitor cancer control activities in the country.

The Research Group for Population-based Cancer Registration in Japan has reported annually cancer incidence numbers and rates in all Japan based on data from registries of relatively good quality since 1975. However, survival of cancer patients had not been reported from the Group. Cancer survival has been reported only from some registries including the Osaka Cancer Registry which have reported survival data since 1975 with active follow-up using a residential register of municipalities. In 2000, the Group decided to estimate survival of cancer patients in all Japan as another collaborative study of participating registries, because patient survival is important information which the population-based cancer registry can provide as a measure of evaluating cancer control activities.

Methods

Data on cancer cases diagnosed in 1993 and their follow-up data were collected from twelve registries participating in the Group. Cancer registries participating in the survival collaborative study are shown in Fig.1. Follow-up methods were different by registries, *i.e.*, active follow-up using residential register of municipalities: 4 registries, passive follow-up by collation with death certificate files with names and addresses: 5 registries and passive follow-up by collation with death certificate files without names and addresses: 3 registries.

According to the methods of the EUROCARE study (*2*), DCO cases and *in situ* cancer (including mucosal cancer of colon and rectum) cases were excluded from the

1-3-3 Nakamichi, Higashinari-ku, Osaka 537-8511, Japan

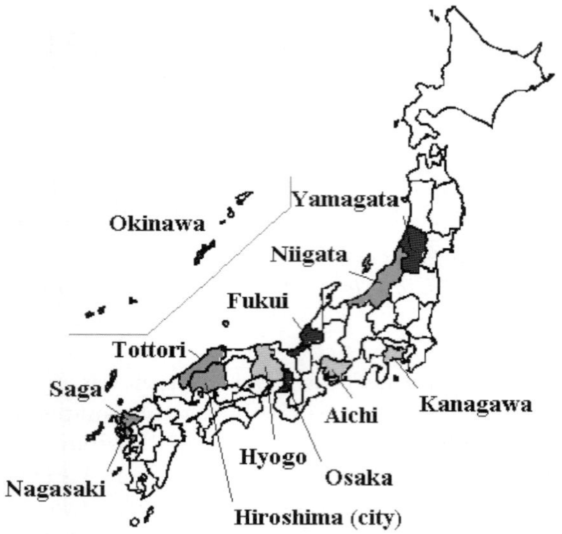

FIG. 1. Cancer registries participating in the survival collaborative study. ■, active follow-up using residential register of municipalities (4); ■, passive follow-up by collation to death certificates file with names and addresses (5); ■, passive follow-up by collation to death certificates file without names and addresses (3).

analysis. In the case of multiple cancers only the first-diagnosed tumor was analyzed. Number of cancer cases for the analysis was 80,607 in total. This corresponds to about 19% of estimated cancer incidence cases in 1993 in Japan (432,990). Relative five-year survival was calculated by the standard method (*1*).

Results

Table I shows the five-year relative survival of cancer patients diagnosed in 1993 in 12 registries in Japan for major sites. Survival of cancer patients of all sites was 46.0%, 56.3% and 50.4% for males, females and total, respectively. Survival of cancers of breast and uterus was high, *i.e.*, over 70% and that of cancers of liver and lung was low, *i.e.*, below 20%. The difference by sex was not large in each site.

Table II shows the five-year relative survival of cancer patients of relatively minor sites. Survival of cancers of testis and thyroid was high, *i.e.*, over 90%, but that of can-

TABLE I. Five-year Relative Survival in Japan for Major Sites (Cancer Cases Diagnosed in 1993, 12 Cancer Registries in Japan)

Site	Number of cases analyzed	5-year relative survival (Male) (%)	5-year relative survival (Female) (%)	5-year relative survival (Total) (%)
All sites	80,607	46.0	56.3	50.4
Stomach	18,754	58.4	55.3	57.3
Colon & Rectum	13,180	67.2	63.6	65.7
Liver	6,712	17.7	18.2	17.8
Lung	9,183	19.0	24.3	20.5
Breast	6,218	—	84.0	84.0
Uterus	2,543	—	72.7	72.7

TABLE II. Five-year Relative Survival in Japan for Minor Sites (Cases Diagnosed in 1993, 12 Cancer Registries in Japan)

Site	Number of cases analyzed	5-year relative survival (%)	Site	Number of cases analyzed	5-year relative survival (%)
Esophagus	1,959	22.7	Testis	204	90.8
Gallbladder	2,341	20.9	Kidney	1,540	61.3
Pancreas	2,385	7.6	Bladder	1,973	76.0
Larynx	697	77.6	Thyroid	1,185	90.4
Ovary	1,015	45.5	Lymphoma	1,911	45.8
Prostate	1,719	62.7	Leukemia	1,242	31.1

TABLE III. Five-year Relative Survivals by Site from Osaka Cancer Registry and SEER Program

Site (ICD-10)	Osaka Cancer Registry (%)	SEER program (%)
All sites (C00–C96)	40.6	62.4
Oral cavity and Pharynx (C00–C14)	48.7	57.4
Esophagus (C15)	18.5	13.2
Stomach (C16)	47.2	21.8
Colon (C18)	57.6	61.2
Rectum (C19–C21)	53.6	61.8
Liver (C22)	14.9	5.6
Gallbladder (C23–C24)	11.7	15.8
Pancreas (C25)	4.4	4.2
Larynx (C32)	75.0	64.2
Lung (C33–C34)	13.0	14.9
Breast (females) (C50)	79.7	86.4
Cervix uteri (C53)	66.5	72.5
Corpus uteri (C54)	68.6	84.9
Ovary (C56)	34.9	52.2
Prostate (C61)	52.8	97.2
Testis (C62)	89.4	95.7
Urinary bladder (C67)	67.3	82.3
Thyroid (C73)	84.7	96.0
Hodgkin's disease (C81)	42.9	82.8
Non-Hodgkin's lymphoma (C82–C85)	37.9	53.3
Leukemia (C91–C95)	27.7	47.1

Osaka Cancer Registry: cancer patients in Osaka Prefecture including Osaka City diagnosed during 1993–95; 59,227 cases, lost to follow-up: 677 cases, 1.14%.
SEER program: cancer cases diagnosed during 1993–95; 282,329 cases, lost to follow-up: 4,804 cases,1.70%.
(Sources: Osaka Cancer Registry, and National Cancer Institute SEER* Stat 5.0, 2003)

cers of esophagus and gallbladder was low, *i.e.*, around 20%, and survival of pancreas cancer was very low, *i.e.*, below 10%.

Discussion

Survival of cancer patients diagnosed in Japan was estimated based on 80,607 cases from 12 registries by the collaborative study of the Research Group for Population-based Cancer Registration in Japan. This collaborative study has just started and the data shown in this preliminary report should be regarded as tentative because there might be some problems found in the methodology. It should be taken into consideration that the quality level of participating registries is not high from the viewpoint of international standards. Data from five of the participating twelve registries appeared in "*Cancer Incidence in Five Continents Volume 8*" (*3*), but ∗ marks on the data from four of these, with the exception of the Hiroshima Tumor Registry, indicate that because of the high proportion of cases registered solely on the basis of a death there is a certain degree of uncertainty. Moreover, there are problems about the follow-up methods. As described in "*Methods*," passive follow-up was conducted by collation to the death certificate file without names and addresses in 3 registries. In these registries some dead cases were dealt with as living because of imperfect follow-up.

Despite these difficulties, the data shown in this report were based on over 80,000 cancer cases and some comparisons can be made among the present report and the report from the Osaka Cancer Registry and the SEER (Surveillance, Epidemiology and End Results) program with the following reservations.

The figures in this report were moderately higher than those survivals reported from the Osaka Cancer Registry as shown in Table III. This suggests that the level of cancer diagnosis and treatment in Osaka in total is not as good as the level in other places. However, it should be taken into consideration that passive follow-up methods were conducted in 8 registries and that the completeness of some of the participating registries was not as good as that of the Osaka Cancer Registry. It should also be taken into consideration that some registries are collecting systematically screen-detected cancer cases with the collaboration of cancer detection centers.

Compared with those in the SEER program series which are also shown in Table III, the relative survivals of ovary, testis, lymphoma and leukemia are lower in those in the Japanese and Osaka series. This seems to be due to the relatively low level of dissemination of the best-practice chemotherapy in Japan.

The Research Group is going to continue the collaborative study in order to establish the estimation methods of survival for cancer patients throughout Japan, to monitor cancer control activities in the country, and to conduct international comparison studies. The Group is also going to continue the collaborative study in order to standardize survival calculation methods and to clarify regional differences in survival and related factors in Japan.

Acknowledgments

The authors would like to thank the following registries which participated in the collaborative survival study and all those who are associated with them: Yamagata Cancer Registry, Niigata Cancer Registry, Kanagawa Cancer Registry, Aichi Cancer Registry, Fukui Cancer Registry, Osaka Cancer Registry, Hyogo Cancer Registry, Hiroshima City Tumor Registry, Saga Caner Registry, Nagasaki Cancer Registry, and Okinawa Cancer Registry. This study was supported in part by a Grant-in-Aid from the Ministry of Health, Labour and Welfare, Japan (14-2).

REFERENCES

1. Ajiki, W., Matsuda, T., Sato, Y., Fujita, M., Yamazaki, S., Murakami, R., Tsukuma, H., and Oshima, A. A standard method of calculating survival rates in population-based cancer registries. *Jpn J. Cancer Clin.*, **44**, 981–993 (1998).
2. Berrino, F., Esteve, J., and Coleman, M.P. Basic issues in estimating and comparing the survival of cancer patients. *In* "Survival of Cancer Patients in Europe. EURO-

CARE study," ed. F. Berrino, A. Sant, R. Verdecchia, R. Capocaccia, T. Hakulinen, and J. Esteve, pp. 1–14 (1995). International Agency for Research on Cancer, Lyon.

3. Parkin, D.M., Whelan, S.L., Ferlay, J., Teppo, L., and Thomas, D.B. "Cancer Incidence in Five Continents," vol. 8 (2002). International Agency for Research on Cancer, Lyon.

TRENDS IN CANCER INCIDENCE AND SURVIVAL IN OSAKA

Wakiko AJIKI, Hideaki TSUKUMA, and Akira OSHIMA

Department of Cancer Control and Statistics, Osaka Medical Center for Cancer and Cardiovascular Diseases

Cancer incidence in Osaka has been tabulated over a long period of time. Comparison of time trends between incidence and mortality would provide important clues to evaluate cancer control in this area.

Survival of cancer patients as determined from population-based cancer registries is also an important measure in evaluating cancer control in a population. Time trends of relative five-year survival were presented according to primary site and year of diagnosis during the period 1975–1995, as well as according to stage at diagnosis in 1993–1995. Survival for all sites in 1993–1995 was 42.6% among all incident cases and 75.0% for localized cases for both sexes in Osaka.

Trends in the Age-standardized Incidence Rates in Osaka (1966–1999)

The Osaka Cancer Registry (OCR) is one of four registries (others are Miyagi, Hiroshima City, and Nagasaki City) that can prepare long-term trends of incidence for more than 30 years with an assurance of accuracy. Of all population-based cancer registries in Japan, it covers the largest population (8.8 million in the 2000 census). In 1993, the monograph "*Cancer Incidence and Mortality in Osaka 1963–1989*" was issued in commemoration of the 30th anniversary of the OCR (*2*). This report shows time trends of age-standardized incidence and mortality for major sites during the period 1966-1999.

Figure 1 shows age-standardized incidence rates (ASIR) per 100,000 population standardized to the Japanese 1985 model population. Rates during 1966–1998 were averages for each three-year period, those in 1999 being the latest results in the OCR. ASIR in 1999 was 358.1 for males and 201.6 for females. The decrease in ASIR for stomach and uterus cancer has been remarkable during these periods. ASIR for lung and liver cancer had increased in 1969-1983, but the increase has slowed since 1984. A decrease in ASIR for liver has been remarkable especially for males since the early 1990s. A rapid and continuous increase in ASIR for colon and breast cancer was observed during these periods.

Figure 2 shows age-standardized mortality rates (ASMR). ASMR in 1999 was 252.8 for males and 119.8 for females. A decrease in stomach and uterus cancer and an increase in liver, lung and colon cancer were also observed in ASMR. The slope for stomach and uterus cancer (mainly cervical cancer) in ASMR, however, was steeper than that in ASIR, which suggests that secondary preventive measures and/or the

3-3 Nakamichi 1-chome, Higashinari-ku, Osaka 537-8511, Japan

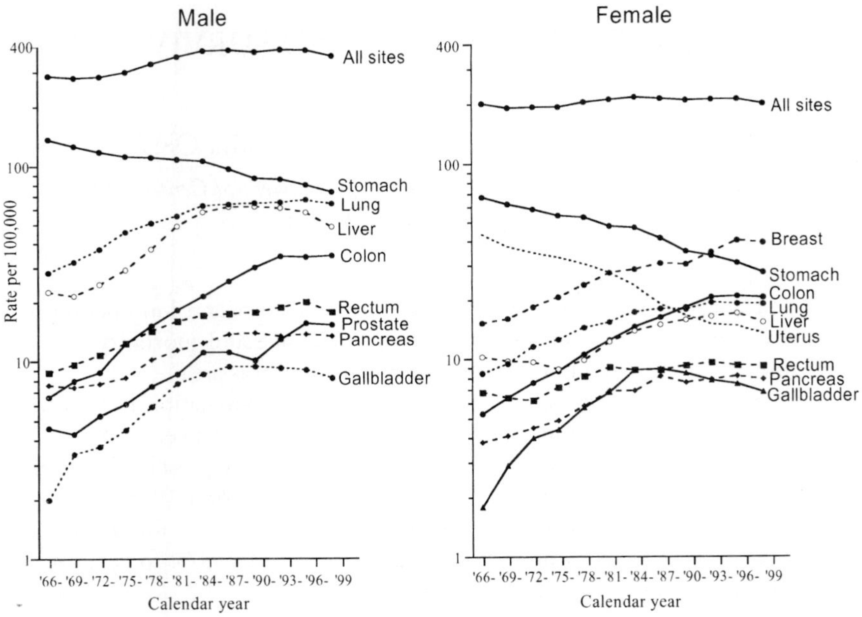

FIG. 1. Trends of age-standardized incidence rates for major sites in Osaka, 1966–99

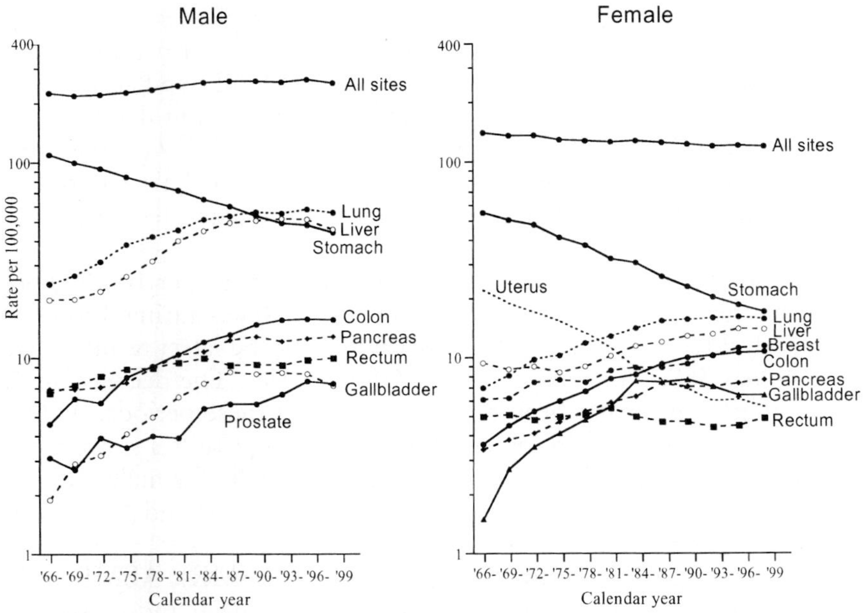

FIG 2. Trends of age-standardized mortality rates for major sites in Osaka, 1966–99

progress in treatment have been effective for these two cancers.

A high incidence of and mortality for liver cancer, especially among males, has been characteristic of Osaka, and is suggested to be attributable to the high prevalence of HCV(hepatitis C virus) carriers in the area (*4*).

Trends in the Survival Rate of Cancer by Site in Osaka (1975–1995)

Information on survival of cancer patients from cancer registries is also an important measure of evaluating cancer control. Cancer survival for major sites has been reported using a data bank for site-specific registry in Japan (*5*). However, cases registered in the data bank have been restricted to those who received treatment in a limited number of university or large hospitals. The overall prognosis of cancer patients could not be assessed by using these reports. Survival data from the population-based cancer registries are essential to evaluate the progress of cancer diagnosis and treatment in the population as a whole.

OCR is one of three population-based cancer registries (others are Yamagata and Fukui) in Japan that has been routinely calculating cancer survival using data based on an active follow-up survey to confirm the vital status of cancer patients. Survival data of these patients diagnosed in Osaka during 1975–1989 were re-examined and re-calculated according to the standardized methods (*1*) and published in 1998 as a monograph titled "*Survival of Cancer Patients in Osaka 1975–89*" (*3*).

Data on survival of cancer patients diagnosed in 1995 are now available. This report summarizes the survival of these patients in Osaka in 1975-1995 according to major site and stage at diagnosis.

1. Methods

To obtain information on the prognosis of registered cases, OCR has used the following three steps: 1) collation with the cancer death file, 2) collation with the death certificate file, and 3) confirmation of the cases' living status by referring to registers of inhabitants in local municipality offices. The final step had been conducted for those residing in Osaka Prefecture excluding Osaka City for cases diagnosed in 1975–1992. Therefore, the subjects for survival analysis had been restricted to those who resided in Osaka Prefecture excluding Osaka City at diagnosis. Now the final step is conducted for those residing in the entire prefecture. The percentage of cases lost to follow-up five years after diagnosis was 2.2–4.7% in 1975–1983 and less than 2.0% in 1984–1995.

Subjects were those who met all of the following criteria: (1) all malignant tumors excluding carcinomas *in situ* and mucosal cancers of the colorectum, (2) first primary tumors, and (3) those registered with clinical information from medical institutions. Cases registered by death certificates only were excluded from the analysis. A total of 211,627 cases diagnosed during 1975–1995 were included in this report.

Relative five-year survival (RSR) was calculated by standard methods (*1*): cumulative survival was calculated by the actuarial method, and then was divided by the expected survival of the patient groups calculated by the Ederer II method using "cohort survival tables," which have been prepared annually by the National Cancer Center using life tables in the Japanese population.

Details about the subjects and methods can be found in the monograph (*3*).

TABLE I. Relative Five-year Survival (%) by Primary Site and Period of Diagnosis in Osaka Prefecture excluding Osaka City, Both Sexes

Primary site	ICD-10	1975–77		1978–80		1981–83		1984–86		1987–89		1990–92		1993–95	
		No.	RSR	No.	RSR	No.	RSR	No.	RSR	No.	RSR	No.	RSR	No.	RSR
All sites	C00–C96	17,927	30.4	22,112	34.0	26,458	36.9	31,247	38.2	34,961	41.2	37,207	41.3	41,715	42.6
Esophagus	C15	403	5.7	476	9.6	576	12.6	687	10.8	773	14.7	880	13.5	1,020	19.7
Stomach	C16	5,866	27.9	6,719	33.8	7,326	38.9	8,366	43.1	8,410	47.2	8,175	46.2	8,889	48.9
Colon	C18	770	35.3	1,056	36.7	1,428	41.0	1,906	45.5	2,529	53.3	3,378	55.0	3,969	59.7
Rectum	C19–C21	703	28.1	977	38.1	1,203	43.9	1,389	45.4	1,674	52.4	1,917	55.3	2,167	55.6
Liver	C22	1,029	1.6	1,452	3.3	2,329	3.5	2,986	7.8	3,725	9.1	4,469	13.0	4,827	15.7
Gallbladder *etc.*	C23, C24	242	2.6	413	7.0	615	6.8	805	7.4	926	11.3	1,014	12.3	1,025	11.9
Pancreas	C25	397	3.3	557	2.4	748	2.7	870	2.9	1,097	4.9	1,138	4.1	1,271	4.5
Lung	C33, C34	1,751	6.2	2,301	9.8	2,649	10.3	3,381	11.2	3,945	11.7	4,128	13.1	5,040	13.8
Female breast	C50	1,165	67.6	1,505	70.0	1,911	80.1	2,226	78.4	2,708	83.6	2,860	80.7	3,367	80.0
Uterus	C53–C55	1,638	61.5	1,701	63.8	1,745	68.3	1,696	71.4	1,502	67.0	1,323	71.0	1,241	66.7
Ovary	C56	197	20.2	309	32.0	394	31.0	458	34.4	491	37.5	527	43.4	528	36.4
Prostate	C61	166	49.2	228	48.1	303	54.7	456	44.1	518	51.9	480	49.1	727	55.5
Bladder	C67	348	51.2	505	59.7	547	66.0	737	63.7	847	75.0	777	69.2	870	70.7
Lymphatic tissue	C81–C90, C96	499	17.5	574	27.0	806	28.6	961	31.6	1,010	34.8	1,159	35.4	1,281	37.1
Leukemia	C91–C95	471	10.3	539	15.5	644	19.9	696	20.9	696	23.2	705	24.2	816	29.6

RSR: relative five-year survival.

2. *Results*

Table I shows RSR in Osaka Prefecture excluding Osaka City for both sexes, together with the number of cases observed according to primary site and year of diagnosis. Survival for all sites increased from 30.4% in 1975–1977 to 42.6% in 1993–1995. The time trends of RSR are illustrated in Fig. 3. Female breast, bladder, and

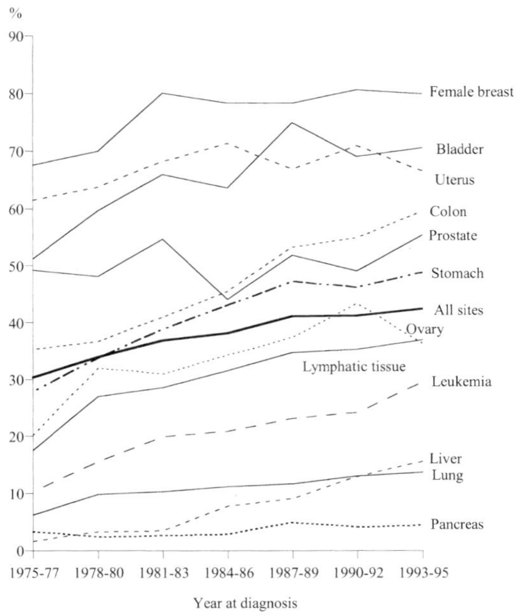

FIG. 3. Time-trends of relative 5-year survival by selected site for both sexes in Osaka, 1975–95

TABLE II. Relative Five-year Survival (%) by Primary Site and Clinical Stage in Osaka, 1993–95

Primary site	ICD-10	Localized		Regional		Distant		Stage unknown	
		No.	RSR	No.	RSR	No.	RSR	No.	RSR
All sites	C00–C96	22,243	75.0	17,379	33.9	12,452	7.8	7,153	24.0
Esophagus	C15	344	45.8	737	13.3	275	1.3	159	24.1
Stomach	C16	5,268	88.6	3,968	29.7	2,266	1.3	1,098	32.5
Colon	C18	2,444	93.4	1,611	54.0	1,048	5.8	452	49.8
Rectum	C19–C21	1,304	86.9	1,109	47.1	468	5.2	201	45.5
Liver	C22	3,328	24.4	898	5.3	910	3.9	1,943	6.1
Gallbladder *etc.*	C23, C24	280	45.0	654	6.9	336	0.0	274	6.5
Pancreas	C25	175	30.4	719	2.7	699	0.7	299	3.7
Lung	C33, C34	1,158	52.0	2,790	11.6	2,780	2.1	775	4.9
Female breast	C50	2,384	96.0	1,686	75.3	249	18.9	228	77.8
Uterus	C53–55	981	91.2	644	48.6	129	13.1	99	39.7
Ovary	C56	182	82.2	238	26.1	189	12.3	68	34.5
Prostate	C61	334	89.1	144	64.9	376	27.9	83	43.4
Bladder	C67	807	86.9	139	28.4	83	3.1	99	47.8

Localized: confined to the original organ.
Regional: spread to regional lymph-nodes and/or spread to immediately adjacent tissues.
Distant: metastatsis to distant organs.
RSR: relative five-year survival.

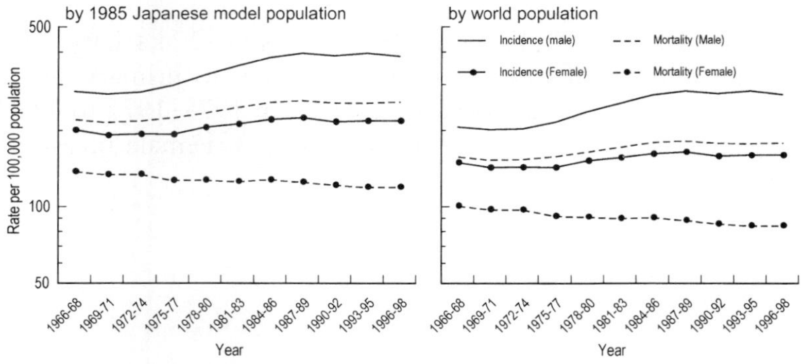

FIG. 4-1. Trends of incidence, mortality, and survival —all cancer—
Age-standardized incidence of and mortality from all cancer by sex, 1966–98

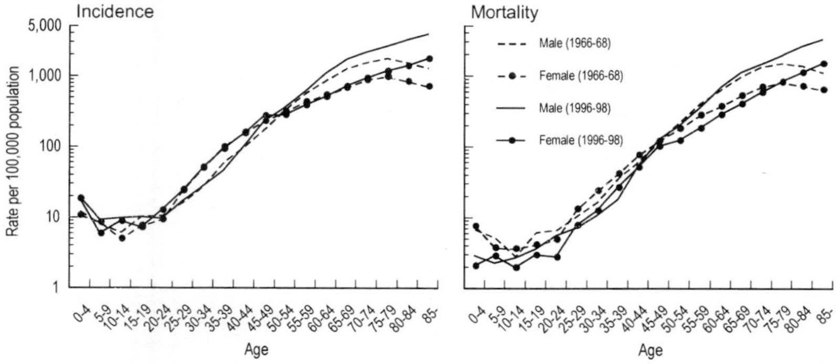

FIG. 4-2. Trends of incidence, mortality, and survival —all cancer—
Age-specific incidence of and mortality from all cancer by sex, 1966–68 and 1996–98

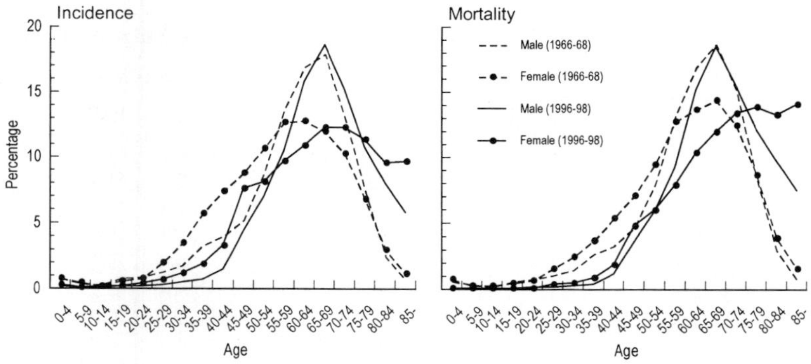

FIG. 4-3. Trends of incidence, mortality, and survival —all cancer—
Incidence of and mortality from all cancer: frequency distribution by age-group, 1966–68 and 1996–98

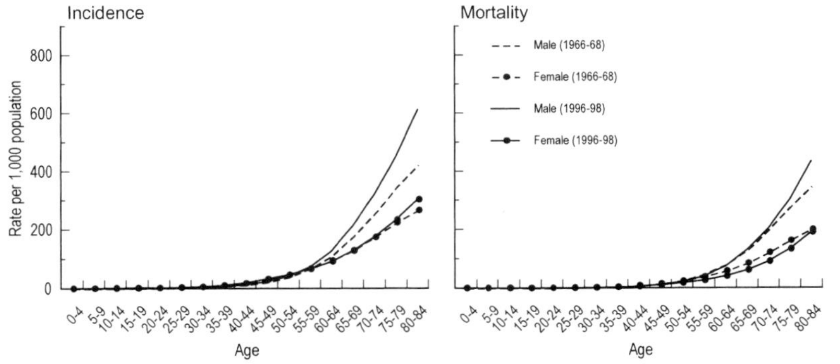

FIG. 4-4. Trends of incidence, mortality, and survival —all cancer—
Cumulative rate of incidence of and mortality from all cancer by age and sex, 1966–68 and 1996–98

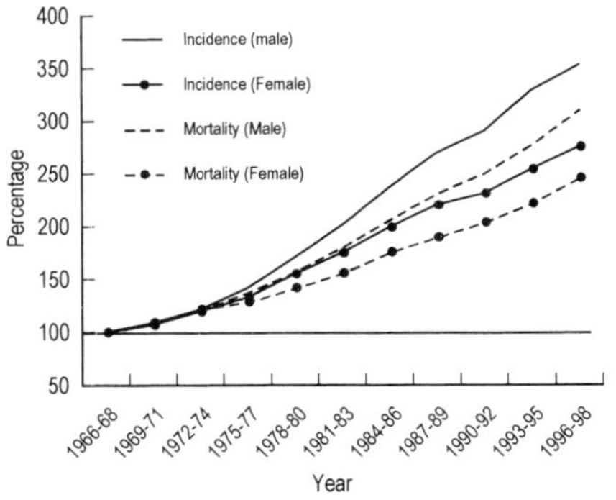

FIG. 4-5. Trends of incidence, mortality, and survival —all cancer—
The numbers of new cases of and deaths from all cancer by sex, 1966–98 (1966–68=100)

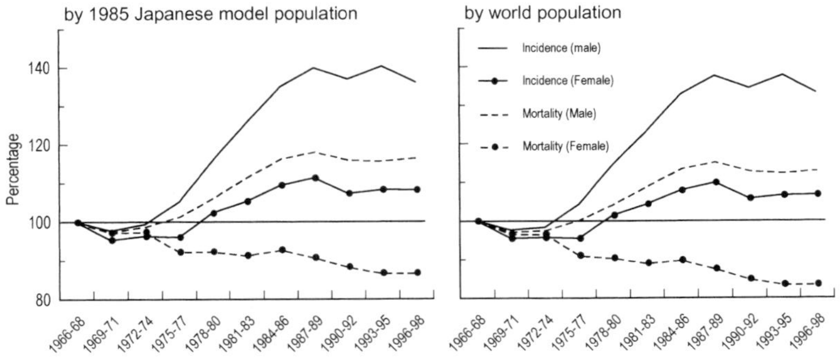

FIG. 4-6. Trends of incidence, mortality, and survival —all cancer—
Age-standardized incidence of and mortality from all cancer by sex, 1966–98 (1966–68=100)

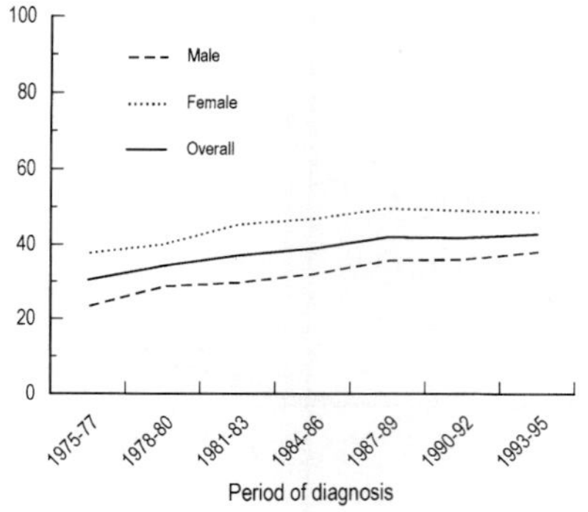

FIG. 4-S1. Trends of incidence, mortality, and survival —all cancer—
Relative 5-year survival (%), 1975–95

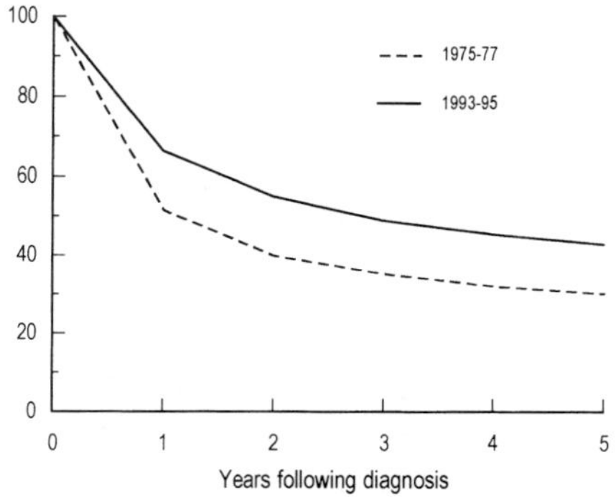

FIG. 4-S2. Trends of incidence, mortality, and survival —all cancer—
Relative survival (%), 1975–77 and 1993–95

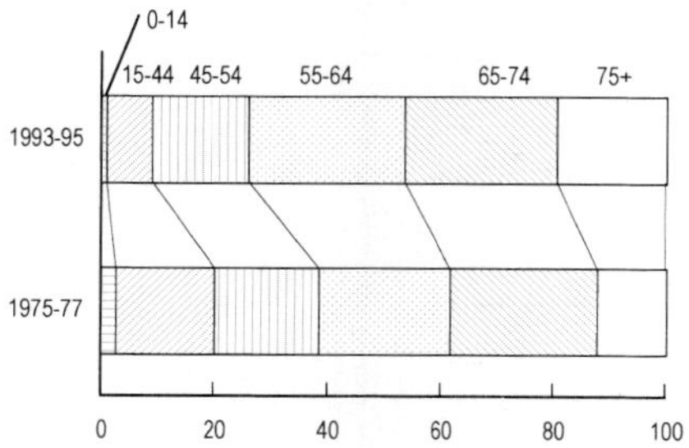

FIG. 4-S3. Trends of incidence, mortality, and survival —all cancer—
Age-distribution (%) in 1975–77 and 1993–95

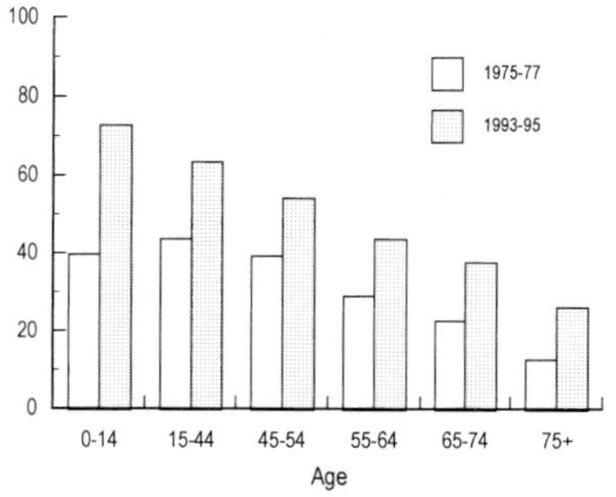

FIG. 4-S4. Trends of incidence, mortality, and survival —all cancer—
Relative 5-year survival (%) by age-group, 1975–77 and 1993–95

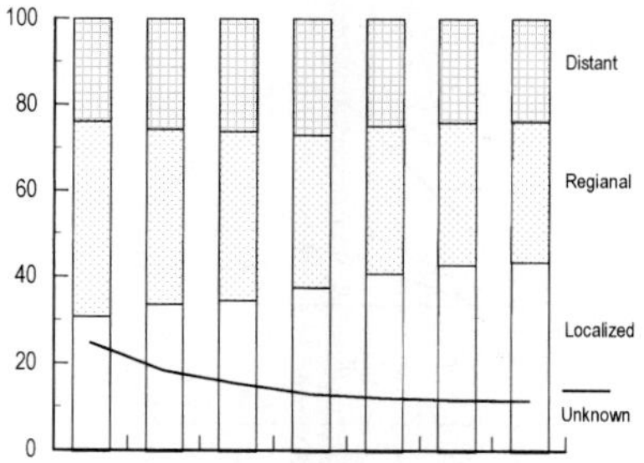

FIG. 4-S5. Trends of incidence, mortality, and survival —all cancer—
Stage-distribution (%), 1975–95

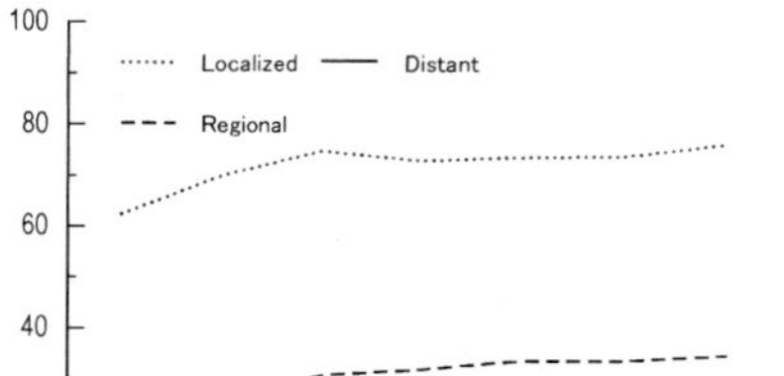

FIG. 4-S6. Trends of incidence, mortality, and survival —all cancer—
Relative 5-year survival (%) by stage, 1975–95

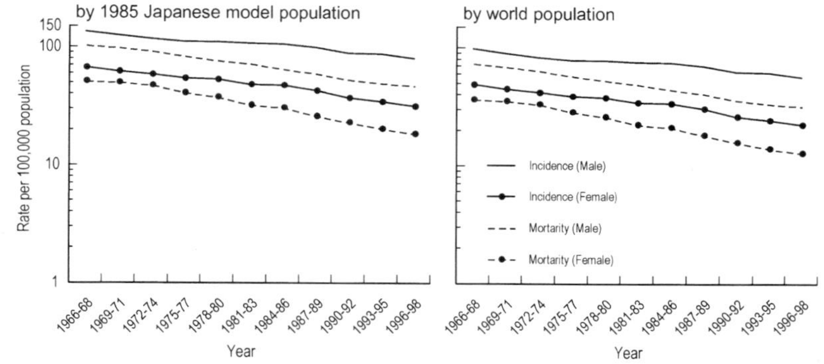

FIG. 5-1. Trends of incidence, mortality, and survival —stomach cancer—
Age-standardized incidence of and mortality from stomach cancer by sex, 1966–98

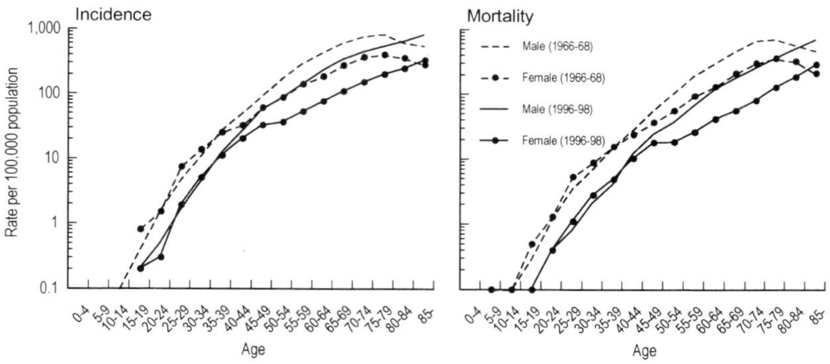

FIG. 5-2. Trends of incidence, mortality, and survival —stomach cancer—
Age-specific incidence of and mortality from stomach cancer by sex, 1966–68 and 1996–98

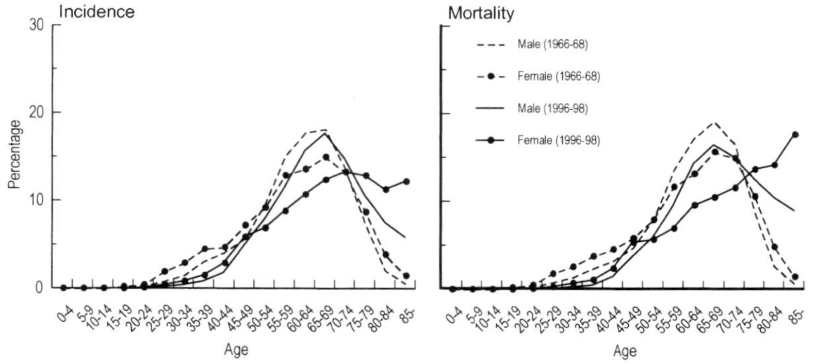

FIG. 5-3. Trends of incidence, mortality, and survival —stomach cancer—
Incidence of and mortality from stomach cancer: frequency distribution by age-group, 1966–68 and 1996–98

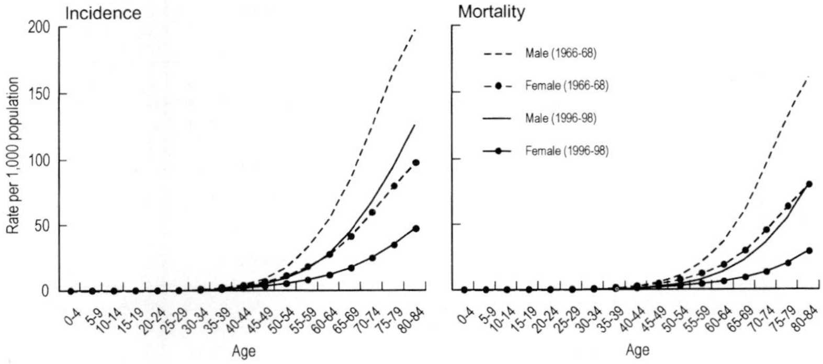

FIG. 5-4. Trends of incidence, mortality, and survival —stomach cancer—
Cumulative rate of incidence of and mortality from stomach cancer by age and sex, 1966–68 and 1996–98

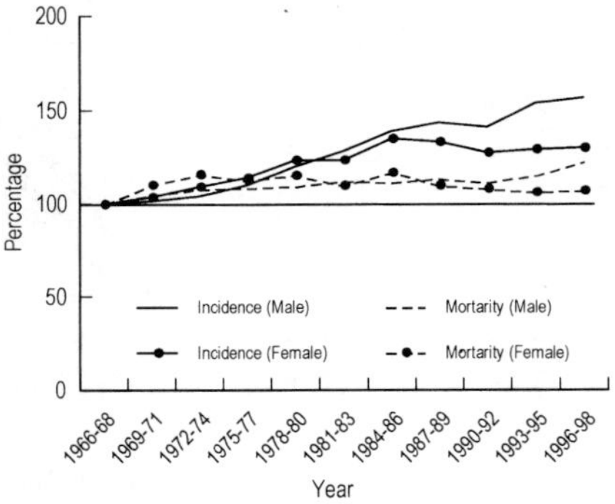

FIG. 5-5. Trends of incidence, mortality, and survival —stomach cancer—
The numbers of new cases of and deaths from stomach cancer by sex, 1966–98 (1966–68=100)

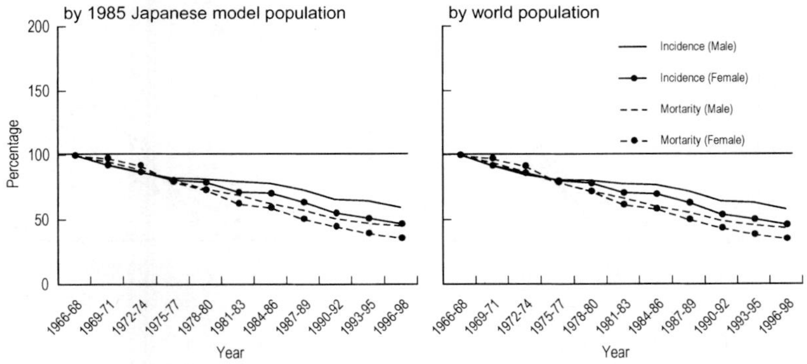

FIG. 5-6. Trends of incidence, mortality, and survival —stomach cancer—
Age-standardized incidence of and mortality from stomach cancer by sex, 1966–98 (1966–68=100)

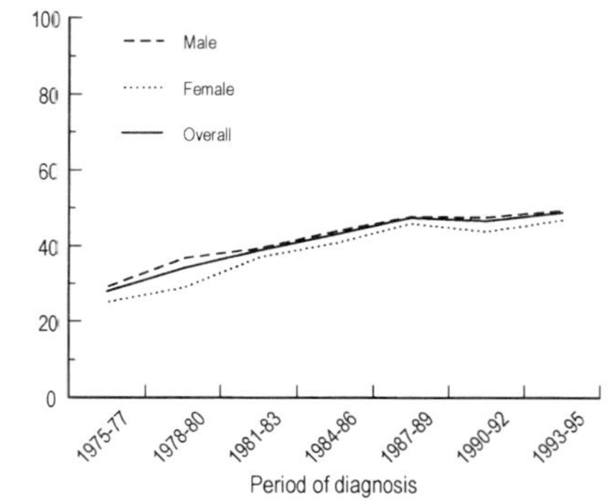

FIG. 5-S1. Trends of incidence, mortality, and survival —stomach cancer—
Relative 5-year survival (%), 1975–95

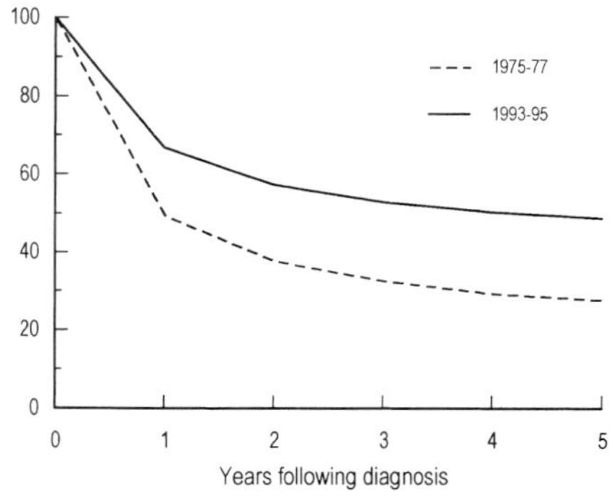

FIG. 5-S2. Trends of incidence, mortality, and survival —stomach cancer—
Relative survival (%), 1975–77 and 1993–95

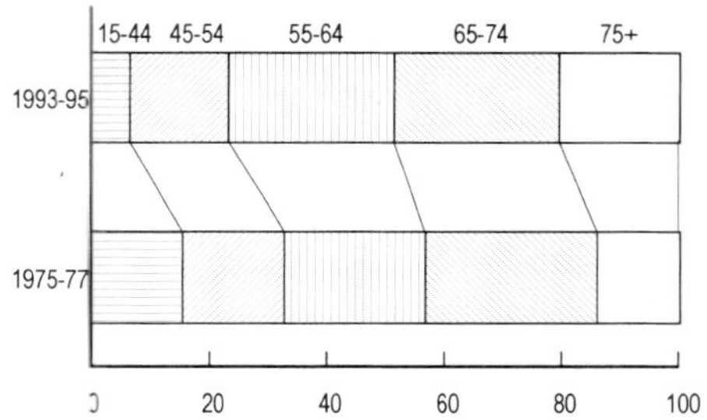

FIG. 5-S3. Trends of incidence, mortality, and survival —stomach cancer—
Age-distribution (%) in 1975–77 and 1993–95

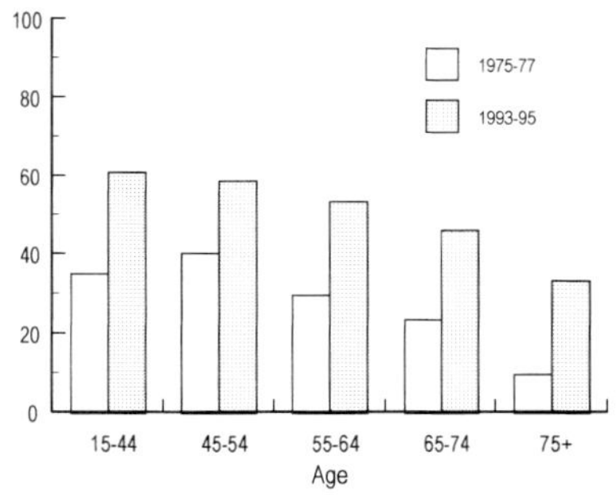

FIG. 5-S4. Trends of incidence, mortality, and survival —stomach cancer—
Relative 5-year survival (%) by age-group, 1975–77 and 1993–95

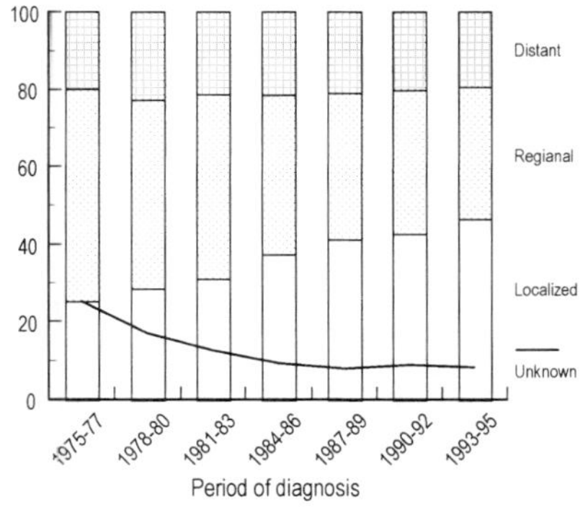

FIG. 5-S5. Trends of incidence, mortality, and survival —stomach cancer—
Stage-distribution (%), 1975–95

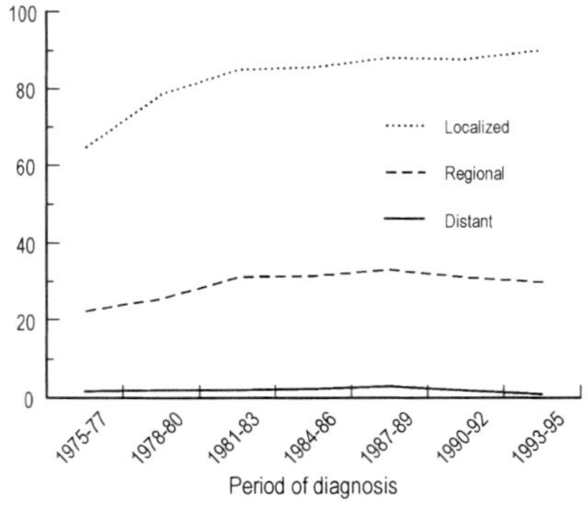

FIG. 5-S6. Trends of incidence, mortality, and survival —stomach cancer—
Relative 5-year survival (%) by stage, 1975–95

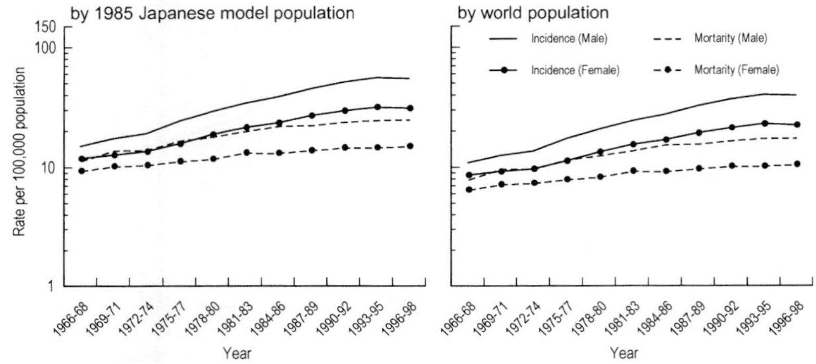

FIG. 6-1. Trends of incidence, mortality, and survival —colorectal cancer—
Age-standardized incidence of and mortality from colorectal cancer by sex, 1966–98

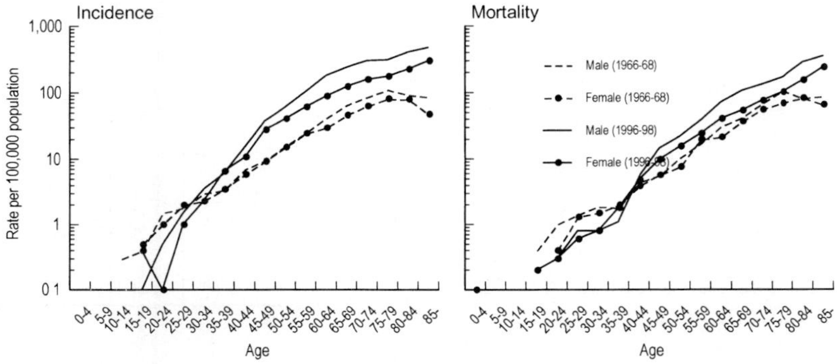

FIG. 6-2. Trends of incidence, mortality, and survival —colorectal cancer—
Age-specific incidence of and mortality from colorectal cancer by sex, 1966–68 and 1996–98

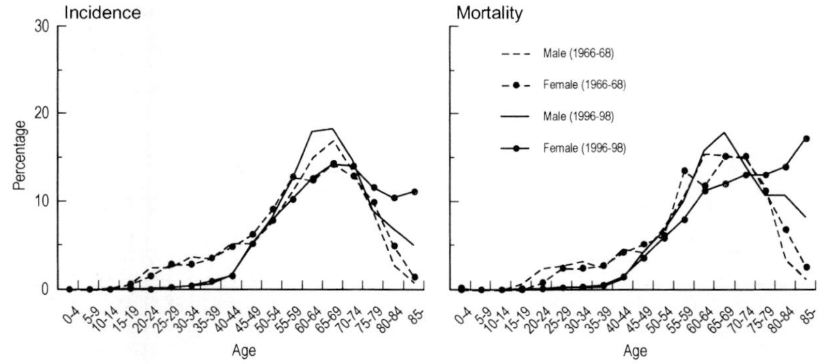

FIG. 6-3. Trends of incidence, mortality, and survival —colorectal cancer—
Incidence of and mortality from colorectal cancer: frequency distribution by age group, 1966–68 and 1996–98

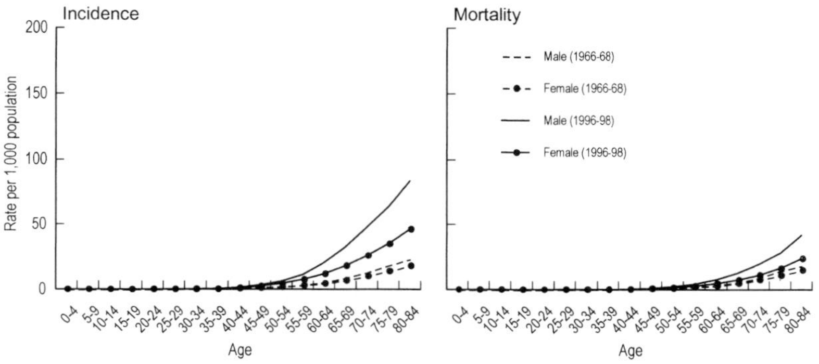

FIG. 6-4. Trends of incidence, mortality, and survival —colorectal cancer—
Cumulative rate of incidence of and mortality from colorectal cancer by age and sex, 1966–68 and 1996–98

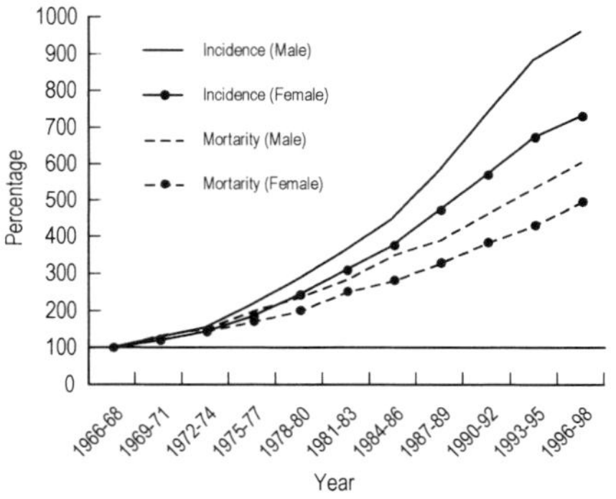

FIG. 6-5. Trends of incidence, mortality, and survival —colorectal cancer—
The numbers of new cases of and deaths from colorectal cancer by sex, 1966–98 (1966–68=100)

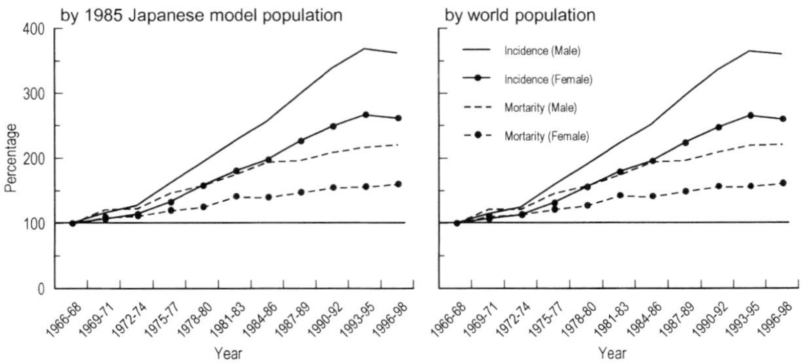

FIG. 6-6. Trends of incidence, mortality, and survival —colorectal cancer—
Age-standardized incidence of and mortality from colorectal cancer by sex, 1966–98 (1966–68=100)

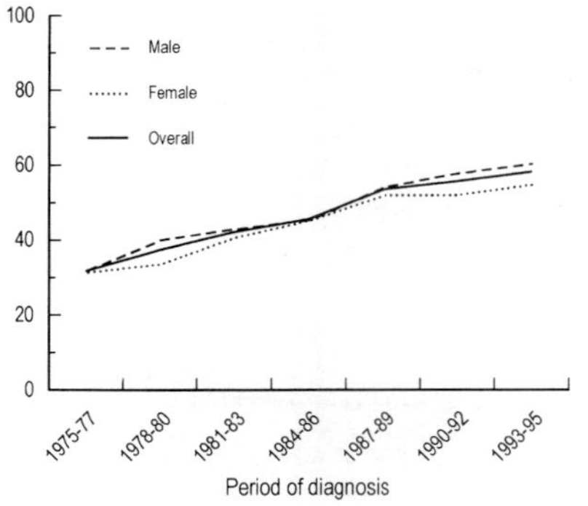

FIG. 6-S1. Trends of incidence, mortality, and survival —colorectal cancer—
Relative 5-year survival (%), 1975–95

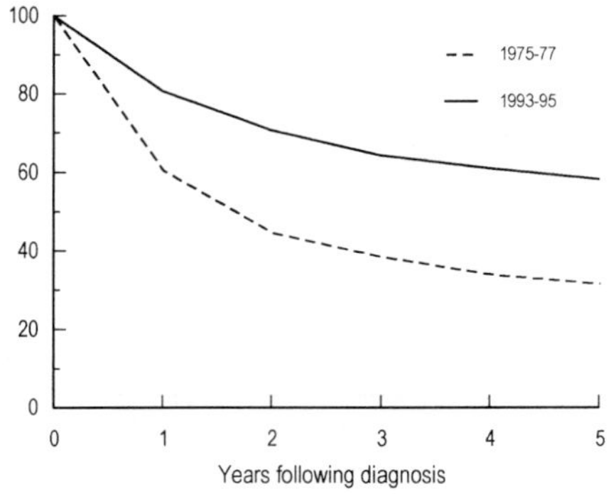

FIG. 6-S2. Trends of incidence, mortality, and survival —colorectal cancer—
Relative survival (%), 1975–77 and 1993–95

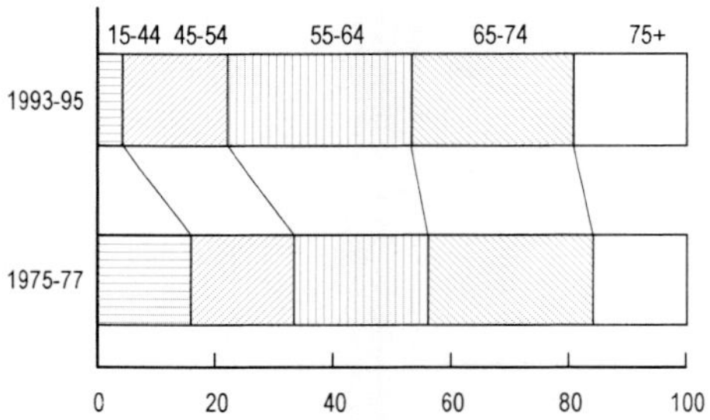

FIG. 6-S3. Trends of incidence, mortality, and survival —colorectal cancer—
Age-distribution (%) in 1975–77 and 1993–95

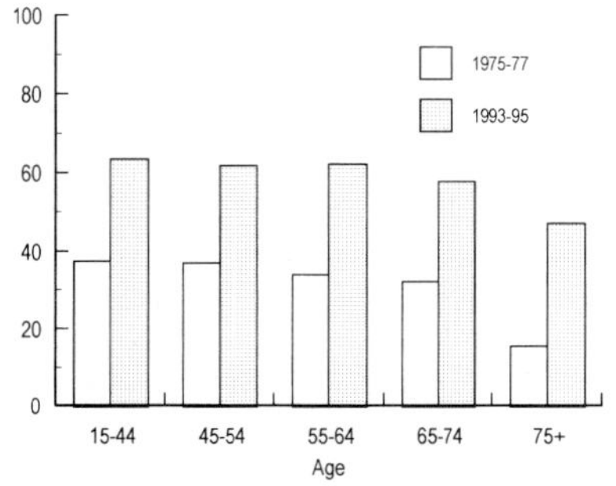

FIG. 6-S4. Trends of incidence, mortality, and survival —colorectal cancer—
Relative 5-year survival (%) by age-group, 1975–77 and 1993–95

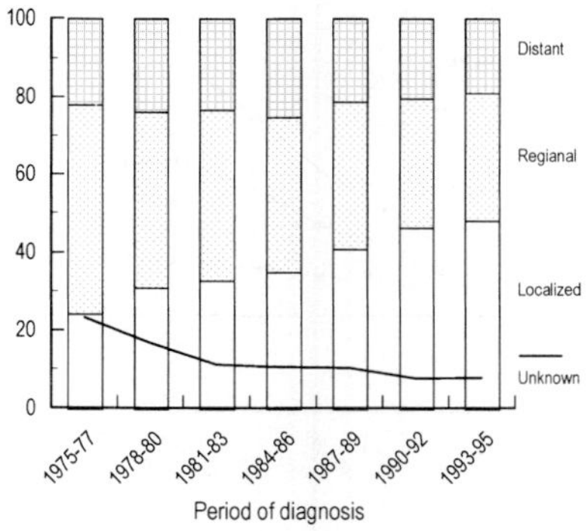

FIG. 6-S5. Trends of incidence, mortality, and survival —colorectal cancer—
Stage-distribution (%), 1975–95

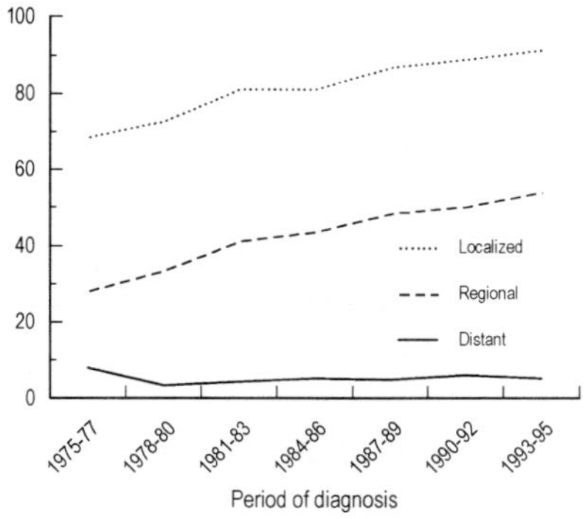

FIG. 6-S6. Trends of incidence, mortality, and survival —colorectal cancer—
Relative 5-year survival (%) by stage, 1975–95

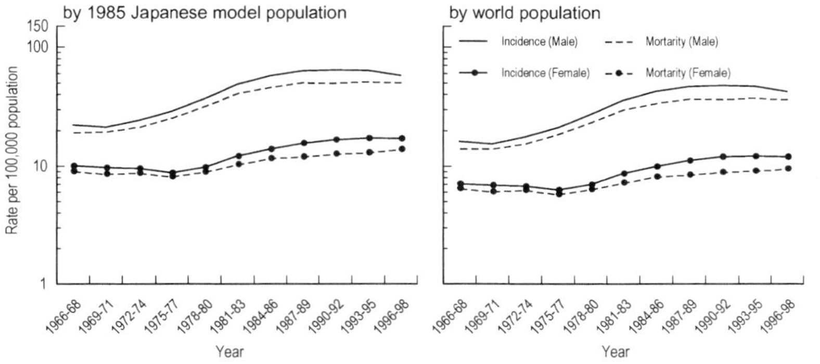

FIG. 7-1. Trends of incidence, mortality, and survival —liver cancer—
Age-standardized incidence of and mortality from liver cancer by sex, 1966–98

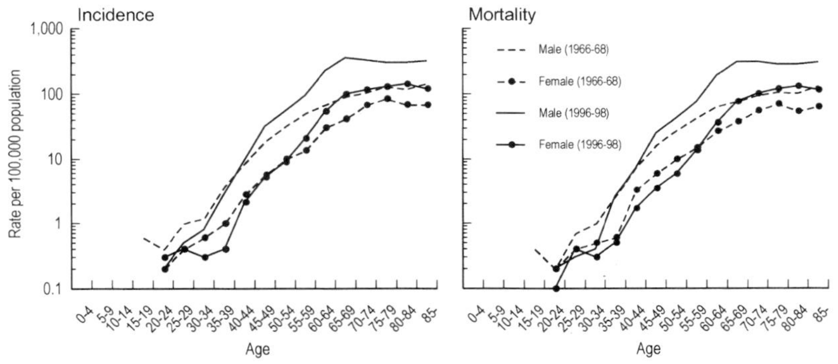

FIG. 7-2. Trends of incidence, mortality, and survival —liver cancer—
Age-specific incidence of and mortality from liver cancer by sex, 1966–68 and 1996–98

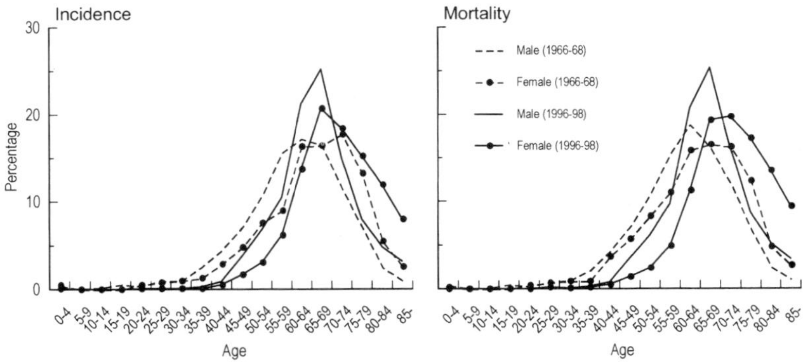

FIG. 7-3. Trends of incidence, mortality, and survival —liver cancer—
Incidence of and mortality from liver cancer: frequency distribution by age-group, 1966–68 and 1996–98

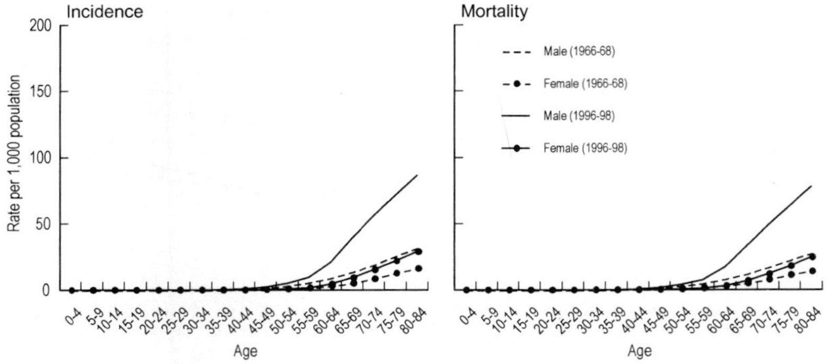

FIG. 7-4. Trends of incidence, mortality, and survival —liver cancer—
Cumulative rate of incidence of and mortality from liver cancer by age and sex, 1966–68 and 1996–98

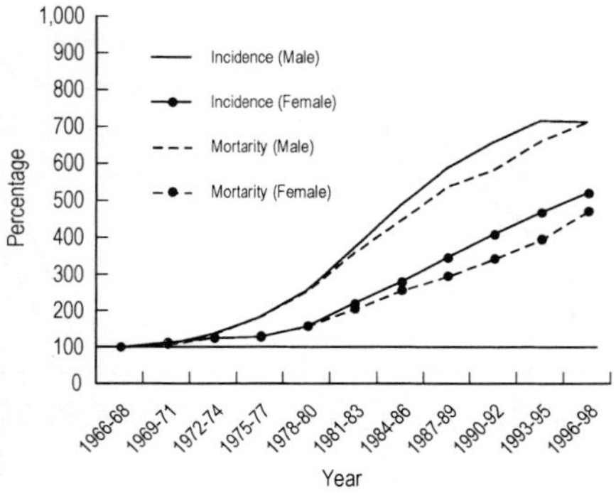

FIG. 7-5. Trends of incidence, mortality, and survival —liver cancer—
The numbers of new cases of and deaths from liver cancer by sex, 1966–98 (1966–68=100)

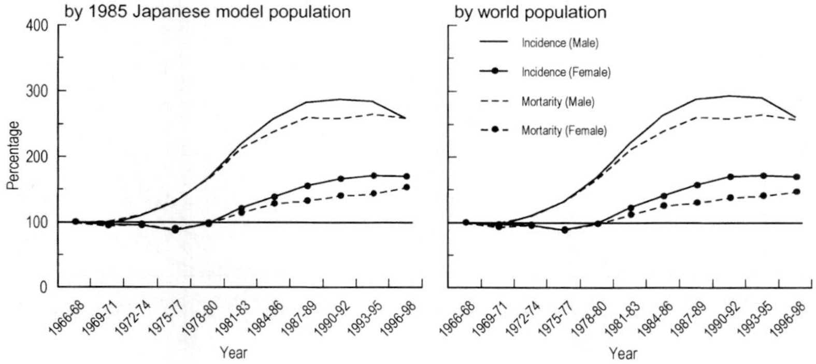

FIG. 7-6. Trends of incidence, mortality, and survival —liver cancer—
Age-standardized incidence of and mortality from liver cancer by sex, 1966–98 (1966–68=100)

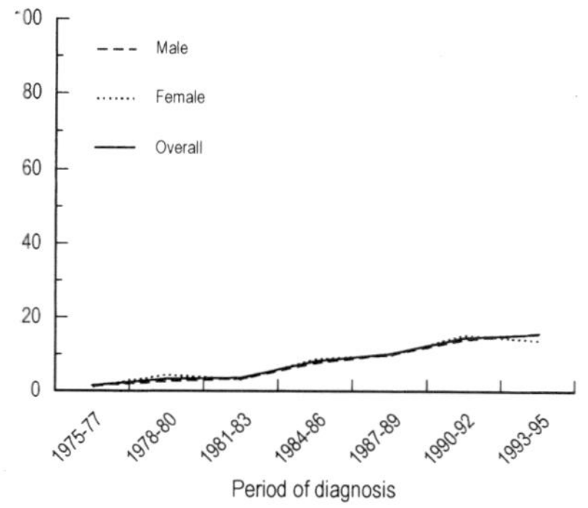

FIG. 7-S1. Trends of incidence, mortality, and survival —liver cancer—
Relative 5-year survival (%), 1975–95

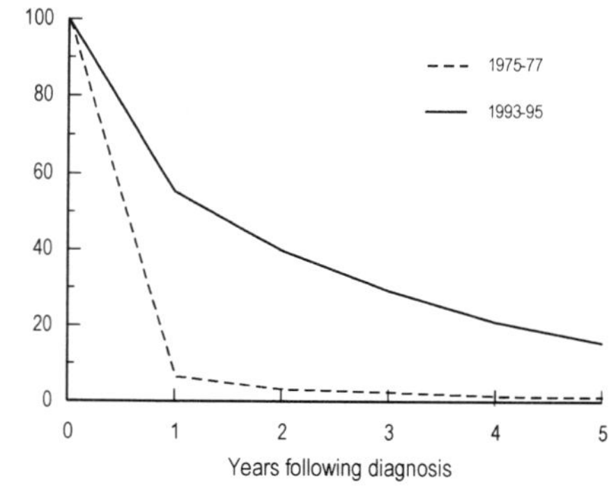

FIG. 7-S2. Trends of incidence, mortality, and survival —liver cancer—
Relative survival (%), 1975–77 and 1993–95

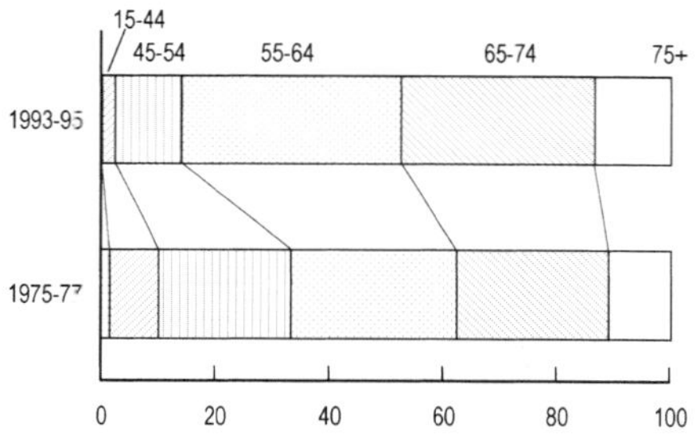

FIG. 7-S3. Trends of incidence, mortality, and survival —liver cancer—
Age-distribution (%) in 1975–77 and 1993–95

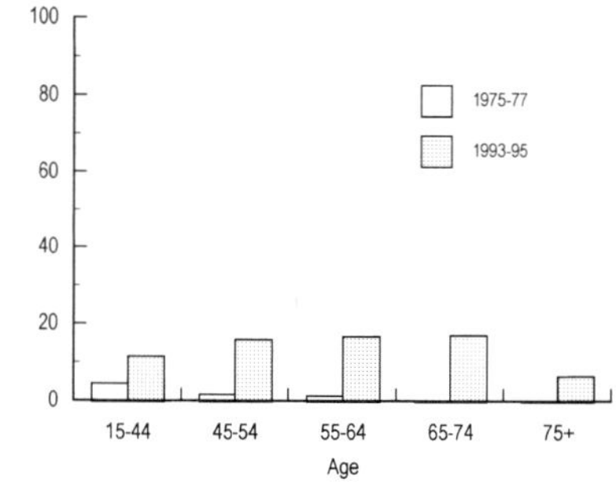

FIG. 7-S4. Trends of incidence, mortality, and survival —liver cancer—
Relative 5-year survival (%) by age-group, 1975–77 and 1993–95

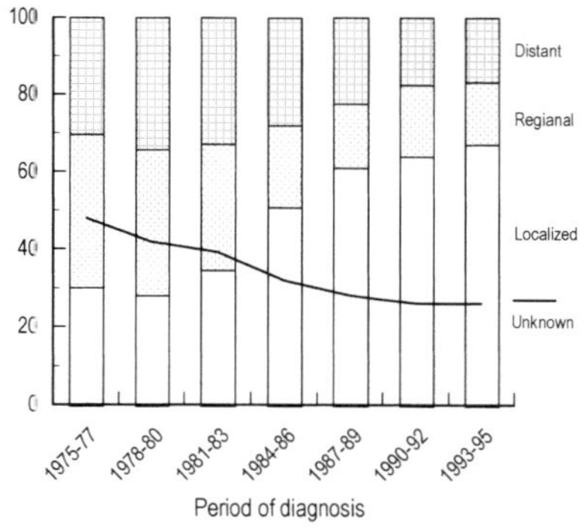

FIG. 7-S5. Trends of incidence, mortality, and survival —liver cancer—
Stage-distribution (%), 1975–95

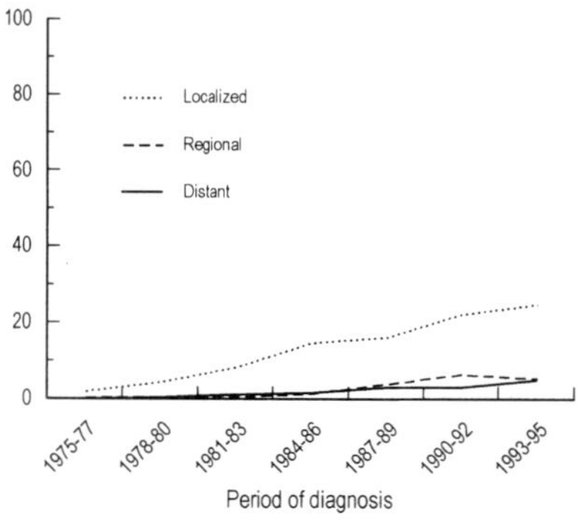

FIG. 7-S6. Trends of incidence, mortality, and survival —liver cancer—
Relative 5-year survival (%) by stage, 1975–95

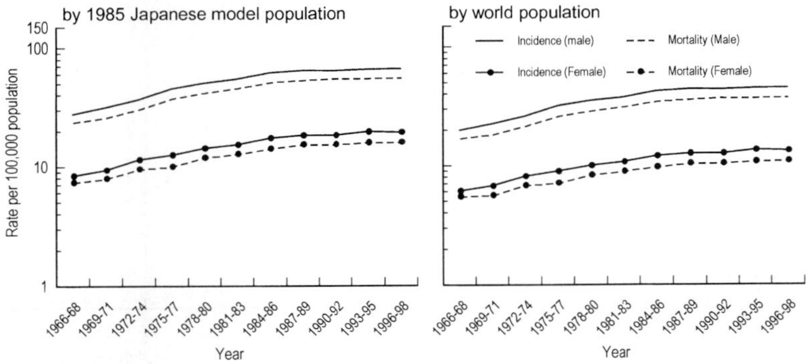

FIG. 8-1. Trends of incidence, mortality, and survival —lung cancer—
Age-standardized incidence of and mortality from lung cancer by sex, 1966–98

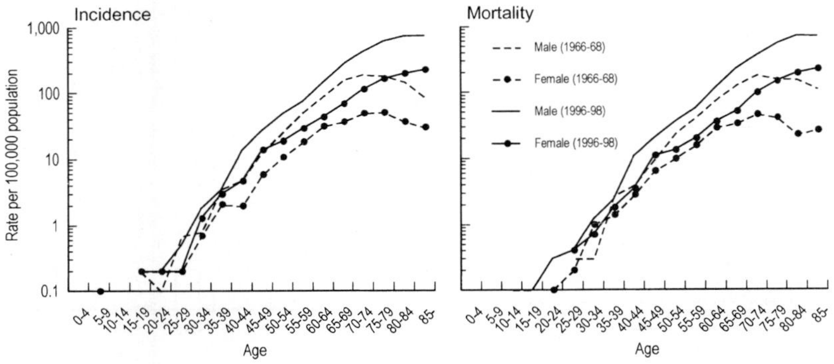

FIG. 8-2. Trends of incidence, mortality, and survival —lung cancer—
Age-specific incidence of and mortality from lung cancer by sex, 1966–68 and 1996–98

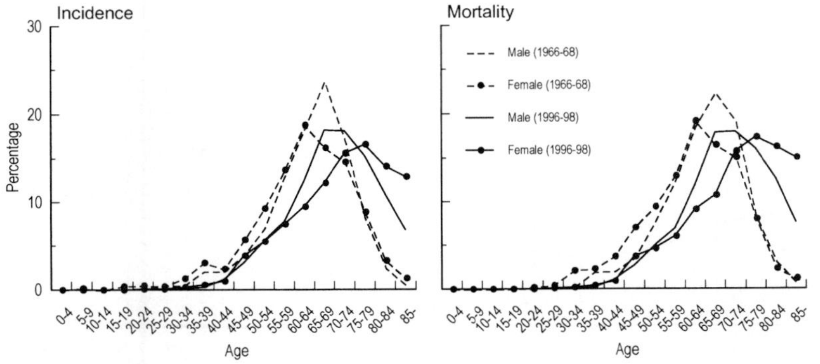

FIG. 8-3. Trends of incidence, mortality, and survival —lung cancer—
Incidence of and mortality from lung cancer: frequency distribution by age-group, 1966–68 and 1996–98

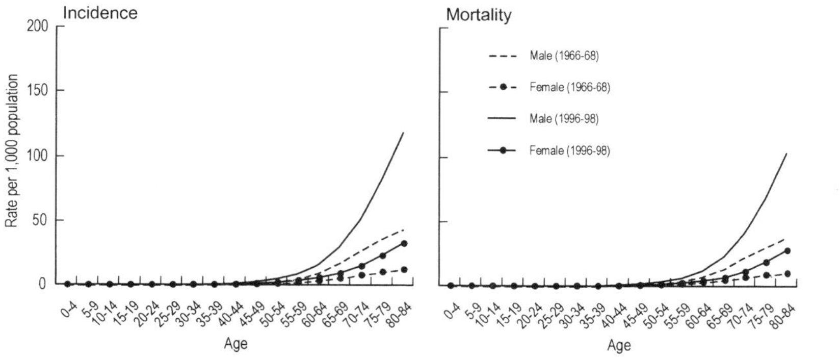

FIG. 8-4. Trends of incidence, mortality, and survival —lung cancer—
Cumulative rate of incidence of and mortality from lung cancer by age and sex, 1966–68 and 1996–98

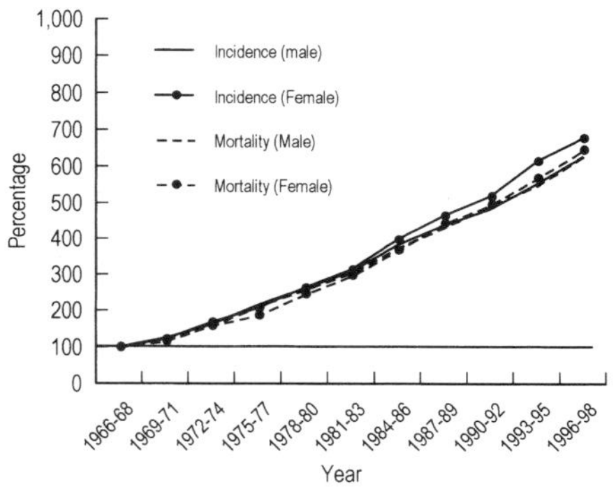

FIG. 8-5. Trends of incidence, mortality, and survival —lung cancer—
The numbers of new cases of and deaths from lung cancer by sex, 1966–98 (1966–68=100)

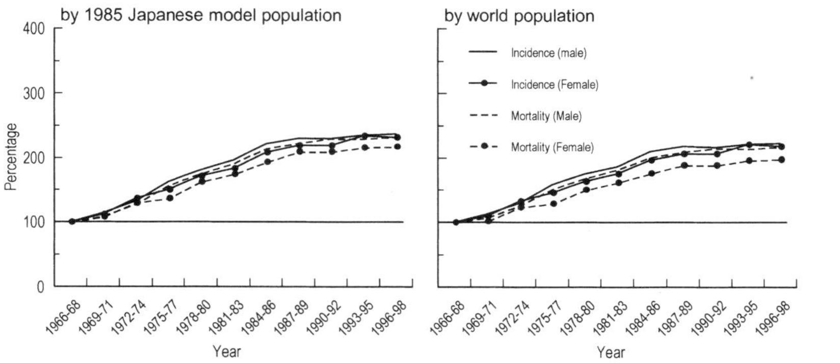

FIG. 8-6. Trends of incidence, mortality, and survival —lung cancer—
Age-standardized incidence of and mortality from lung cancer by sex, 1966–98 (1966–68=100)

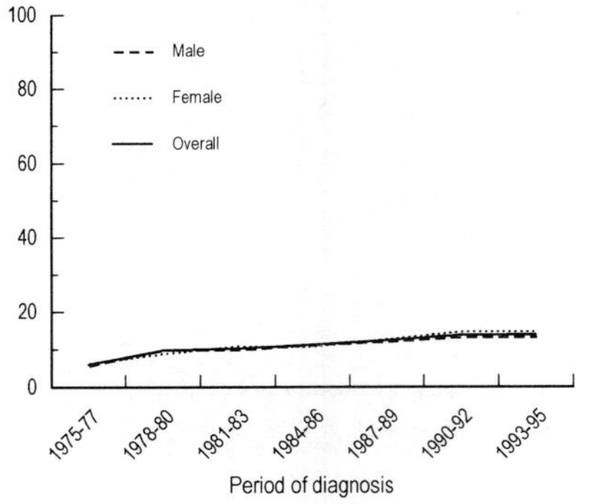

FIG. 8-S1. Trends of incidence, mortality, and survival —lung cancer—
Relative 5-year survival (%), 1975–95

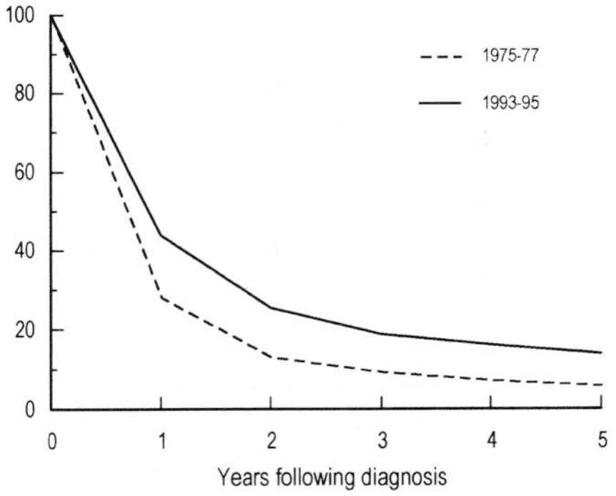

FIG. 8-S2. Trends of incidence, mortality, and survival —lung cancer—
Relative survival (%), 1975–77 and 1993–95

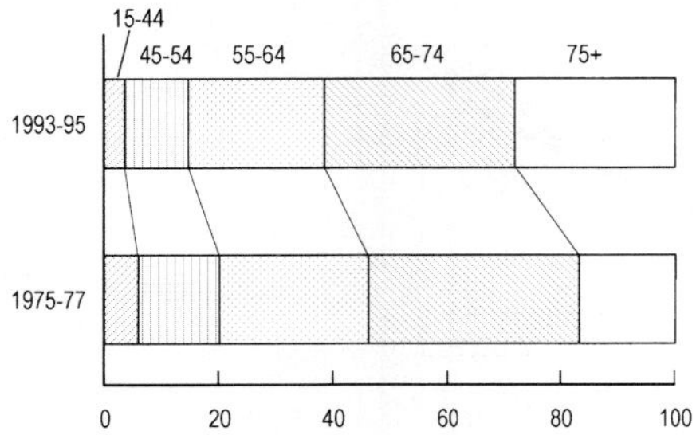

FIG. 8-S3. Trends of incidence, mortality, and survival —lung cancer—
Age-distribution (%) in 1975–77 and 1993–95

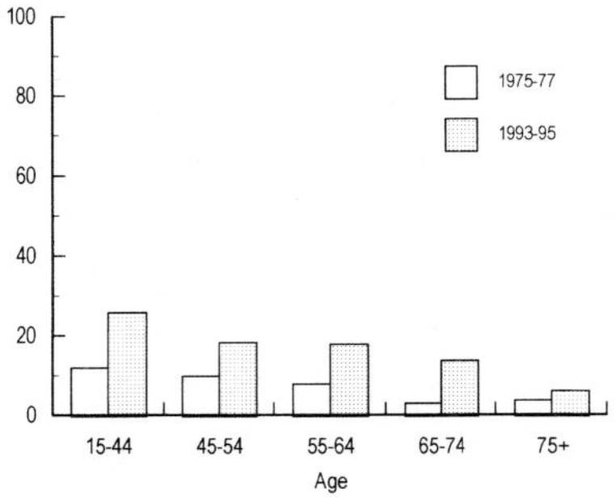

FIG. 8-S4. Trends of incidence, mortality, and survival —lung cancer—
Relative 5-year survival (%) by age-group, 1975–77 and 1993–95

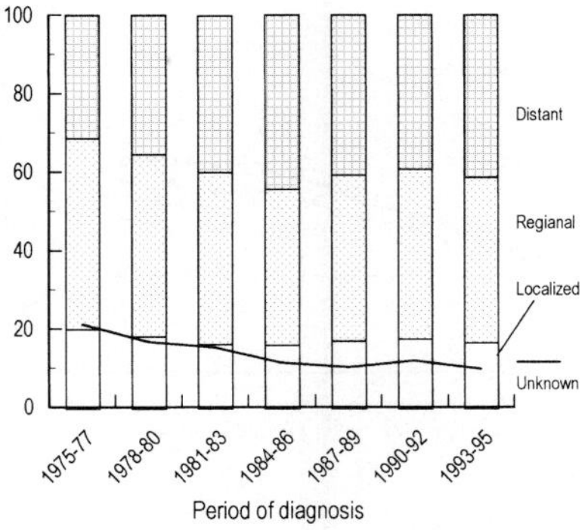

FIG. 8-S5. Trends of incidence, mortality, and survival —lung cancer—
Stage-distribution (%), 1975–95

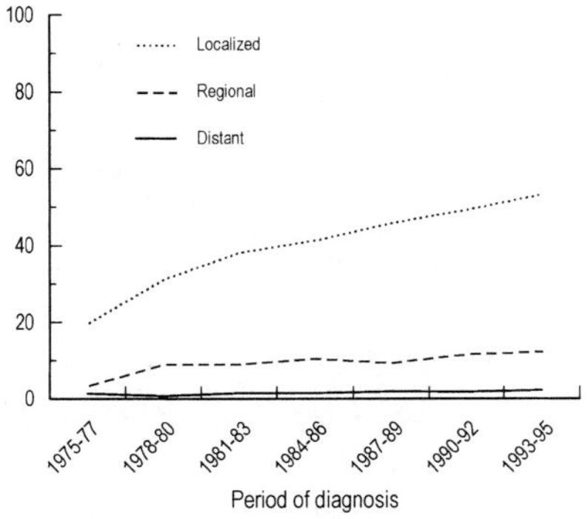

FIG. 8-S6. Trends of incidence, mortality, and survival —lung cancer—
Relative 5-year survival (%) by stage, 1975–95

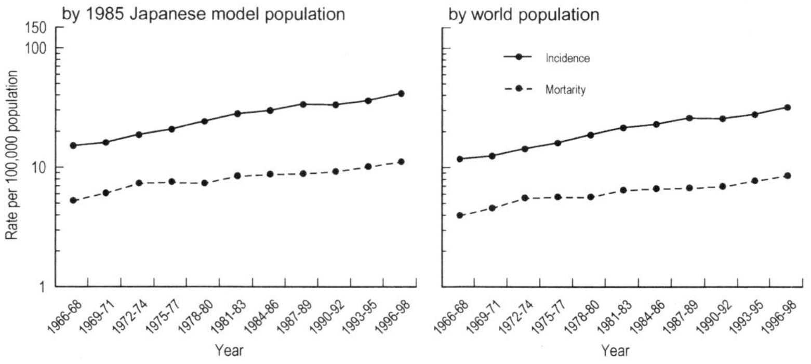

FIG. 9-1. Trends of incidence, mortality, and survival —breast cancer for female—
Age-standardized incidence of and mortality from breast cancer by sex, 1966–98

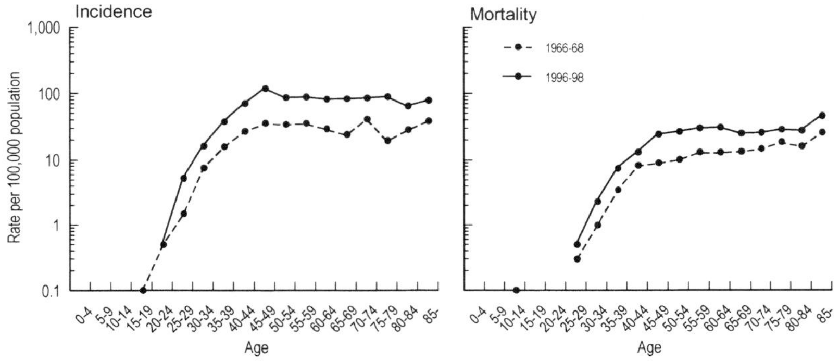

FIG. 9-2. Trends of incidence, mortality, and survival —breast cancer for female—
Age-specific incidence of and mortality from breast cancer by sex, 1966–68 and 1996–98

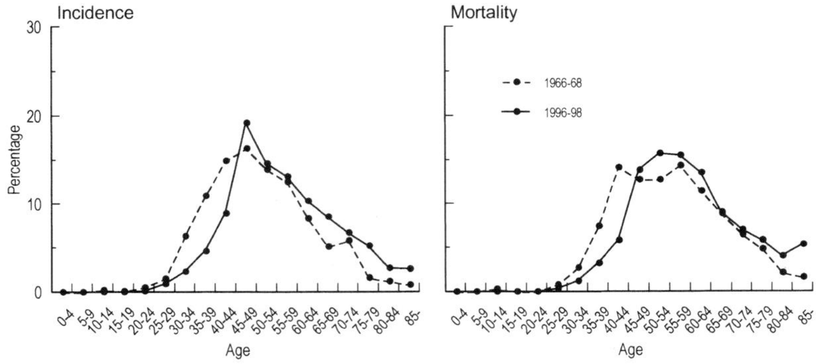

FIG. 9-3. Trends of incidence, mortality, and survival —breast cancer for female—
Incidence of and mortality from breast cancer: frequency distribution by age-group, 1966–68 and 1996–98

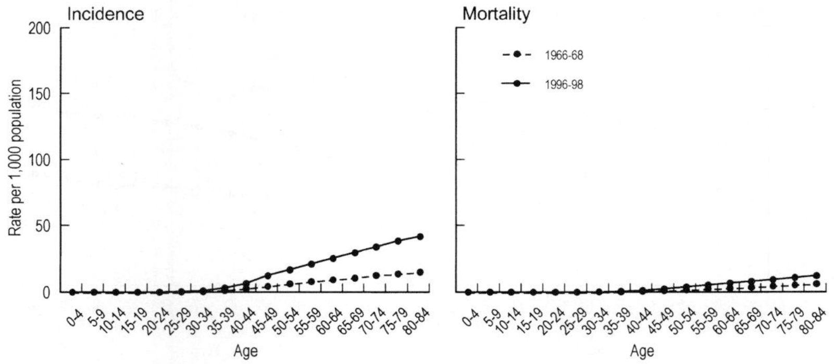

FIG. 9-4. Trends of incidence, mortality, and survival —breast cancer for female—
Cumulative rate of incidence of and mortality from breast cancer by age and sex, 1966–68 and 1996–98

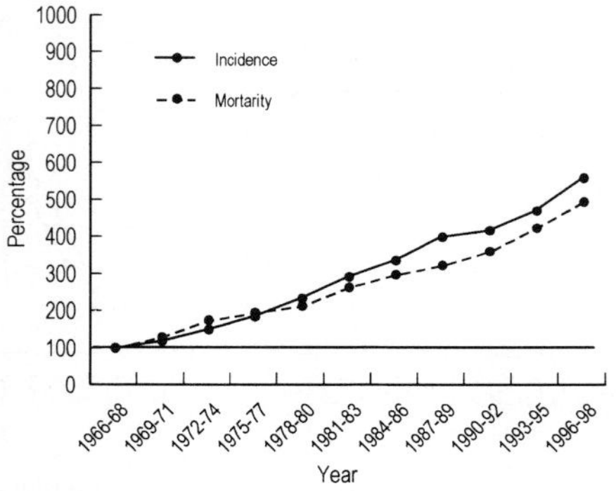

FIG. 9-5. Trends of incidence, mortality, and survival —breast cancer for female—
The numbers of new cases of and deaths from breast cancer by sex, 1966–98 (1966–68=100)

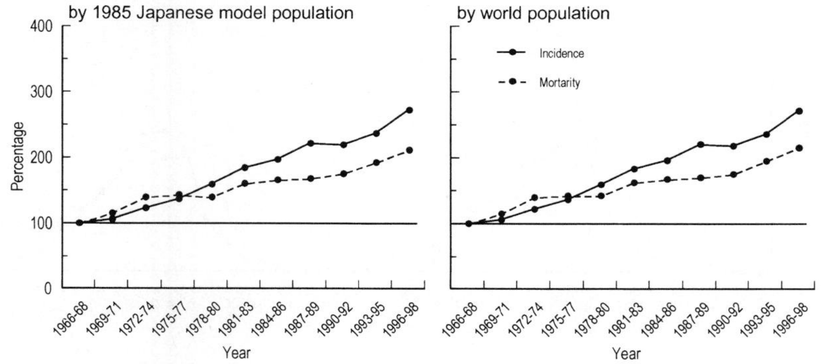

FIG. 9-6. Trends of incidence, mortality, and survival —breast cancer for female—
Age-standardized incidence of and mortality from breast cancer by sex, 1966–98 (1966–68=100)

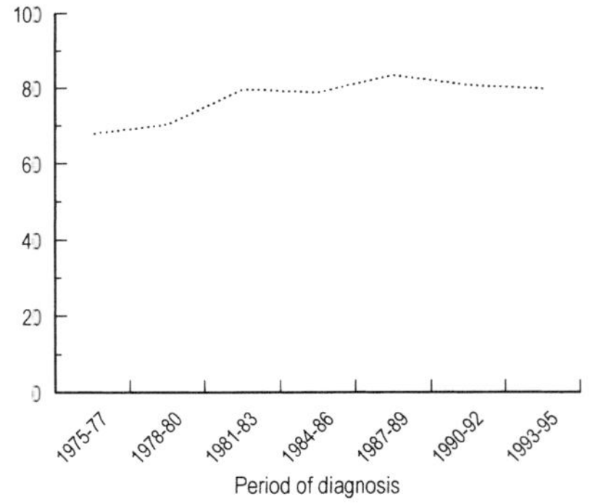

FIG. 9-S1. Trends of incidence, mortality, and survival —breast cancer for female—
Relative 5-year survival (%), 1975–95

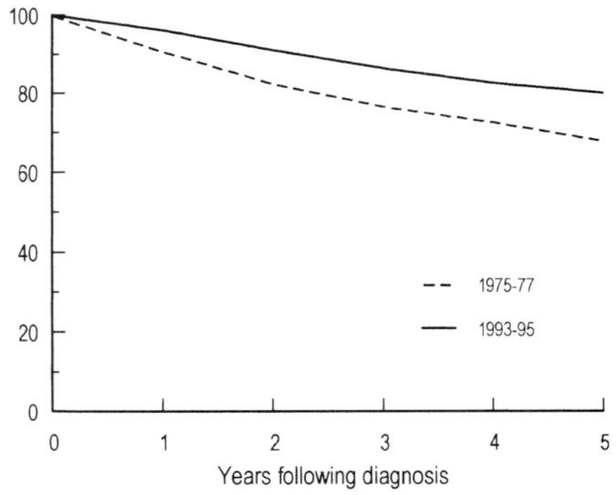

FIG. 9-S2. Trends of incidence, mortality, and survival —breast cancer for female—
Relative survival (%), 1975–77 and 1993–95

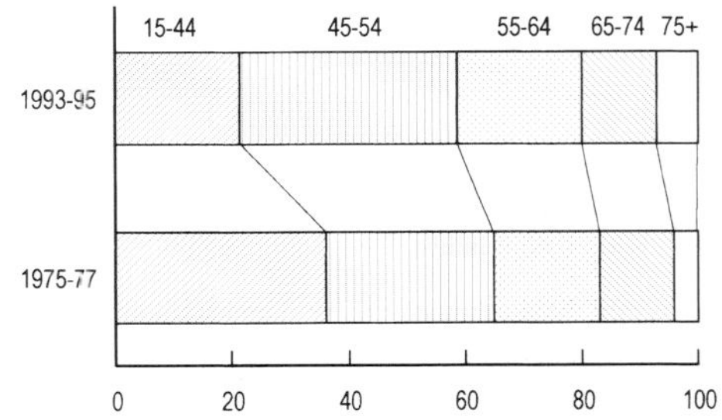

FIG. 9-S3. Trends of incidence, mortality, and survival —breast cancer for female—
Age-distribution (%) in 1975–77 and 1993–95

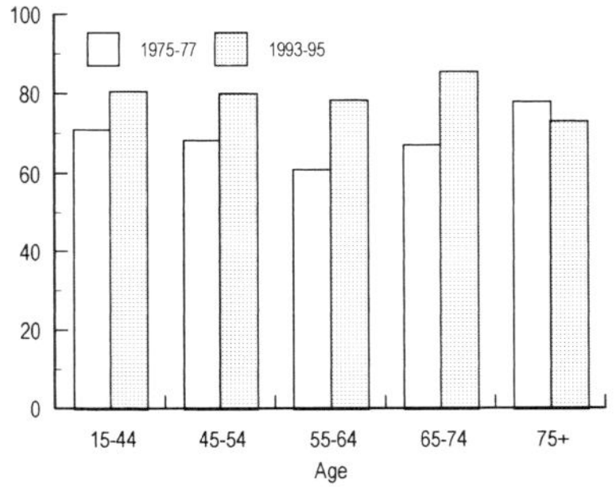

FIG. 9-S4. Trends of incidence, mortality, and survival —breast cancer for female—
Relative 5-year survival (%) by age-group, 1975–77 and 1993–95

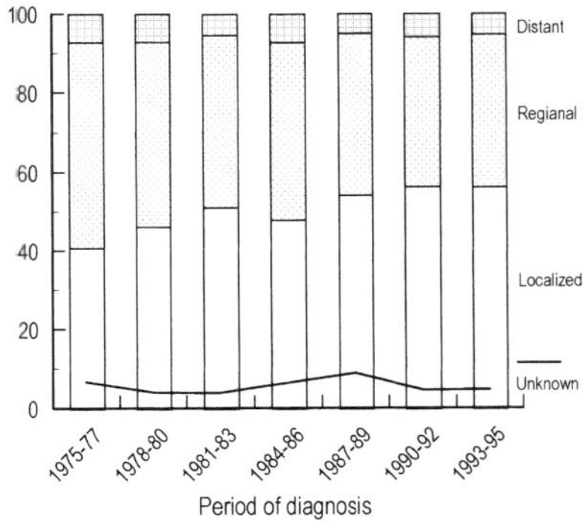

FIG. 9-S5. Trends of incidence, mortality, and survival —breast cancer for female—
Stage-distribution (%), 1975–95

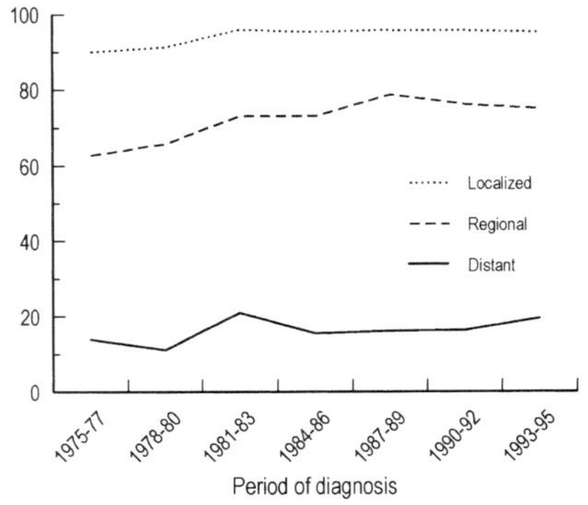

FIG. 9-S6. Trends of incidence, mortality, and survival —breast cancer for female—
Relative 5-year survival (%) by stage, 1975–95

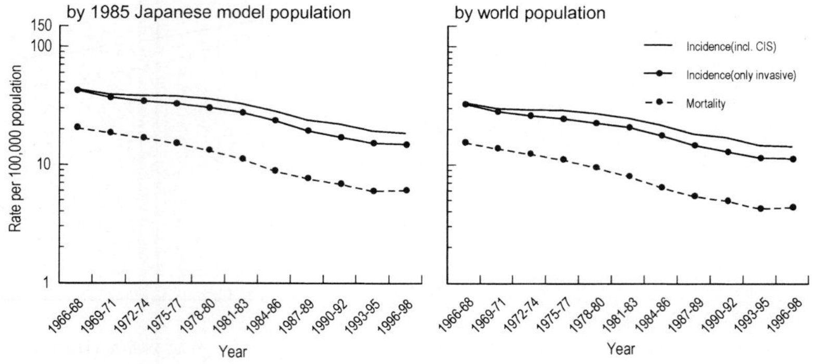

FIG. 10-1. Trends of incidence, mortality, and survival —uterus cancer—
Age-standardized incidence of and mortality from uterus cancer by sex, 1966–98

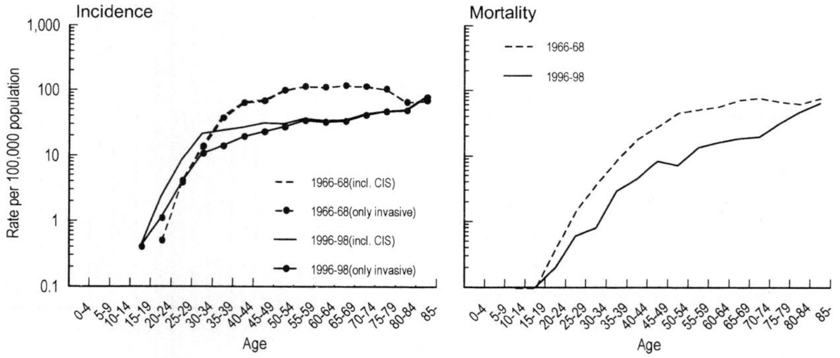

FIG. 10-2. Trends of incidence, mortality, and survival —uterus cancer—
Age-specific incidence of and mortality from uterus cancer by sex, 1966–68 and 1996–98

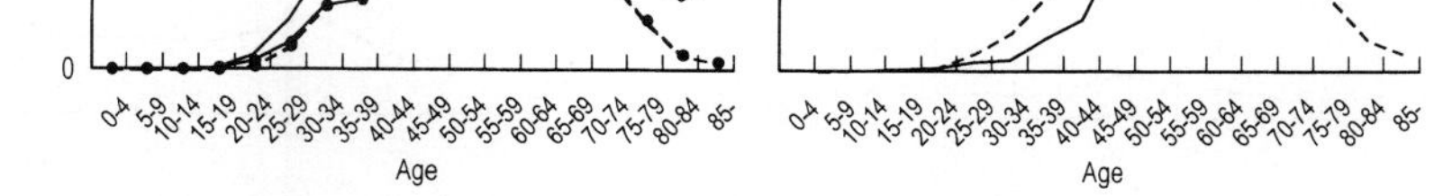

FIG. 10-3. Trends of incidence, mortality, and survival —uterus cancer—
Incidence of and mortality from uterus cancer: frequency distribution by age group, 1966–68 and 1996–98

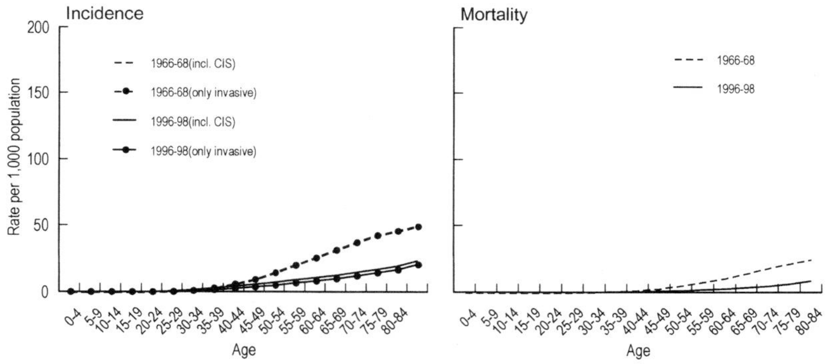

FIG. 10-4. Trends of incidence, mortality, and survival —uterus cancer—
Cumulative rate of incidence of and mortality from uterus cancer by age and sex, 1966–68 and 1996–98

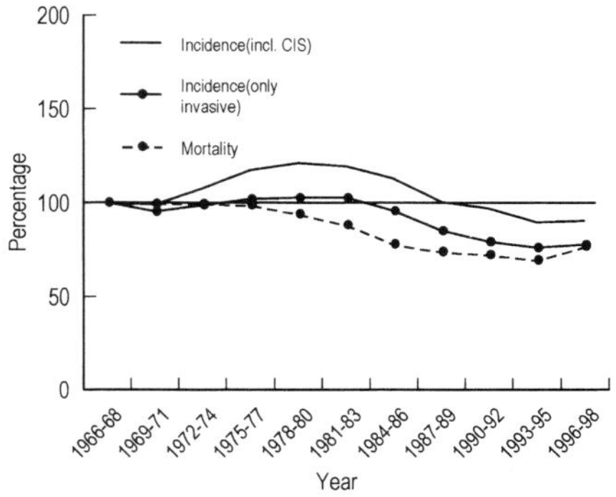

FIG. 10-5. Trends of incidence, mortality, and survival —uterus cancer—
The numbers of new cases of and deaths from uterus cancer by sex, 1966–98 (1966–68=100)

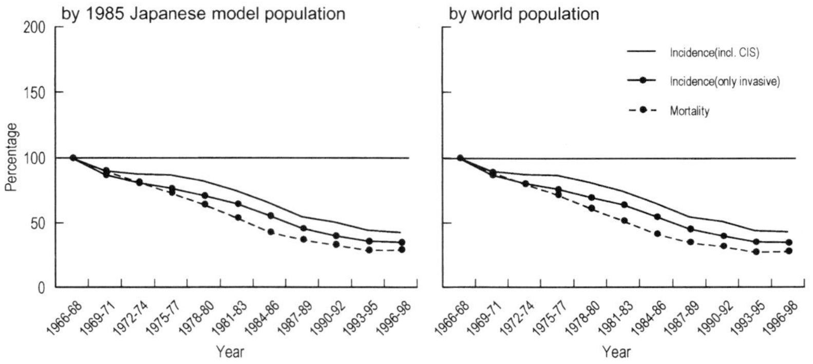

FIG. 10-6. Trends of incidence, mortality, and survival —uterus cancer—
Age-standardized incidence of and mortality from uterus cancer by sex, 1966–98 (1966–68=100)

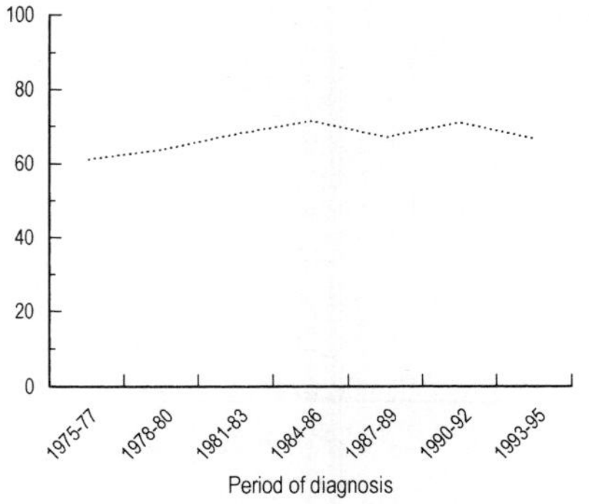

FIG. 10-S1. Trends of incidence, mortality, and survival —uterus cancer—
Relative 5-year survival (%), 1975–95

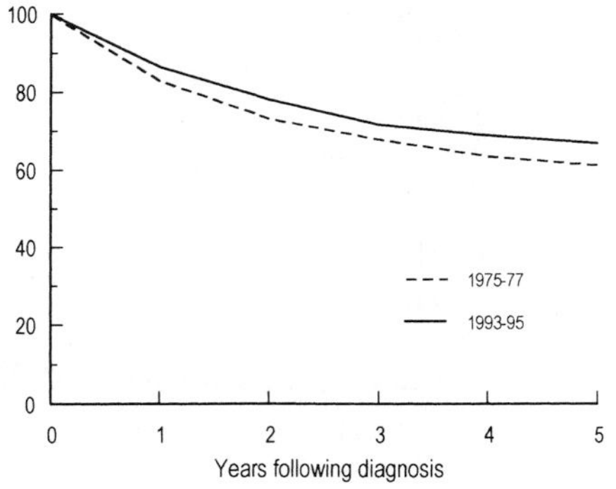

FIG. 10-S2. Trends of incidence, mortality, and survival —uterus cancer—
Relative survival (%), 1975–77 and 1993–95

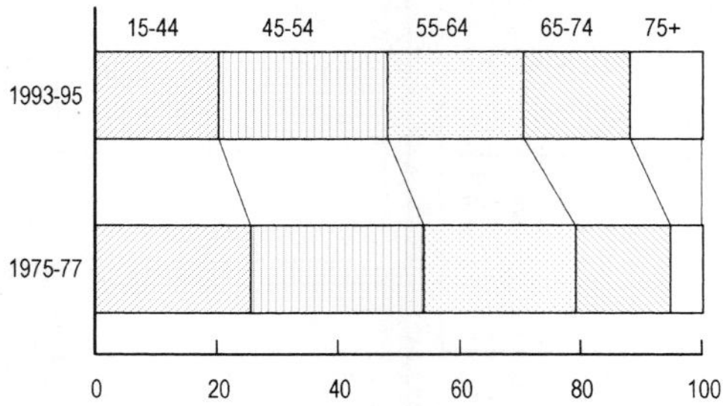

FIG. 10-S3. Trends of incidence, mortality, and survival —uterus cancer—
Age-distribution (%) in 1975–77 and 1993–95

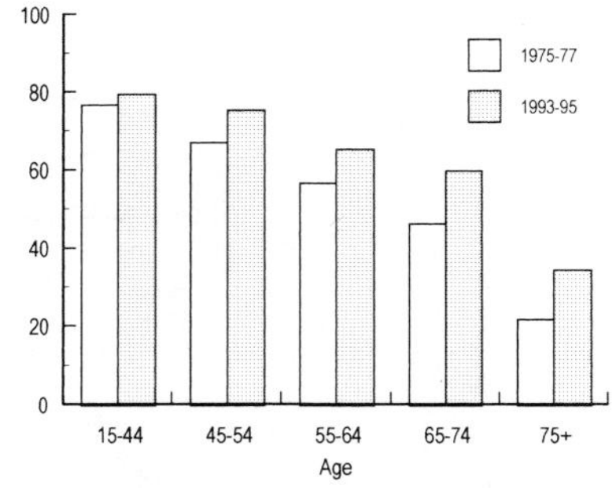

FIG. 10-S4. Trends of incidence, mortality, and survival —uterus cancer—
Relative 5-year survival (%) by age-group, 1975–77 and 1993–95

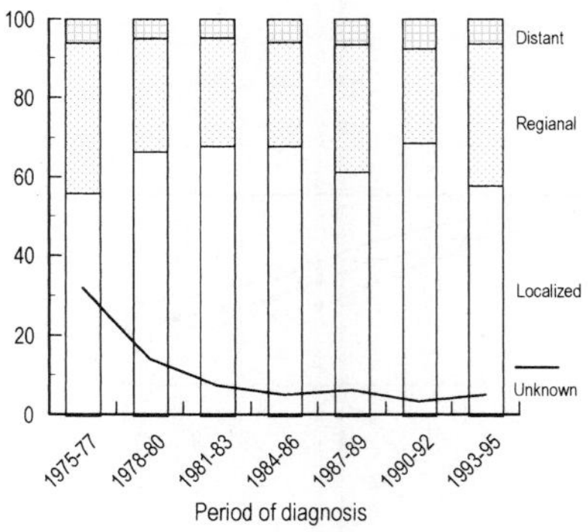

FIG. 10-S5. Trends of incidence, mortality, and survival —uterus cancer—
Stage-distribution (%), 1975–95

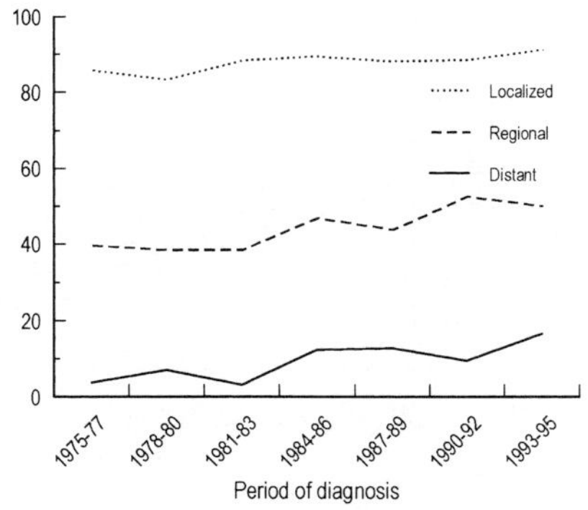

FIG. 10-S6. Trends of incidence, mortality, and survival —uterus cancer—
Relative 5-year survival (%) by stage, 1975–95

uterus showed RSR higher than 66% in 1993–1995. RSR for the colon, rectum, prostate, stomach, lymphatic tissue, and ovary were distributed from 36% to 60%. RSR for the lung, gallbladder, esophagus, liver, and pancreas were below 16%.

Table II shows RSR for cancer diagnosed in 1993–1995 according to stage at diagnosis: localized, regional and distant. The subjects for this table included those who resided in Osaka City at diagnosis. The prognosis for localized and regional cases has improved, while that for distant cases has changed little for most sites during these 21 years.

Trends of Incidence, Mortality, and Survival in Osaka

Trends of incidence, mortality, and survival for all sites, stomach, colorectal, liver, lung, female breast and uterus cancer are presented in Figs. 4–10. These figures include trends in age-standardized rates, age-specific rates, frequency distribution by age group, cumulative rate, changes in numbers (1966–68=100), changes in age-standardized rates (1966–68=100), RSR by sex, relative survival curves, age distribution, RSR by age-group, stage distribution, and RSR by stage.

Acknowledgments

The authors would like to acknowledge the Osaka Prefectural Government, the Osaka Medical Association, all medical institutions and health centers in Osaka Prefecture, and the Health Departments of Osaka City, Sakai City, and Higashi-osaka City. This study was supported in part by a grant-in-aid from the Ministry of Health, Labour and Welfare, Japan (14-2) .

REFERENCES

1. Ajiki, W., Matsuda, T., Sato, Y., Fujita, M., Yamazaki, S., Murakami, R., Tsukuma, H., and Oshima, A. Standard method of calculating survival rates in population-based cancer registries. *Jpn. J. Cancer Clin.*, **44**, 981–993 (1998).
2. Fujimoto, I., Hanai, A., Hiyama, T., Tsukuma, H., Takasugi, Y., and Sugaya, T. "Cancer Incidence and Mortality in Osaka 1963–1989" (1993). Shinohara Publishing Inc., Tokyo.
3. Oshima, A., Tsukuma, H., Ajiki, W., Kitano, M., Kitagawa, T., Tanaka, A., Sakamoto, M., Yahata, M., and Sasai, Y. "Survival of Cancer Patients in Osaka 1975–89" (1993). Shinohara Publishing, Inc., Tokyo.
4. Tanaka, H. and Tsukuma, H. Hepatitis C virus. *In* "Cancer Surveys vol. 33: Infections and Human Cancer," ed. R. Newton, V. Beral, and R. A. Weiss, pp. 213-235 (1999). Cold Spring Harbor Laboratory Press, New York.
5. Watanabe, S., Tominaga, S., and Kakizoe, T. (eds.). "Cancer Treatment and Survival," Gann Monograph on Cancer Research No. 43, p. 250 (1995). Japan Sci. Soc. Press, Tokyo/CRC Press, Boca Raton.

CANCER MORTALITY STATISTICS IN 30 COUNTRIES (1953–1997)

Tetsuo KUROISHI,[*1,*2] Kaoru HIROSE,[*1] Toshiro TAKEZAKI,[*3]
Suketami TOMINAGA,[*4] Kunio AOKI,[*1,*5] and Kazuo TAJIMA,[*1]

Division of Epidemiology and Cancer Prevention, Aichi Cancer Center Research Institute[*1], *Nagoya Preventive Medical Institute,*[*2] *School of Medicine, Kagoshima University,*[*3] *Foundation of Aichi Health Promotion,*[*4] *and Nagoya University*[*5]

Cancer mortality statistics from 1953–57 to 1993–97 in 30 countries of the world were compiled and calculated from data downloaded from the Mortality Data Base in the WHO (World Health Organization) Internet Web-site.

This report includes the following cancer mortality statistics:

1) Age-adjusted death rates for malignant neoplasms for 19 sites by sex and year for 30 countries of the world (1953–57 to 1993–97) (Tables I-1 to I-19).
2) Bar graphs showing age-adjusted death rates for malignant neoplasms for 19 sites by sex for 30 countries (1993–1997) (Figs. I-1 to I-19).
3) Line graphs for trends in age-adjusted death rates for malignant neoplasms for 19 sites by sex for 30 countries (1953–57 to 1993–1997) (Fig. II-1 to Fig. II-19).

The monograph "*Cancer Mortality and Morbidity Statistics—Japan and the World—*" (GANN Monograph on Cancer Research, No. 26) was published in 1981 by some of the present authors (*5*, *2*). This monograph included a chapter entitled; "World cancer mortality statistics in 56 countries from 1950 to 1975" (*5*). Since then, four monographs of "*Cancer Mortality Statistics*" have been published as UICC publications: in 1984, 1989, 1992 and 1998. The first one included cancer mortality statistics in 24 countries from 1950 to 1979, with age-specific death rates for 1978–1979 (*4*). The second was a revised edition of the first with data updated from 1980 to 1985 (*3*). The third was a monograph entitled "*Death Rates for Malignant Neoplasm for Selected Sites by Sex and Five-Year Age Groups in 33 Countries 1953–57 to 1983–87*" which included limited graphic illustrations and was compiled for use in time trend or cohort analyses of cancer mortality (*1*). The fourth was to update the third one with data from 1988 to 1992 (*7*).

To present more detailed graphical materials showing international comparisons of recent cancer mortality rates, together with time trends of cancer mortality by site

[*1] 1-1 Kanokoden, Chikusa-ku, Nagoya 464-8681, Japan
[*2] 4-23 Nagaosa-cho, Nakamura-ku, Nagoya 453-8521, Japan
[*3] 8-35-1 Sakuragaoda, Kagoshima 890-8520, Japan
[*4] 1-1 Gengoyama, Morioka, Higashiura-cho, Nagoya 462-0844, Japan
[*5] 65 Tsurumai-cho, Showa-ku, Nagoya 466-8550, Japan

TABLE A. Standard Population for Age-adjusted Death Rates (World Population)

All ages	100
0–4	12
5–9	10
10–14	9
15–19	9
20–24	8
25–29	8
30–34	6
35–39	6
40–44	6
45–49	6
50–54	5
55–59	4
60–64	4
65–69	3
70–74	2
75–79	1
80–84	0.5
85–	0.5

in each country, the report "Cancer Mortality in 33 Countries of the World (1953–1987)" was published in 1994 as one chapter in the monograph "*Cancer Mortality and Morbidity Statistics —Japan and the World— 1994*" (*6*). To update the data from 1988-1992, the report "Cancer Mortality in 33 Countries of the World (1953–1992)" was published in 1999 in the monograph "*Cancer Mortality and Morbidity Statistics —Japan and the World— 1999*" (*8*).

The main aim of this report is to update the data from 1993–1997, and to pro-

Site of malignant neoplasm	ICD				
	6th revision	7th revision	8th revision	9th revision	10th revision
All sites	140–205	140–205	140–209	140–208	C00–C97
Lip, oral cavity and pharynx	140–148	140–148	140–149	140–149	C00–C14
Esophagus	150	150	150	150	C15
Stomach	151	151	151	151	C16
Intestine, except rectum	152, 153	152, 153	152, 153	152, 153	C17, C18
Rectum, rectosigmoid junction and anus	154	154	154	154	C19–C21
Liver and intrahepatic bile ducts			155, 197.8	155	C22
Gallbladder and extrahepatic bile ducts		155.1	156	156	C23, C24
Pancreas	157	157	157	157	C25
Larynx	161	161	161	161	C32
Trachea, bronchus and lung	162, 163	162,163	162	162	C33, C34
Skin	190, 191	190, 191	172, 173	172, 173	C43, C44
Female breast	170	170	174	174	C50
Uterus (all parts)	171–174	171–174	180–182	179–182	C53–C55, C58
Ovary and other uterine adnexa	175	175	183	183	C56
Prostate	177	177	185	185	C61
Bladder	181	181	188	188	C67
Thyroid gland	194	194	193	193	C73
Leukemia	204	204	204–207	204–208	C91–C95

vide graphical material showing international comparisons and secular trends in cancer mortality rates by site and by sex. The original data on cancer mortality and population for each country of the world were downloaded from the Mortality Data Base in the WHO Internet Web-site. No recent mortality data in the former Czechoslovakia, the former Germany, Fed. Rep., the former Yugoslavia, England and Wales of the United Kingdom, Northern Ireland (UK) or Scotland (UK) were found in the Mortality Data Base on the WHO server. Neither those among Whites and Non-whites in the United States were found in the Mortality Data Base. So, mortality data in these countries and of races have been omitted from this report. Mortality data in Bulgaria, Germany, and Iceland are included in this paper. Age-adjusted death rates were calculated using the age distribution of Segi-Doll's World Population as a standard (Table A). Nineteen sites of malignant neoplasm were selected on the basis of frequency of disease and common interest. The International Classification of Diseases (ICD) category corresponding to each type of malignant neoplasm in the 6th to 10th revisions are listed as follows:

Age-adjusted death rates from malignant neoplasm by site in 30 countries (1953–57 to 1993–97).

Age-adjusted death rates for 19 selected sites of malignant neoplasm including all sites, from 1953–57 to 1993–97 in 30 countries, are given in Tables I-1 to I-19 Age-adjusted death rates for 1993–97 (the latest 5 year period) are illustrated by sex and site in Figs. I-1 to I-19 as a bar graph, in descending order. Trends in age-adjusted death rates for countries from 1953–1957 to 1993–1997 are illustrated by sex and site in Figs. II-1 to II-19. To avoid unduly complex figures, the trends in some coun-

			Site of malignant neoplasm	ICD (10th revision)
Table I-1	Fig. 1-1	Fig. 2-1	All sites	C00–C97
Table I-2	Fig. 1-2	Fig. 2-2	Lip, oral cavity and pharynx	C00–C14
Table I-3	Fig. 1-3	Fig. 2-3	Esophagus	C15
Table I-4	Fig. 1-4	Fig. 2-4	Stomach	C16
Table I-5	Fig. 1-5	Fig. 2-5	Intestine, except rectum	C17, C18
Table I-6	Fig. 1-6	Fig. 2-6	Rectum	C19–C21
Table I-7	Fig. 1-7	Fig. 2-7	Liver	C22
Table I-8	Fig. 1-8	Fig. 2-8	Biliary passages	C23, C24
Table I-9	Fig. 1-9	Fig. 2-9	Pancreas	C25
Table I-10	Fig. 1-10	Fig. 2-10	Larynx	C32
Table I-11	Fig. 1-11	Fig. 2-11	Trachea, bronchus and lung	C33, C34
Table I-12	Fig. 1-12	Fig. 2-12	Skin	C43, C44
Table I-13	Fig. 1-13	Fig. 2-13	Female breast	C50
Table I-14	Fig. 1-14	Fig. 2-14	Uterus (all parts)	C53–C55, C58
Table I-15	Fig. 1-15	Fig. 2-15	Ovary and other uterine adnexa	C56
Table I-16	Fig. 1-16	Fig. 2-16	Prostate	C61
Table I-17	Fig. 1-17	Fig. 2-17	Urinary Bladder	C67
Table I-18	Fig. 1-18	Fig. 2-18	Thyroid gland	C73
Table I-19	Fig. 1-19	Fig. 2-19	Leukemia	C91–C95

tries were omitted.

The contents of the tables and figures in this report are summarized in the following table.

Acknowledgments

We wish to acknowledge the support and assistance of the Statistical Information Office of the World Health Organization. We would like to express our thanks to Dr. J. L. Duppenthaler of WHO, for accessing and downloading the Mortality Data Base from the WHO Web-site. We would also like to extend our deep appreciation to the Japanese National Committee of the UICC for financial support.

REFERENCES

1. Aoki, K., Kurihara, M., Hayakawa, N., and Suzuki, S. (eds.) "Death Rates for Malignant Neoplasms for Selected Sites by Sex and Five-year Age Group in 33 countries 1953–57 to 1983–87," (1992). International Union against Cancer, The University of Nagoya Coop Press, Nagoya.
2. Aoki, K., Tominaga, S., and Kuroishi, T. Age-adjusted death rates for cancer by site (ICD, 8th revision) in 50 countries in 1975. *In* "Cancer Mortality and Morbidity Statistics: Japan and the World," ed. M. Segi *et al.*, GANN Monograph on Cancer Research No. 26, (1981). Japan Scientific Societies Press, Tokyo.
3. Kurihara, M., Aoki, K., and Hisamichi, S. (eds.) "Cancer Mortality Statistics in the World 1950–1985," (1989). The University of Nagoya Press, Nagoya.
4. Kurihara, M., Aoki, K., and Tominaga, S. (eds) "Cancer Mortality Statistics in the World 1950–1979," (1984). The University of Nagoya Press, Nagoya.
5. Segi, M., Aoki, K., and Kurihara, M. World cancer mortality. *In* "Cancer Mortality and Morbidity Statistics: Japan and the World," ed. M. Segi *et al.*, GANN Monograph on Cancer Research No. 26, (1981). Japan Scientific Societies Press, Tokyo.
6. Tominaga, S., Aoki, K., Fujimoto, I., and Kurihara, M. (eds.) *In* "Cancer Mortality and Morbidity Statistics —Japan and the World— 1994," GANN Monograph on Cancer Research No. 41, (1994). Japan Scientific Societies Press, Tokyo.
7. Tominaga, S., Kuroishi, T., and Aoki, K. (eds.) "Cancer Mortality Statistics in 33 Countries 1953–1992," (1998). International Union against Cancer, Roppo Shupan Co. Ltd., Nagoya.
8. Tominaga, S., and Oshima, A. (eds.) *In* "Cancer Mortality and Morbidity Statistics —Japan and the World— 1999," GANN Monograph on Cancer Research No. 47, (1999). Japan Scientific Societies Press, Tokyo.

TABLE I-1. Age-adjusted Death Rates of Cancer

1. All sites (male)

	Country	1953–1957	1958–1962	1963–1967	1968–1972	1973–1977	1978–1982	1983–1987	1988–1992	1993–1997
1	Australia	130.4	135.7	143.6	156.9	161.6	163.4	164.9	161.1	153.5
2	Austria	189.0[a]	193.5	195.0	193.4	187.8	184.8	177.8	174.3	163.2
3	Belgium	154.0[b]	169.0	183.5	193.8	202.1	213.3	209.2	200.5	194.2[h]
4	Bulgaria	—	—	138.9[f]	132.1	126.6	125.3	134.8	139.7	145.9
5	Canada	134.3	139.2	145.4	155.2	160.4	164.7	167.5	168.0	155.2
6	Chile	141.8[a]	150.7	155.9	162.8	153.6	145.1	141.9	140.4	143.0[i]
7	Costa Rica	—	142.2[c]	146.8	134.9	129.5	136.0	146.8	147.0	132.9[j]
8	Denmark	152.4	161.3	165.2	165.6	167.9	178.3	183.5	179.1	177.7
9	Finland	188.5	192.5	189.0	192.6	184.5	178.5	165.6	153.0	142.3
10	France	151.7	166.2	180.2	183.6	193.7	199.8	203.6	199.2	187.5
11	Germany	—	—	—	—	—	—	—	177.8[g]	171.1
12	Greece	—	108.1[c]	123.3	125.4	137.7	142.8	144.0	143.4	145.2
13	Hong Kong	—	128.1[d]	156.1	169.9	180.1	184.2	178.4	174.0	163.9
14	Hungary	137.4[a]	151.9	163.5	178.0	193.0	211.0	227.4	250.2	267.9
15	Iceland	141.0	149.7	130.2	129.6	130.9	126.5	135.6	144.8	136.5
16	Ireland	130.2	135.7	142.0	155.4	164.3	164.2	171.3	174.9	170.2
17	Italy	124.2	138.9	154.4	169.0	173.7	183.2	192.7	189.5	174.8
18	Japan	124.6	136.1	141.6	143.1	142.9	146.3	149.8	150.4	152.8
19	Mexico	—	48.2	49.0	54.3	59.1	66.7	75.6	82.8	84.4[j]
20	Netherlands	149.7	161.2	176.0	187.2	195.1	199.6	199.7	192.9	181.6
21	New Zealand	138.5	141.8	149.3	163.7	173.5	171.7	173.1	168.7	160.4
22	Norway	125.7	125.7	127.5	135.3	136.9	143.2	146.8	147.1	147.0
23	Poland	—	114.7[e]	142.2	154.8	164.2	177.2	194.6	203.3	205.0[h]
24	Portugal	95.0[a]	103.8	116.1	125.2	131.2	137.2	140.3	145.0	155.2
25	Singapore	110.1[a]	148.8	168.5	164.1	188.9	189.1	186.8	167.1	158.7
26	Spain	103.6	120.6	132.1	134.3	146.2	150.8	158.3	168.4	171.7
27	Sweden	118.8	128.8	128.8	136.1	147.0	139.5	129.0	128.9	124.2
28	Switzerland	170.8	170.4	171.1	176.5	179.0	176.0	177.2	170.2	151.0
29	U.K.	172.0	179.1	185.5	190.5	189.8	186.3	185.2	180.5	166.0
30	U.S.	138.1	142.3	149.8	157.0	161.0	164.0	164.2	164.2	157.4

[a]1955–57, [b]1954–57, [c]1958–60, [d]1960–62, [e]1959–62, [f]1964–67, [g]1990–92, [h]1993–96, [i]1993, 94, [j]1993–95.

by Site and Year (1953–57 to 1993–97)
1. All sites (female)

	Country	1953–1957	1958–1962	1963–1967	1968–1972	1973–1977	1978–1982	1983–1987	1988–1992	1993–1997
1	Australia	102.6	98.1	98.5	101.6	101.5	98.8	103.1	101.0	97.7
2	Austria	136.7[a]	133.3	132.3	127.9	121.8	115.0	112.1	107.3	101.1
3	Belgium	124.4[b]	125.0	122.7	118.9	114.3	114.8	110.0	105.5	102.2[h]
4	Bulgaria	—	—	86.8[f]	83.0	80.0	81.4	84.7	84.6	86.5
5	Canada	116.7	113.9	111.6	110.3	108.0	108.0	109.7	109.8	106.4
6	Chile	133.3[a]	137.2	143.7	142.1	125.1	115.2	112.8	109.3	106.4[i]
7	Costa Rica	—	127.9[c]	130.8	118.5	104.1	106.3	109.0	100.0	99.2[j]
8	Denmark	144.1	142.3	138.7	134.1	130.9	134.2	137.6	139.6	139.5
9	Finland	117.9	111.5	107.1	102.9	97.6	94.9	92.6	90.5	85.6
10	France	106.5	105.5	103.9	98.7	96.3	92.6	90.6	87.4	84.6
11	Germany	—	—	—	—	—	—	—	108.3[g]	104.3
12	Greece	—	71.4[c]	75.2	75.4	79.1	81.3	79.6	78.1	78.1
13	Hong Kong	—	88.9[d]	96.3	98.4	99.5	97.8	96.6	92.7	87.2
14	Hungary	116.4[a]	119.5	120.5	123.5	128.1	127.8	127.9	132.5	138.4
15	Iceland	115.5	128.3	125.5	122.3	111.0	109.6	112.7	113.9	117.8
16	Ireland	111.3	111.9	115.2	122.9	127.5	122.9	124.1	126.8	119.4
17	Italy	97.5	99.7	102.0	102.7	100.7	98.8	100.0	98.1	92.7
18	Japan	93.8	97.2	95.9	92.7	88.0	84.3	79.9	76.4	75.1
19	Mexico	—	72.4	68.2	71.7	73.2	74.1	78.7	79.1	79.1[j]
20	Netherlands	125.3	121.0	121.7	119.2	113.1	109.8	109.1	109.1	108.4
21	New Zealand	111.4	111.5	112.0	114.0	121.3	121.8	123.3	123.6	119.1
22	Norway	109.9	104.4	100.5	102.0	100.0	100.6	100.7	100.5	104.2
23	Poland	—	88.2[e]	104.5	103.9	101.7	103.6	106.6	107.7	107.6[h]
24	Portugal	77.3[a]	80.1	85.5	88.8	86.4	85.1	84.9	86.4	84.6
25	Singapore	72.3[a]	84.4	99.6	95.9	101.8	110.0	108.9	99.9	98.6
26	Spain	77.4	86.0	89.7	86.6	87.4	82.1	79.9	80.3	78.7
27	Sweden	111.8	111.6	107.3	109.1	110.6	105.6	98.4	97.6	94.9
28	Switzerland	122.2	117.0	112.3	110.5	104.7	103.0	101.0	97.2	89.2
29	U.K.	117.0	116.3	116.7	120.3	122.3	124.0	127.0	126.0	117.4
30	U.S.	114.0	109.3	108.0	107.4	106.3	106.9	109.5	110.6	108.7

[a] 1955–57, [b] 1954–57, [c] 1958–60, [d] 1960–62, [e] 1959–62, [f] 1964–67, [g] 1990–92, [h] 1993–96, [i] 1993, 94, [j] 1993–95.

TABLE I-2. Age-adjusted Death Rates of Cancer

2. Lip, oral cavity and pharynx (male)

	Country	1953–1957	1958–1962	1963–1967	1968–1972	1973–1977	1978–1982	1983–1987	1988–1992	1993–1997
1	Australia	4.0	3.3	3.5	3.9	4.2	4.3	4.8	4.6	4.1
2	Austria	3.5[a]	2.8	3.9	3.7	4.1	4.6	5.5	6.0	6.0
3	Belgium	2.7[b]	2.9	2.7	2.8	3.0	3.5	4.0	4.7	5.8[g]
4	Bulgaria	—	—	2.0[e]	2.0	1.8	2.1	3.2	4.0	4.6
5	Canada	4.7	4.2	4.2	4.4	4.3	4.4	4.5	4.3	3.8
6	Chile	1.7[a]	2.1	2.3	2.3	2.8	2.7	2.4	2.3	2.2[h]
7	Costa Rica	—	—	3.6	3.6	3.0	3.0	3.6	3.1	2.9[i]
8	Denmark	2.5	2.2	2.0	2.2	2.1	3.1	3.4	4.0	4.5
9	Finland	4.3	3.2	3.0	2.6	2.3	2.5	2.0	2.3	2.2
10	France	6.7	8.3	9.9	12.2	14.9	15.6	15.0	13.2	11.3
11	Germany	—	—	—	—	—	—	—	6.6[f]	6.5
12	Greece	—	—	1.4	1.5	1.5	1.7	1.8	1.7	1.9
13	Hong Kong	—	15.4[c]	17.9	18.8	19.6	17.7	15.6	14.0	11.6
14	Hungary	4.3[a]	4.1	4.1	4.5	5.5	7.9	11.1	15.4	19.2
15	Iceland	1.7	3.1	1.9	2.6	2.6	1.9	2.3	2.0	2.1
16	Ireland	7.6	6.1	4.6	4.5	4.2	4.0	4.4	4.4	4.7
17	Italy	5.1	5.4	5.6	6.0	5.9	6.2	6.6	6.0	5.3
18	Japan	1.3	1.3	1.4	1.6	1.7	1.9	2.1	2.3	2.9
19	Mexico	—	1.3	1.4	1.3	1.5	1.6	1.7	1.9	1.9[i]
20	Netherlands	1.9	1.8	1.8	1.9	1.9	2.0	2.4	2.8	2.8
21	New Zealand	3.6	3.4	2.6	3.3	3.3	4.0	3.9	3.7	3.0
22	Norway	3.2	2.9	2.7	3.1	2.8	2.5	3.0	3.1	3.0
23	Poland	—	2.5[d]	3.5	4.3	4.8	4.8	5.5	6.3	6.3[g]
24	Portugal	4.4[a]	4.5	4.9	4.9	5.0	5.0	5.1	5.7	6.5
25	Singapore	—	—	12.7	13.8	15.9	14.8	14.5	12.4	11.6
26	Spain	2.5	2.7	2.9	2.9	3.8	4.2	5.4	6.6	6.9
27	Sweden	2.2	2.3	2.3	2.3	2.5	2.7	2.7	2.5	2.2
28	Switzerland	6.4	6.9	6.8	6.0	6.6	6.5	6.8	6.4	5.2
29	U.K.	4.9	3.9	3.2	3.0	2.8	2.8	2.9	3.0	2.9
30	U.S.	4.7	4.7	4.7	4.8	4.7	4.5	4.0	3.6	3.3

[a] 1955–57, [b] 1954–57, [c] 1960–62, [d] 1959–62, [e] 1964–67, [f] 1990–92, [g] 1993–96, [h] 1993, 94, [i] 1993–95.

by Site and Year (1953–57 to 1993–97)
2. Lip, oral cavity and pharynx (female)

	Country	1953–1957	1958–1962	1963–1967	1968–1972	1973–1977	1978–1982	1983–1987	1988–1992	1993–1997
1	Australia	1.1	1.1	1.2	1.2	1.2	1.3	1.4	1.3	1.3
2	Austria	0.9[a]	0.8	1.0	0.8	0.7	0.6	0.9	0.9	1.1
3	Belgium	0.7[b]	0.7	0.7	0.6	0.7	0.8	1.0	1.0	1.3[g]
4	Bulgaria	—	—	0.7[e]	0.7	0.6	0.7	0.7	0.6	0.8
5	Canada	1.2	1.2	1.1	1.3	1.3	1.3	1.4	1.3	1.2
6	Chile	0.8[a]	0.9	0.8	0.9	0.8	0.6	0.6	0.6	0.6[h]
7	Costa Rica	—	—	1.2	1.1	0.9	0.8	1.3	1.0	1.1[i]
8	Denmark	0.9	1.0	1.0	1.0	1.0	1.4	1.4	1.4	1.5
9	Finland	1.8	1.6	1.1	1.1	1.1	1.2	0.9	0.8	1.0
10	France	0.7	0.8	0.8	1.0	1.1	1.2	1.3	1.3	1.3
11	Germany	—	—	—	—	—	—	—	1.1[f]	1.2
12	Greece	—	—	0.6	0.5	0.6	0.6	0.6	0.5	0.6
13	Hong Kong	—	6.8[c]	7.1	7.1	6.8	6.1	4.8	4.1	3.4
14	Hungary	1.0[a]	0.9	0.8	0.9	1.0	1.2	1.5	1.9	2.4
15	Iceland	2.1	1.9	2.0	1.4	1.5	1.1	0.8	0.9	1.0
16	Ireland	2.5	2.1	1.9	1.9	1.8	1.4	1.5	1.0	1.2
17	Italy	0.9	0.9	0.9	0.9	0.9	0.9	1.0	1.0	1.0
18	Japan	0.6	0.6	0.6	0.6	0.7	0.7	0.6	0.6	0.8
19	Mexico	—	0.6	0.5	0.6	0.7	0.7	0.7	0.7	0.7[i]
20	Netherlands	0.9	0.9	0.8	0.6	0.7	0.8	0.8	1.0	1.1
21	New Zealand	1.5	1.5	1.2	1.0	1.3	1.3	1.3	1.3	1.0
22	Norway	1.5	1.4	1.4	1.0	0.9	0.9	1.0	1.0	1.1
23	Poland	—	0.8[d]	1.0	1.0	1.0	1.0	1.0	1.0	1.1[g]
24	Portugal	0.9[a]	1.1	1.1	1.1	0.9	0.9	0.8	0.9	0.8
25	Singapore	—	—	5.2	4.8	5.4	5.3	5.1	4.0	3.6
26	Spain	0.5	0.5	0.6	0.6	0.6	0.6	0.7	0.8	0.9
27	Sweden	1.7	1.6	1.4	1.1	1.1	0.9	1.0	0.9	0.9
28	Switzerland	1.0	1.0	0.9	1.0	1.0	1.1	1.2	1.2	1.1
29	U.K.	1.7	1.6	1.5	1.4	1.3	1.3	1.3	1.2	1.1
30	U.S.	1.2	1.3	1.3	1.5	1.5	1.5	1.4	1.3	1.2

[a] 1955–57, [b] 1954–57, [c] 1960–62, [d] 1959–62, [e] 1964–67, [f] 1990–92, [g] 1993–96, [h] 1993, 94, [i] 1993–95.

TABLE I-3. Age-adjusted Death Rates of Cancer

3. Esophagus (male)

	Country	1953–1957	1958–1962	1963–1967	1968–1972	1973–1977	1978–1982	1983–1987	1988–1992	1993–1997
1	Australia	3.4	3.3	3.5	3.8	4.4	4.2	4.4	4.9	4.9
2	Austria	4.6[a]	4.4	4.3	4.3	3.8	3.9	3.8	3.7	3.7
3	Belgium	3.8[b]	3.7	3.9	3.7	3.8	4.3	4.8	4.8	5.5[g]
4	Bulgaria	—	—	1.6[e]	1.2	1.1	1.3	1.4	3.1	3.3
5	Canada	3.0	3.1	3.3	3.4	3.7	3.7	4.2	4.3	4.4
6	Chile	8.9[a]	8.6	10.4	10.9	10.0	9.2	8.3	7.7	7.4[h]
7	Costa Rica	—	—	5.7	4.3	4.6	2.9	4.1	4.3	3.7[i]
8	Denmark	3.6	3.1	2.8	2.7	3.2	3.5	4.5	5.1	5.7
9	Finland	8.5	6.8	5.6	4.7	3.7	3.6	2.9	3.0	3.0
10	France	10.8	12.6	14.3	14.2	14.3	13.3	12.4	11.0	9.2
11	Germany	—	—	—	—	—	—	—	5.0[f]	5.2
12	Greece	—	—	1.7	1.8	2.0	1.9	1.7	1.5	1.4
13	Hong Kong	—	9.4[c]	11.1	10.9	11.5	12.3	11.2	10.1	8.6
14	Hungary	2.6[a]	2.4	2.7	2.5	2.9	4.1	5.7	7.6	8.9
15	Iceland	8.0	6.5	5.7	4.6	4.1	3.1	4.7	4.0	5.7
16	Ireland	4.3	5.1	4.9	5.2	5.8	6.1	6.4	7.3	8.0
17	Italy	3.8	4.3	4.4	4.7	4.6	4.8	4.7	4.2	3.6
18	Japan	6.9	6.9	7.3	7.8	7.3	7.0	6.9	7.0	7.3
19	Mexico	—	1.3	1.3	1.5	1.6	1.6	1.8	2.0	2.0
20	Netherlands	3.7	3.2	3.0	2.9	3.1	3.4	4.2	5.3	6.2
21	New Zealand	3.7	3.5	4.0	3.8	5.1	4.7	4.7	5.3	5.8
22	Norway	3.2	3.0	2.5	2.5	2.6	2.6	2.4	3.0	2.9
23	Poland	—	4.4[d]	5.0	4.7	4.2	4.2	4.9	4.9	4.9[g]
24	Portugal	4.6[a]	4.7	5.5	5.5	6.0	5.8	6.0	5.5	5.4
25	Singapore	—	—	13.9	14.3	13.9	10.6	8.8	7.2	5.7
26	Spain	2.5	3.3	3.8	4.5	5.2	5.4	5.5	5.6	5.5
27	Sweden	2.8	2.5	2.5	2.8	2.9	2.9	2.9	2.9	2.9
28	Switzerland	12.8	11.2	9.5	8.6	7.4	6.6	5.8	5.4	5.0
29	U.K.	4.7	4.5	4.6	5.1	5.5	6.1	6.9	7.8	8.5
30	U.S.	3.7	3.8	3.9	3.9	4.2	4.4	4.5	4.7	4.9

[a] 1955–57, [b] 1954–57, [c] 1960–62, [d] 1959–62, [e] 1964–67, [f] 1990–92, [g] 1993–96, [h] 1993, 94, [i] 1993–95.

by Site and Year (1953–57 to 1993–97)
3. Esophagus (female)

	Country	1953–1957	1958–1962	1963–1967	1968–1972	1973–1977	1978–1982	1983–1987	1988–1992	1993–1997
1	Australia	1.2	1.3	1.4	1.6	1.7	1.7	1.8	1.7	1.7
2	Austria	0.9[a]	0.8	0.8	0.6	0.6	0.5	0.5	0.4	0.5
3	Belgium	1.3[b]	1.1	1.0	1.0	0.9	1.1	1.1	1.1	1.1[g]
4	Bulgaria	—	—	0.6[e]	0.6	0.4	0.4	0.4	1.1	0.9
5	Canada	1.2	1.2	1.2	1.2	1.1	1.2	1.1	1.2	1.2
6	Chile	3.8[a]	5.0	5.6	5.1	4.6	4.1	3.7	3.3	3.2[h]
7	Costa Rica	—	—	2.1	2.7	1.6	1.6	1.6	1.1	1.0[i]
8	Denmark	1.7	1.4	1.2	1.2	1.1	1.2	1.3	1.4	1.7
9	Finland	5.8	5.2	4.3	3.4	2.6	2.2	1.9	1.4	1.2
10	France	1.1	1.1	1.1	1.1	1.1	1.0	1.0	1.0	1.0
11	Germany	—	—	—	—	—	—	—	0.8[f]	1.0
12	Greece	—	—	0.6	0.7	0.7	0.6	0.5	0.5	0.4
13	Hong Kong	—	2.5[c]	2.4	3.5	2.9	2.3	2.0	1.7	1.4
14	Hungary	0.7[a]	0.5	0.5	0.5	0.5	0.6	0.6	0.7	0.9
15	Iceland	3.7	5.1	3.9	2.3	2.5	2.3	1.7	1.1	2.8
16	Ireland	3.3	3.3	4.0	4.2	4.0	3.9	3.7	3.8	3.5
17	Italy	0.9	0.8	0.8	0.8	0.8	0.8	0.8	0.7	0.6
18	Japan	2.3	2.2	2.2	2.0	1.7	1.4	1.1	1.0	0.9
19	Mexico	—	0.6	0.5	0.7	0.7	0.7	0.8	0.8	0.7[i]
20	Netherlands	1.5	1.4	1.2	1.2	1.1	1.2	1.4	1.6	2.0
21	New Zealand	1.9	1.7	1.8	1.9	2.1	2.0	1.9	2.1	1.9
22	Norway	1.0	0.6	0.8	0.7	0.7	0.6	0.6	0.7	0.7
23	Poland	—	1.3[d]	1.3	1.1	0.9	0.8	0.8	0.7	0.8[g]
24	Portugal	1.6[a]	1.7	1.9	2.0	1.8	1.6	1.4	1.1	0.9
25	Singapore	—	—	4.0	5.2	3.7	3.0	2.5	1.9	1.5
26	Spain	0.7	1.0	1.1	1.1	1.0	0.8	0.7	0.6	0.5
27	Sweden	1.4	1.1	1.0	0.9	0.9	0.8	0.8	0.9	0.8
28	Switzerland	1.5	1.4	1.1	1.1	0.9	0.9	1.0	1.1	1.0
29	U.K.	2.4	2.4	2.5	2.6	2.8	2.9	3.1	3.2	3.4
30	U.S.	0.9	0.9	1.0	1.1	1.1	1.2	1.2	1.1	1.1

[a] 1955–57, [b] 1954–57, [c] 1960–62, [d] 1959–62, [e] 1964–67, [f] 1990–92, [g] 1993–96, [h] 1993, 94, [i] 1993–95.

TABLE I-4. Age-adjusted Death Rates of Cancer

4. Stomach (male)

	Country	1953–1957	1958–1962	1963–1967	1968–1972	1973–1977	1978–1982	1983–1987	1988–1992	1993–1997
1	Australia	22.5	19.1	16.1	14.9	12.5	10.7	9.2	7.2	6.2
2	Austria	46.9[a]	46.2	41.8	36.4	29.9	25.5	20.6	16.5	13.3
3	Belgium	33.2[b]	31.0	27.6	23.4	19.0	16.4	13.0	10.0	8.3[g]
4	Bulgaria	—	—	39.8[e]	33.5	28.8	24.7	21.9	19.9	17.1
5	Canada	23.5	20.2	17.5	15.0	12.5	10.5	8.7	7.5	6.1
6	Chile	69.4[a]	67.8	62.1	62.1	52.0	42.7	35.3	33.7	32.4[h]
7	Costa Rica	—	—	60.4	52.6	48.3	45.7	45.9	46.8	37.9[i]
8	Denmark	31.2	26.8	21.6	17.2	14.7	12.2	9.9	7.5	6.4
9	Finland	59.6	49.1	38.8	31.3	24.7	20.2	16.0	12.5	10.0
10	France	27.6	25.2	22.0	18.0	15.2	12.5	10.6	8.7	7.1
11	Germany	—	—	—	—	—	—	—	14.2[f]	12.2
12	Greece	—	—	16.0	14.4	13.6	12.0	10.5	9.3	8.4
13	Hong Kong	—	18.6[c]	19.3	18.0	16.4	13.9	11.5	11.4	9.9
14	Hungary	47.3[a]	47.2	42.6	40.6	35.9	31.6	25.9	23.9	20.5
15	Iceland	69.9	59.1	42.2	34.3	31.6	20.5	21.7	17.4	11.2
16	Ireland	28.7	25.2	24.3	22.6	19.6	16.2	14.1	12.1	10.5
17	Italy	36.0	34.6	34.0	30.9	25.8	22.6	20.4	17.1	13.9
18	Japan	69.4	70.3	68.3	63.6	55.8	47.8	40.8	34.5	30.5
19	Mexico	—	8.6	9.0	10.2	9.5	9.5	9.7	10.2	9.9[j]
20	Netherlands	36.0	31.4	28.1	24.1	21.1	17.5	15.0	12.7	10.2
21	New Zealand	21.6	19.5	16.9	14.9	14.3	12.3	10.7	8.8	6.6
22	Norway	37.5	30.2	26.2	22.5	17.5	14.6	12.9	10.9	9.1
23	Poland	—	40.1[d]	43.7	39.7	35.0	30.4	26.8	22.7	19.3[h]
24	Portugal	29.3[a]	31.4	34.2	34.9	33.9	29.8	26.5	24.4	21.6
25	Singapore	—	—	39.0	31.3	33.5	26.4	23.9	19.4	16.4
26	Spain	28.2	29.9	31.1	27.3	24.6	19.2	16.1	14.2	12.5
27	Sweden	30.5	26.8	21.8	17.9	16.0	12.8	10.1	8.6	6.6
28	Switzerland	38.3	31.9	27.0	22.6	18.3	14.3	11.5	9.4	7.2
29	U.K.	28.0	26.3	23.9	21.6	19.4	16.9	14.8	12.4	9.7
30	U.S.	15.2	12.4	10.1	8.3	7.1	6.2	5.5	5.1	4.4

[a] 1955–57, [b] 1954–57, [c] 1960–62, [d] 1959–62, [e] 1964–67, [f] 1990–92, [g] 1993–96, [h] 1993, 94, [i] 1993–95.

by Site and Year (1953–57 to 1993–97)

4. Stomach (female)

	Country	1953–1957	1958–1962	1963–1967	1968–1972	1973–1977	1978–1982	1983–1987	1988–1992	1993–1997
1	Australia	12.2	9.7	8.1	7.6	6.2	4.7	4.0	3.3	2.8
2	Austria	28.0[a]	25.7	23.2	19.4	15.5	12.3	10.0	8.1	7.0
3	Belgium	19.9[b]	18.4	15.3	11.9	9.9	7.8	6.2	4.7	3.5[g]
4	Bulgaria	—	—	25.2[e]	19.9	16.3	14.2	12.0	10.7	8.7
5	Canada	12.1	9.9	8.1	6.9	5.6	4.6	3.9	3.3	2.8
6	Chile	45.2[a]	42.4	39.2	34.9	25.3	18.8	14.7	13.3	11.9[h]
7	Costa Rica	—	—	32.4	31.7	22.2	21.5	22.5	19.3	18.0[i]
8	Denmark	20.5	16.3	12.7	9.4	7.6	6.2	5.0	4.1	3.1
9	Finland	34.9	27.3	20.0	15.8	12.3	10.5	8.9	6.7	5.0
10	France	14.6	12.9	10.7	8.4	6.8	5.4	4.3	3.4	2.7
11	Germany	—	—	—	—	—	—	—	7.5[f]	6.4
12	Greece	—	—	9.5	8.3	7.7	6.6	5.5	4.9	4.3
13	Hong Kong	—	11.4[c]	11.2	8.9	7.7	6.8	6.5	5.4	5.0
14	Hungary	27.2[a]	25.7	22.7	20.3	17.1	14.0	11.3	10.1	9.2
15	Iceland	28.9	27.3	18.8	10.8	15.2	8.1	6.2	7.2	5.6
16	Ireland	19.2	17.0	16.1	14.8	11.9	8.8	7.0	5.9	5.0
17	Italy	20.7	18.7	17.5	15.2	12.6	10.7	9.5	8.1	6.6
18	Japan	37.0	37.0	35.3	33.2	28.5	23.6	19.0	15.2	12.6
19	Mexico	—	8.7	7.8	9.0	8.5	7.9	7.6	7.5	7.2[j]
20	Netherlands	22.5	17.1	15.1	11.9	9.6	7.4	6.1	4.9	4.2
21	New Zealand	12.8	9.9	8.2	6.9	6.3	5.5	4.8	4.1	3.3
22	Norway	21.6	17.5	14.4	11.8	9.0	7.4	6.3	5.0	4.2
23	Poland	—	19.6[d]	20.8	17.4	14.0	11.6	9.8	8.1	6.9[h]
24	Portugal	17.5[a]	17.8	19.5	19.2	17.4	14.5	12.9	11.9	10.0
25	Singapore	—	—	17.1	14.7	15.0	13.1	11.3	9.8	8.7
26	Spain	17.0	17.6	17.4	15.0	12.8	9.6	7.7	6.5	5.4
27	Sweden	19.3	14.8	11.8	9.8	8.1	6.7	5.3	4.3	3.6
28	Switzerland	23.4	19.0	14.9	11.6	9.0	7.0	5.3	4.2	3.2
29	U.K.	15.5	13.8	11.8	10.3	8.9	7.5	6.2	5.1	3.9
30	U.S.	7.8	6.3	5.0	4.0	3.3	2.9	2.5	2.3	2.1

[a] 1955–57, [b] 1954–57, [c] 1960–62, [d] 1959–62, [e] 1964–67, [f] 1990–92, [g] 1993–96, [h] 1993, 94, [i] 1993-95.

TABLE I-5. Age-adjusted Death Rates of Cancer

5. Intestine, except rectum (male)

	Country	1953–1957	1958–1962	1963–1967	1968–1972	1973–1977	1978–1982	1983–1987	1988–1992	1993–1997
1	Australia	13.2	12.6	12.7	13.6	14.9	15.1	15.7	14.9	14.8
2	Austria	11.0[a]	9.7	10.6	12.7	13.8	14.0	13.5	14.5	14.5
3	Belgium	11.1[b]	12.2	12.8	13.4	13.2	14.2	13.6	14.1	13.8[g]
4	Bulgaria	—	—	3.2[e]	3.7	4.2	5.0	5.4	6.8	7.0
5	Canada	13.7	13.9	14.1	14.8	14.9	13.9	13.3	13.1	12.1
6	Chile	2.9[a]	3.2	3.7	4.6	4.5	4.5	4.2	4.2	4.7[h]
7	Costa Rica	—	—	3.6	2.6	3.6	3.6	4.3	5.0	5.4[i]
8	Denmark	12.4	13.4	13.5	11.8	12.9	13.9	14.2	14.2	14.6
9	Finland	4.9	5.0	5.7	5.9	6.1	6.3	7.0	7.2	7.2
10	France	11.1	11.7	12.2	12.7	13.3	12.2	12.4	12.8	12.5
11	Germany	—	—	—	—	—	—	—	14.1[f]	14.1
12	Greece	—	—	4.6	4.8	5.6	5.0	4.9	6.0	7.0
13	Hong Kong	—	6.4[c]	7.5	8.3	8.4	8.3	9.4	9.9	11.0
14	Hungary	6.0[a]	6.6	7.8	9.6	11.8	12.8	14.1	17.1	18.7
15	Iceland	6.2	7.5	6.4	11.7	8.8	9.0	9.0	10.8	11.3
16	Ireland	12.9	12.1	12.4	14.2	15.5	14.8	15.7	17.0	16.0
17	Italy	5.8	7.4	8.6	10.2	11.0	9.0	9.8	10.2	11.2
18	Japan	2.4	2.8	3.3	4.1	5.2	6.3	7.8	9.3	10.4
19	Mexico	—	1.7	1.6	1.9	2.0	1.7	2.2	2.5	2.7[i]
20	Netherlands	9.5	9.7	10.9	11.4	12.4	12.7	13.8	13.8	14.0
21	New Zealand	13.0	12.7	13.3	15.9	16.3	15.8	15.8	15.7	15.1
22	Norway	7.3	8.0	8.3	9.7	8.8	10.0	11.0	12.7	12.4
23	Poland	—	2.8[d]	4.1	4.8	5.2	5.1	5.7	6.7	8.0[g]
24	Portugal	6.1[a]	6.5	7.9	8.4	8.8	8.6	8.8	9.9	12.1
25	Singapore	—	—	6.3	7.1	9.4	9.9	11.2	11.4	13.6
26	Spain	4.4	5.7	6.2	6.3	6.9	6.1	7.4	9.9	12.1
27	Sweden	9.6	9.8	10.0	10.9	11.8	10.4	10.0	9.8	9.1
28	Switzerland	11.5	11.2	11.8	12.5	12.4	12.3	12.7	12.6	11.2[g]
29	U.K.	14.5	12.9	12.5	13.0	12.9	12.2	12.7	13.0	11.9
30	U.S.	12.8	13.1	13.6	14.2	14.9	15.2	15.2	14.3	13.1

[a] 1955–57, [b] 1954–57, [c] 1960–62, [d] 1959–62, [e] 1964–67, [f] 1990–92, [g] 1993–96, [h] 1993, 94, [i] 1993–95.

by Site and Year (1953–57 to 1993–97)

5. Intestine, except rectum (female)

	Country	1953–1957	1958–1962	1963–1967	1968–1972	1973–1977	1978–1982	1983–1987	1988–1992	1993–1997
1	Australia	14.2	13.6	13.3	13.6	13.5	12.7	12.6	11.2	10.6
2	Austria	9.7[a]	8.3	9.2	10.3	11.0	10.2	10.0	9.5	8.7
3	Belgium	12.1[b]	13.1	12.8	13.0	12.4	11.8	10.7	10.5	9.8[g]
4	Bulgaria	—	—	3.0[e]	3.4	3.6	4.0	4.2	5.2	5.0
5	Canada	16.0	15.9	15.1	14.6	13.9	11.9	10.6	9.4	8.5
6	Chile	3.7[a]	4.3	4.6	5.3	5.1	4.4	4.5	4.4	4.6[h]
7	Costa Rica	—	—	4.5	2.7	4.3	4.3	4.2	5.5	5.6[i]
8	Denmark	13.5	13.8	13.3	12.7	12.2	12.7	12.4	12.3	11.7
9	Finland	5.4	5.6	5.7	6.3	6.1	6.0	5.9	5.6	5.5
10	France	11.3	11.0	10.5	10.0	9.9	8.3	8.0	7.9	7.5
11	Germany	—	—	—	—	—	—	—	10.8[f]	10.3
12	Greece	—	—	4.7	4.8	5.7	4.6	4.5	5.0	5.3
13	Hong Kong	—	5.1[c]	4.9	5.5	6.0	6.3	6.9	7.6	8.0
14	Hungary	6.2[a]	7.3	8.2	9.2	10.5	10.8	10.9	11.8	12.4
15	Iceland	8.3	7.3	8.1	11.3	8.9	8.9	7.8	7.8	8.1
16	Ireland	13.1	13.2	13.5	15.1	15.3	13.2	13.4	12.1	10.4
17	Italy	5.9	6.7	7.5	8.3	9.0	6.8	6.9	7.0	7.4
18	Japan	2.5	2.9	3.3	3.8	4.5	5.2	5.9	6.6	7.0
19	Mexico	—	2.6	2.2	2.5	2.5	2.0	2.2	2.4	2.8[i]
20	Netherlands	11.2	11.4	11.9	12.1	11.6	11.4	11.4	10.8	10.3
21	New Zealand	15.1	14.3	14.5	14.9	17.0	15.6	15.5	13.9	12.6
22	Norway	7.2	7.6	8.1	8.8	8.6	9.7	9.7	9.6	10.6
23	Poland	—	2.6[d]	3.9	4.1	4.3	4.1	4.6	5.1	5.9[g]
24	Portugal	7.2[a]	7.6	8.8	8.5	8.2	7.1	6.7	7.3	7.7
25	Singapore	—	—	5.3	6.0	7.7	9.9	10.9	10.4	10.7
26	Spain	5.2	6.5	6.9	6.6	6.6	5.2	5.6	6.9	7.7
27	Sweden	8.9	9.7	9.1	9.4	9.7	9.1	8.0	8.1	7.5
28	Switzerland	9.5	9.2	9.2	8.8	8.8	8.6	8.6	8.0	6.7[g]
29	U.K.	14.1	13.0	12.2	12.3	11.9	10.8	10.5	10.0	8.6
30	U.S.	13.5	13.3	13.0	12.6	12.3	11.6	11.0	10.0	9.2

[a] 1955–57, [b] 1954–57, [c] 1960–62, [d] 1959–62, [e] 1964–67, [f] 1990–92, [g] 1993–96, [h] 1993, 94, [i] 1993–95.

TABLE I-6. Age-adjusted Death Rates of Cancer

6. Rectum (Male)

	Country	1953–1957	1958–1962	1963–1967	1968–1972	1973–1977	1978–1982	1983–1987	1988–1992	1993–1997
1	Australia	6.4	6.1	5.9	6.1	6.2	6.3	6.3	6.0	5.5
2	Austria	8.5[a]	8.6	9.0	9.8	10.0	9.5	8.8	8.6	7.9
3	Belgium	9.6[b]	9.9	9.2	8.8	7.9	7.1	6.6	5.2	4.5[g]
4	Bulgaria	—	—	3.7[e]	4.5	5.5	6.9	8.8	9.0	10.5
5	Canada	7.8	7.2	7.0	7.0	6.4	5.9	5.2	4.6	4.0
6	Chile	2.2[a]	2.2	2.4	2.7	2.5	2.5	2.6	2.2	2.2[h]
7	Costa Rica	—	—	1.9	1.9	1.2	1.7	2.5	2.1	1.9[i]
8	Denmark	12.5	12.3	11.2	10.5	10.2	10.5	9.6	8.7	8.6
9	Finland	4.6	4.6	5.3	5.7	5.8	5.9	5.7	5.7	5.4
10	France	6.9	7.1	7.2	7.0	7.1	6.7	5.9	5.0	4.3
11	Germany	—	—	—	—	—	—	—	7.4[f]	7.1
12	Greece	—	—	0.6	0.8	0.7	0.9	0.8	0.9	1.0
13	Hong Kong	—	3.9[c]	4.4	4.9	4.9	5.6	5.7	5.7	6.3
14	Hungary	5.6[a]	6.0	7.1	7.8	9.1	11.0	12.3	13.1	14.7
15	Iceland	2.0	3.1	4.0	4.7	3.3	4.1	2.5	3.1	2.4
16	Ireland	8.5	7.4	7.4	8.0	8.3	7.8	7.1	6.2	6.2
17	Italy	4.0	4.5	5.4	6.0	6.2	6.0	5.9	5.5	5.0
18	Japan	4.3	4.4	4.8	5.3	5.9	6.1	6.2	6.4	6.7
19	Mexico	—	0.9	0.8	0.8	0.7	0.7	0.8	0.8	0.8[i]
20	Netherlands	7.3	7.1	6.9	6.9	7.0	6.3	5.6	4.8	4.4
21	New Zealand	7.8	7.6	7.9	8.6	9.3	10.0	10.6	10.4	9.7
22	Norway	5.1	4.6	5.4	6.2	7.0	8.1	8.2	8.1	8.0
23	Poland	—	2.3[d]	3.3	4.4	5.6	7.1	8.0	8.8	8.7[g]
24	Portugal	3.4[a]	3.7	3.9	4.9	6.2	6.0	5.3	5.6	6.2
25	Singapore	—	—	6.8	6.2	8.2	7.4	7.4	7.4	7.2
26	Spain	2.2	2.7	3.0	3.5	4.2	4.4	4.2	4.3	4.5
27	Sweden	6.3	6.8	6.3	6.4	6.9	6.1	5.4	5.3	5.1
28	Switzerland	9.0	8.4	7.7	8.3	7.2	6.5	6.1	5.5	4.9[g]
29	U.K.	11.0	10.0	9.4	9.3	9.0	8.6	8.2	7.7	6.6
30	U.S.	6.6	6.0	5.4	4.9	4.2	3.4	2.9	2.6	2.6

[a] 1955–57, [b] 1954–57, [c] 1960–62, [d] 1959–62, [e] 1964–67, [f] 1990–92, [g] 1993–96, [h] 1993, 94, [i] 1993–95.

by Site and Year (1953–57 to 1993–97)
6. Rectum (female)

	Country	1953–1957	1958–1962	1963–1967	1968–1972	1973–1977	1978–1982	1983–1987	1988–1992	1993–1997
1	Australia	4.0	3.8	3.6	3.7	3.7	3.6	3.4	3.0	2.8
2	Austria	4.9[a]	4.9	5.5	5.5	5.6	5.4	5.0	4.7	3.9
3	Belgium	6.0[b]	5.9	5.8	5.3	4.7	4.3	3.7	2.8	2.4[g]
4	Bulgaria	—	—	2.9[e]	3.4	3.7	4.7	5.8	5.9	6.7
5	Canada	4.7	4.7	4.5	4.1	3.5	3.3	2.8	2.3	2.0
6	Chile	2.3[a]	2.1	2.3	2.4	2.1	2.2	2.1	1.7	1.8[h]
7	Costa Rica	—	—	2.0	1.7	1.8	2.4	2.1	1.8	1.4[i]
8	Denmark	7.2	6.9	6.7	6.3	6.2	5.9	5.6	5.1	4.8
9	Finland	3.6	3.6	4.3	4.0	4.1	3.6	3.6	3.3	3.0
10	France	3.8	3.8	3.8	3.6	3.4	3.4	2.9	2.5	2.3
11	Germany	—	—	—	—	—	—	—	4.5[f]	4.1
12	Greece	—	—	0.6	0.6	0.7	0.6	0.7	0.6	0.8
13	Hong Kong	—	2.8[c]	2.8	2.9	2.9	3.7	3.6	3.5	3.7
14	Hungary	4.2[a]	4.6	4.8	5.4	5.7	6.9	7.0	6.8	6.8
15	Iceland	2.6	2.0	2.8	1.8	3.2	2.5	2.1	2.1	1.6
16	Ireland	4.2	4.3	4.0	4.5	4.4	4.1	3.4	2.9	2.8
17	Italy	2.8	3.1	3.3	3.7	3.8	3.7	3.4	3.2	2.8
18	Japan	3.2	3.4	3.5	3.8	3.9	3.7	3.4	3.3	3.0
19	Mexico	—	1.0	0.9	0.9	0.7	0.7	0.7	0.7	0.6[i]
20	Netherlands	5.1	4.7	4.6	4.4	4.0	3.6	3.1	2.6	2.6
21	New Zealand	4.8	5.2	5.1	5.1	6.1	6.3	5.6	5.6	5.3
22	Norway	3.1	3.0	3.4	4.0	4.5	4.9	4.9	4.5	4.7
23	Poland	—	1.7[d]	2.5	3.2	4.0	5.1	5.6	5.5	5.4[g]
24	Portugal	2.4[a]	2.6	2.8	3.5	4.0	3.2	2.9	3.0	2.9
25	Singapore	—	—	3.1	3.5	4.8	5.5	4.5	4.2	4.2
26	Spain	1.9	2.2	2.4	2.5	2.9	2.9	2.7	2.6	2.4
27	Sweden	3.8	3.8	3.9	3.9	4.0	3.5	3.5	3.3	3.1
28	Switzerland	4.6	4.1	3.8	3.9	3.7	3.6	3.2	2.7	2.9[g]
29	U.K.	6.0	5.7	5.5	5.4	5.2	4.8	4.5	4.0	3.3
30	U.S.	4.5	3.9	3.4	3.0	2.5	2.0	1.7	1.5	1.5

[a] 1955–57, [b] 1954–57, [c] 1960–62, [d] 1959–62, [e] 1964–67, [f] 1990–92, [g] 1993–96, [h] 1993, 94, [i] 1993–95.

TABLE I-7. Age-adjusted Death Rates of Cancer

7. Liver and intrahepatic bile ducts (male)

	Country	1953–1957	1958–1962	1963–1967	1968–1972	1973–1977	1978–1982	1983–1987	1988–1992	1993–1997
1	Australia	—	—	—	1.6	1.7	—	2.4	2.7	3.2
2	Austria	—	—	—	—	5.0	5.6	6.2	6.7	7.0
3	Belgium	—	—	—	5.3[a]	4.5	—	—	—	4.2[j]
4	Bulgaria	—	—	—	—	—	—	—	—	—
5	Canada	—	—	—	2.4[a]	2.3	2.3	2.7	3.2	3.6
6	Chile	—	—	—	—	—	—	—	—	—
7	Costa Rica	—	—	—	—	—	—	—	—	—
8	Denmark	—	—	—	3.3[a]	3.1	2.8[d]	—	3.3	3.5
9	Finland	—	—	—	3.6[a]	3.8	3.7	4.3[g]	—	—
10	France	—	—	—	7.3	7.1	7.4	8.6	10.1	11.0
11	Germany	—	—	—	—	—	—	—	4.4[i]	4.6
12	Greece	—	—	—	16.7	18.2	17.8	15.9	14.1	12.0
13	Hong Kong	—	—	—	—	—	—	—	—	—
14	Hungary	—	—	—	7.3[b]	7.9	8.2[e]	8.0	8.4	8.2
15	Iceland	—	—	—	—	3.0	1.7	2.4	3.1	3.0
16	Ireland	—	—	—	2.5[c]	2.9	2.2	2.8	2.8	3.1
17	Italy	—	—	—	10.9	10.2	9.6	11.1	12.9	13.0
18	Japan	—	—	—	12.4	12.7	15.5	18.8	20.6	21.9
19	Mexico	—	—	—	—	—	—	—	—	—
20	Netherlands	—	—	—	—	2.3	1.8	1.7	1.8	2.1
21	New Zealand	—	—	—	2.0	2.1	2.4	2.5	2.9	3.1
22	Norway	—	—	—	1.9[a]	1.5	1.6	1.6	1.4	1.4
23	Poland	—	—	—	—	—	—	—	—	—
24	Portugal	—	—	—	—	—	—	4.3[h]	4.4	5.0
25	Singapore	—	—	—	24.2[a]	26.3	28.5[f]	24.5	—	19.8
26	Spain	—	—	—	—	9.9	9.3	8.8	8.8	8.4
27	Sweden	—	—	—	—	—	—	—	4.1	4.0
28	Switzerland	—	—	—	4.1[a]	4.2	—	5.2	5.3	5.8
29	U.K.	—	—	—	—	—	1.7[e]	1.9	2.2	2.5
30	U.S.	—	—	—	—	—	2.5[e]	2.7	3.2	3.9

[a] 1969–72, [b] 1970–72, [c] 1968, 69, 71, 72, [d] 1978–81, [e] 1979–82, [f] 1978, 79, 81, 82, [g] 1983–86, [h] 1984–87, [i] 1990–92, [j] 1993–95.

by Site and Year (1953–57 to 1993–97)
7. Liver and intrahepatic bile ducts (female)

	Country	1953–1957	1958–1962	1963–1967	1968–1972	1973–1977	1978–1982	1983–1987	1988–1992	1993–1997
1	Australia	—	—	—	0.7	0.8	—	0.9	1.0	1.2
2	Austria	—	—	—	—	2.3	2.3	2.2	2.0	2.2
3	Belgium	—	—	—	3.8[a]	2.9	—	—	—	1.8[j]
4	Bulgaria	—	—	—	—	—	—	—	—	—
5	Canada	—	—	—	1.4[a]	1.3	1.2	1.3	1.5	1.5
6	Chile	—	—	—	—	—	—	—	—	—
7	Costa Rica	—	—	—	—	—	—	—	—	—
8	Denmark	—	—	—	2.1[a]	2.0	2.2[d]	—	2.0	2.2
9	Finland	—	—	—	1.9[a]	2.0	2.4	2.1[g]	—	—
10	France	—	—	—	4.0	3.1	2.4	2.1	2.0	2.1
11	Germany	—	—	—	—	—	—	—	1.9[i]	1.8
12	Greece	—	—	—	9.1	8.9	8.4	7.3	6.4	5.2
13	Hong Kong	—	—	—	—	—	—	—	—	—
14	Hungary	—	—	—	5.3[b]	4.7	3.9[e]	3.8	3.7	3.8
15	Iceland	—	—	—	—	1.2	1.3	2.3	1.2	1.6
16	Ireland	—	—	—	2.0[c]	2.2	1.3	1.9	1.6	1.6
17	Italy	—	—	—	7.7	6.7	5.5	5.2	5.1	4.7
18	Japan	—	—	—	6.2	5.4	5.2	5.2	5.3	6.0
19	Mexico	—	—	—	—	—	—	—	—	—
20	Netherlands	—	—	—	—	1.4	1.0	0.8	0.8	1.0
21	New Zealand	—	—	—	1.0	1.0	1.1	1.0	1.2	1.2
22	Norway	—	—	—	1.0[a]	0.8	0.9	0.9	0.9	0.8
23	Poland	—	—	—	—	—	—	—	—	—
24	Portugal	—	—	—	—	—	—	2.4[h]	1.9	2.0
25	Singapore	—	—	—	8.3[a]	7.3	8.0[f]	7.7	—	5.7
26	Spain	—	—	—	—	8.3	6.3	4.8	3.9	3.2
27	Sweden	—	—	—	—	—	—	—	2.5	2.4
28	Switzerland	—	—	—	1.5[a]	1.5	—	1.3	1.4	1.6
29	U.K.	—	—	—	—	—	0.8[e]	1.0	1.1	1.3
30	U.S.	—	—	—	—	—	1.2[e]	1.3	1.4	1.7

[a] 1969–72, [b] 1970–72, [c] 1968, 69, 71, 72, [d] 1978–81, [e] 1979–82, [f] 1978, 79, 81–82, [g] 1983–86, [h] 1984–87, [i] 1990–92, [j] 1993–95.

TABLE I-8. Age-adjusted Death Rates of Cancer

8. Gallbladder and extrahepatic bile ducts (male)

	Country	1953–1957	1958–1962	1963–1967	1968–1972	1973–1977	1978–1982	1983–1987	1988–1992	1993–1997
1	Australia	—	—	—	1.5	1.4	1.4	1.2	1.1	0.9
2	Austria	—	—	—	3.2[c]	3.0	3.2	2.6	2.5	2.3
3	Belgium	—	—	—	1.5	1.8	1.8	1.8[h]	—	1.1[m]
4	Bulgaria	—	—	—	1.1	1.0	0.8	0.8[i]	0.6	0.9
5	Canada	—	1.6	1.4	1.5	1.5	1.5	1.3	1.2	0.9
6	Chile	—	—	—	—	—	—	—	—	—
7	Costa Rica	—	—	—	—	—	—	—	—	—
8	Denmark	—	—	—	1.7[c]	1.6	1.6	1.4	1.4	0.9
9	Finland	2.1[a]	1.4	0.9	1.3	1.5	2.1	2.0	1.6[j]	1.5
10	France	0.7[a]	0.9	0.9	1.0	1.1	1.2	1.4	1.5	1.2
11	Germany	—	—	—	—	—	—	—	2.3[k]	2.2
12	Greece	—	—	—	0.3	0.4	0.3	0.3	0.6	0.7
13	Hong Kong	—	—	—	1.6[c]	2.5	3.1[e]	2.9	2.8[l]	2.0
14	Hungary	—	—	—	2.8[d]	3.1	3.5	3.9	3.8	3.6
15	Iceland	—	—	—	—	1.0	1.2	1.8	0.8	0.5
16	Ireland	—	—	—	1.0	1.0	1.3	1.0	0.9	0.7
17	Italy	—	0.9	0.8	1.1	1.2	1.4	1.8	2.0	2.0
18	Japan	—	1.5	2.3	2.9	3.6	4.3	5.3	5.8	5.8
19	Mexico	—	—	—	—	—	—	—	—	—
20	Netherlands	—	—	—	2.3[c]	2.2	2.3	1.9	1.5	1.2
21	New Zealand	—	—	—	1.5	1.7	1.2	1.2	1.0	1.0
22	Norway	—	—	—	1.0[c]	0.9	1.0	1.1	0.8	1.1
23	Poland	—	—	—	—	—	—	—	—	—
24	Portugal	—	—	—	—	—	—	1.3[i]	1.5	1.4
25	Singapore	—	—	—	0.8[c]	0.8	1.1[f]	0.8	0.8	1.2
26	Spain	—	—	—	1.0	0.7	0.9	1.2	1.3	1.3
27	Sweden	—	1.4	1.7[b]	1.9	2.3	2.4	2.5	2.4	2.2
28	Switzerland	—	—	—	1.6[c]	1.7	1.8	1.7	1.5	—
29	U.K.	—	—	—	1.2	1.2	1.0	0.9	0.7	0.5
30	U.S.	—	—	1.4	1.3	1.2	1.1[g]	1.0	0.8	0.7

[a] 1955–57, [b] 1963–66, [c] 1969–72, [d] 1970–72, [e] 1978–81, [f] 1978, 79, 81, 82, [g] 1979–82, [h] 1983, 84, 86, [i] 1984–87, [j] 1989–92, [k] 1990–92, [l] 1988, 89, 91, 92, [m] 1993–96.

by Site and Year (1953–57 to 1993–97)
8. Gallbladder and extrahepatic bile ducts (female)

	Country	1953–1957	1958–1962	1963–1967	1968–1972	1973–1977	1978–1982	1983–1987	1988–1992	1993–1997
1	Australia	—	—	—	2.0	1.9	1.6	1.6	1.4	1.3
2	Austria	—	—	—	5.8[c]	5.2	5.0	4.3	3.6	3.0
3	Belgium	—	—	—	2.1	2.4	2.3	2.2[h]	—	1.3[m]
4	Bulgaria	—	—	—	1.4	1.5	1.4	1.4[i]	1.2	1.1
5	Canada	—	2.7	2.5	2.3	2.1	1.8	1.6	1.4	1.2
6	Chile	—	—	—	—	—	—	—	—	—
7	Costa Rica	—	—	—	—	—	—	—	—	—
8	Denmark	—	—	—	2.9[c]	2.8	2.5	2.4	1.9	1.3
9	Finland	2.1[a]	1.8	1.7	2.5	3.2	3.5	3.5	2.6[j]	2.4
10	France	1.2[a]	1.4	1.4	1.5	1.6	1.7	1.8	1.6	1.4
11	Germany	—	—	—	—	—	—	—	3.5[k]	3.1
12	Greece	—	—	—	0.4	0.5	0.6	0.5	0.7	0.7
13	Hong Kong	—	—	—	1.0[c]	1.7	2.1[e]	2.1	2.2[l]	1.8
14	Hungary	—	—	—	7.1[d]	7.6	8.1	7.8	7.2	6.1
15	Iceland	—	—	—	—	1.1	2.4	1.3	0.9	1.3
16	Ireland	—	—	—	1.9	2.0	1.7	1.4	1.4	1.0
17	Italy	—	1.3	1.3	1.7	1.7	2.1	2.4	2.7	2.6
18	Japan	—	1.5	2.3	3.1	3.8	4.5	5.3	5.4	4.8
19	Mexico	—	—	—	—	—	—	—	—	—
20	Netherlands	—	—	—	4.3[c]	3.7	3.5	2.8	2.1	1.6
21	New Zealand	—	—	—	2.0	1.8	1.7	1.4	1.2	1.0
22	Norway	—	—	—	1.3[c]	1.2	1.2	1.3	1.0	1.2
23	Poland	—	—	—	—	—	—	—	—	—
24	Portugal	—	—	—	—	—	—	1.5[i]	1.5	1.6
25	Singapore	—	—	—	0.8[c]	1.2	1.1[f]	0.9	0.7	1.4
26	Spain	—	—	—	0.9	1.3	1.6	2.0	2.0	1.9
27	Sweden	—	2.5	3.4[b]	3.8	4.0	4.4	4.3	4.1	3.4
28	Switzerland	—	—	—	3.0[c]	3.0	2.9	2.5	2.2	—
29	U.K.	—	—	—	1.4	1.3	1.1	1.0	0.8	0.6
30	U.S.	—	—	2.1	1.8	1.5	1.3[g]	1.2	1.0	0.9

[a] 1955–57, [b] 1963–66, [c] 1969–72, [d] 1970–72, [e] 1978–81, [f] 1978, 79, 81, 82, [g] 1979–82, [h] 1983, 84, 86, [i] 1984–87, [j] 1989–92, [k] 1990–92, [l] 1988, 89, 91, 92, [m] 1993–96.

TABLE I-9. Age-adjusted Death Rates of Cancer

9. Pancreas (male)

	Country	1953–1957	1958–1962	1963–1967	1968–1972	1973–1977	1978–1982	1983–1987	1988–1992	1993–1997
1	Australia	6.1[a]	6.7	7.2	7.8	8.0	7.6	7.0	6.6	6.2
2	Austria	6.1[a]	7.1	7.4	8.1	8.3	8.7	9.0	8.8	9.2
3	Belgium	3.7[a]	4.7	5.5	6.4	7.5[c]	7.9[d]	7.5	7.4	7.4[g]
4	Bulgaria	—	—	—	3.7	4.0	4.9	6.0	6.5	6.9
5	Canada	7.2[a]	7.9	8.4	9.1	8.9	9.0	8.6	7.8	7.1
6	Chile	2.6[a]	3.1	4.0	—	—	—	—	—	—
7	Costa Rica	—	—	—	—	—	—	—	—	—
8	Denmark	6.3[a]	7.2	7.9	9.3	9.3	9.2	9.1	8.5	7.6
9	Finland	5.8[a]	7.3	7.9	9.9	9.9	9.5	9.8	9.0	8.6
10	France	3.9[a]	4.5	5.2	5.9	6.6	7.0	7.1	7.4	7.4
11	Germany	—	—	—	—	—	—	—	8.2[f]	8.2
12	Greece	—	—	—	3.2	4.0	4.8	5.6	6.0	6.0
13	Hong Kong	—	—	—	4.1	4.1	4.5	4.1	4.1	4.0
14	Hungary	—	—	—	7.1[b]	7.9	9.1	9.8	10.8	11.4
15	Iceland	—	—	—	—	10.3	9.1	9.6	9.8	8.2
16	Ireland	5.8[a]	6.0	7.4	8.3	8.8	8.7	9.0	8.8	7.7
17	Italy	2.9[a]	3.5	4.0	4.9	5.6	6.3	7.0	7.5	7.3
18	Japan	2.1[a]	3.0	4.1	5.4	6.0	7.0	8.0	8.4	8.5
19	Mexico	—	—	—	—	—	—	—	—	—
20	Netherlands	4.5[a]	5.8	6.7	8.1	8.8	9.3	8.8	8.1	7.1
21	New Zealand	6.6[a]	7.6	8.1	7.7	8.4	7.7	7.2	6.9	5.9
22	Norway	5.8[a]	5.8	6.8	7.6	7.7	8.1	8.0	7.8	7.3
23	Poland	—	—	3.8	—	—	6.9[e]	7.8	8.2	8.3[g]
24	Portugal	—	—	—	—	—	4.7[e]	5.5	5.6	6.1
25	Singapore	—	—	—	2.3	2.9	3.8	5.1	4.6	4.6
26	Spain	1.2[a]	1.9	2.6	2.9	3.6	4.3	5.0	5.6	5.9
27	Sweden	6.2[a]	7.2	8.2	9.1	9.4	9.2	8.6	8.1	7.7
28	Switzerland	5.0[a]	5.2	5.9	6.5	7.6	7.6	7.7	7.8	—
29	U.K.	—	6.9	—	8.2	8.2	8.2	7.6	7.2	6.5
30	U.S.	7.5[a]	8.0	8.5	8.6	8.4	8.0[d]	7.6	7.5	7.3

[a] 1955–57, [b] 1970–72, [c] 1973–76, [d] 1979–82, [e] 1980–82, [f] 1990–92, [g] 1993–96.

by Site and Year (1953–57 to 1993–97)
9. Pancreas (female)

	Country	1953–1957	1958–1962	1963–1967	1968–1972	1973–1977	1978–1982	1983–1987	1988–1992	1993–1997
1	Australia	3.6[a]	3.6	4.0	4.4	4.6	4.4	4.6	4.6	4.5
2	Austria	4.2[a]	4.5	4.8	5.3	5.3	5.5	5.9	5.9	6.1
3	Belgium	2.5[a]	3.0	3.3	3.5	4.0[c]	4.5[d]	4.3	4.3	4.7[g]
4	Bulgaria	—	—	—	2.2	2.3	2.8	3.2	3.2	3.3
5	Canada	4.7[a]	4.6	4.9	5.3	5.5	5.5	5.6	5.3	5.3
6	Chile	2.5[a]	2.9	3.4	—	—	—	—	—	—
7	Costa Rica	—	—	—	—	—	—	—	—	—
8	Denmark	4.4[a]	4.6	5.6	5.7	6.1	7.1	6.9	6.7	6.2
9	Finland	3.6[a]	4.2	5.2	5.5	6.1	6.5	6.3	6.5	6.2
10	France	2.4[a]	2.6	2.8	3.1	3.1	3.3	3.5	3.8	4.0
11	Germany	—	—	—	—	—	—	—	5.3[f]	5.4
12	Greece	—	—	—	1.8	2.2	2.7	3.1	3.3	3.6
13	Hong Kong	—	—	—	2.2	2.3	2.8	2.8	3.0	2.6
14	Hungary	—	—	—	5.1[b]	5.2	5.8	5.8	6.2	6.7
15	Iceland	—	—	—	—	5.8	5.8	7.8	6.6	7.1
16	Ireland	4.6[a]	5.2	5.0	5.7	6.2	6.0	5.5	5.7	5.4
17	Italy	1.9[a]	2.1	2.4	2.7	3.2	3.5	4.1	4.5	4.7
18	Japan	1.4[a]	1.9	2.6	3.2	3.5	4.0	4.5	4.8	4.8
19	Mexico	—	—	—	—	—	—	—	—	—
20	Netherlands	3.3[a]	3.8	4.4	4.9	5.3	5.5	5.5	5.6	5.3
21	New Zealand	4.6[a]	3.8	4.8	4.2	5.0	4.8	4.7	4.2	4.5
22	Norway	3.1[a]	3.6	3.7	4.6	4.7	5.0	5.4	5.5	5.7
23	Poland	—	—	2.8	—	—	4.3[e]	4.7	4.9	5.0[g]
24	Portugal	—	—	—	—	—	2.7[e]	3.0	3.2	3.3
25	Singapore	—	—	—	1.0	1.9	2.2	3.3	3.2	3.4
26	Spain	1.1[a]	1.4	1.8	2.0	2.3	2.4	2.9	3.2	3.5
27	Sweden	4.2[a]	4.7	5.6	5.8	6.5	6.6	6.6	6.6	6.6
28	Switzerland	3.4[a]	3.4	4.0	4.3	4.6	4.8	5.1	5.2	—
29	U.K.	—	4.4	—	4.8	5.1	5.0	5.1	5.1	4.8
30	U.S.	4.6[a]	4.8	5.0	5.1	5.2	5.2[d]	5.3	5.3	5.3

[a] 1955–57, [b] 1970–72, [c] 1973–76, [d] 1979–82, [e] 1980–82, [f] 1990–92, [g] 1993–96.

TABLE I-10. Age-adjusted Death Rates of Cancer

10. Larynx (male)

	Country	1953–1957	1958–1962	1963–1967	1968–1972	1973–1977	1978–1982	1983–1987	1988–1992	1993–1997
1	Australia	1.7	1.8	1.9	2.0	2.3	2.2	2.2	2.1	1.8
2	Austria	3.5[a]	3.6	3.9	3.2	3.6	3.8	3.5	3.6	3.1
3	Belgium	3.3[b]	4.0	4.8	4.6	4.6	4.7	4.6	4.7	4.0[g]
4	Bulgaria	—	—	3.8[e]	3.8	4.0	3.8	4.1	4.8	5.2
5	Canada	1.7	1.7	2.0	2.1	2.3	2.5	2.5	2.5	2.2
6	Chile	1.4[a]	1.4	1.8	1.9	2.3	2.2	2.2	2.0	2.0[h]
7	Costa Rica	—	—	1.4	1.6	2.3	1.8	3.1	3.0	1.9[i]
8	Denmark	1.0	1.2	1.2	1.7	1.6	2.2	2.6	2.2	2.4
9	Finland	2.8	2.8	3.2	3.0	2.3	2.2	1.5	1.2	0.9
10	France	8.6	9.6	11.0	11.2	11.9	11.1	9.5	7.5	5.5
11	Germany	—	—	—	—	—	—	—	2.7[f]	2.5
12	Greece	—	—	4.4	4.2	4.1	3.9	3.5	3.5	3.1
13	Hong Kong	—	1.9[c]	1.8	2.4	3.9	3.7	3.0	2.8	2.3
14	Hungary	3.8[a]	4.0	4.2	5.1	5.6	6.1	7.3	8.7	9.1
15	Iceland	0.2	0.4	1.0	0.6	1.0	1.4	1.0	0.7	0.4
16	Ireland	2.8	2.4	2.1	2.1	2.1	2.5	2.4	2.4	2.1
17	Italy	3.7	4.5	5.5	6.5	6.6	6.6	6.3	5.3	4.1
18	Japan	1.7	1.6	1.5	1.5	1.4	1.2	1.0	0.9	0.8
19	Mexico	—	1.8	1.9	2.1	2.1	2.3	2.4	2.7	2.5[i]
20	Netherlands	1.5	1.7	1.6	1.8	1.9	1.9	1.7	1.9	1.7
21	New Zealand	2.1	1.3	1.5	1.6	1.8	1.6	1.7	1.4	1.1
22	Norway	0.5	0.5	0.7	1.1	1.0	1.0	1.1	0.9	1.0
23	Poland	—	1.9[d]	3.0	3.5	4.4	5.8	7.0	7.5	7.4[g]
24	Portugal	4.6[a]	5.1	5.4	5.3	5.3	5.5	5.6	5.5	5.4
25	Singapore	—	—	3.5	3.6	4.3	4.5	3.9	3.1	3.2
26	Spain	5.9	6.5	6.8	7.1	7.5	7.6	7.3	7.1	6.4
27	Sweden	0.5	0.6	0.6	0.7	0.9	0.8	0.8	0.7	0.6
28	Switzerland	3.6	3.2	3.3	3.3	3.0	3.0	2.4	2.3	1.6
29	U.K.	2.4	2.1	1.9	1.8	1.7	1.7	1.7	1.7	1.6
30	U.S.	2.1	2.1	2.2	2.3	2.3	2.2	2.0	2.0	1.9

[a] 1955–57, [b] 1954–57, [c] 1960–62, [d] 1959–62, [e] 1964–67, [f] 1990–92, [g] 1993–96, [h] 1993, 94, [i] 1993–95.

by Site and Year (1953–57 to 1993–97)

10. Larynx (female)

	Country	1953–1957	1958–1962	1963–1967	1968–1972	1973–1977	1978–1982	1983–1987	1988–1992	1993–1997
1	Australia	0.3	0.2	0.2	0.2	0.2	0.3	0.2	0.2	0.2
2	Austria	0.2[a]	0.2	0.2	0.2	0.2	0.2	0.2	0.2	0.2
3	Belgium	0.3[b]	0.3	0.4	0.3	0.3	0.4	0.4	0.4	0.4[g]
4	Bulgaria	—	—	0.4[e]	0.4	0.3	0.4	0.3	0.2	0.3
5	Canada	0.3	0.3	0.2	0.3	0.3	0.3	0.4	0.4	0.4
6	Chile	0.4[a]	0.3	0.3	0.3	0.4	0.3	0.3	0.3	0.2[h]
7	Costa Rica	—	—	0.4	0.2	0.5	0.6	0.6	0.6	0.3[i]
8	Denmark	0.2	0.2	0.2	0.2	0.3	0.4	0.4	0.4	0.5
9	Finland	0.3	0.2	0.1	0.1	0.1	0.1	0.1	0.1	0.1
10	France	0.4	0.4	0.4	0.4	0.4	0.4	0.4	0.3	0.3
11	Germany	—	—	—	—	—	—	—	0.2[f]	0.2
12	Greece	—	—	0.4	0.4	0.5	0.2	0.3	0.2	0.2
13	Hong Kong	—	0.1[c]	0.3	0.2	0.4	0.4	0.3	0.3	0.2
14	Hungary	0.5[a]	0.4	0.4	0.5	0.4	0.4	0.5	0.7	0.7
15	Iceland	0.0	0.0	0.4	0.1	0.6	0.2	0.4	0.0	0.1
16	Ireland	1.0	1.1	1.0	1.1	0.8	0.6	0.5	0.5	0.4
17	Italy	0.3	0.3	0.3	0.3	0.3	0.3	0.3	0.2	0.2
18	Japan	0.5	0.4	0.3	0.3	0.2	0.1	0.1	0.1	0.1
19	Mexico	—	0.7	0.6	0.6	0.6	0.6	0.5	0.5	0.5[i]
20	Netherlands	0.3	0.2	0.2	0.2	0.1	0.1	0.2	0.2	0.3
21	New Zealand	0.2	0.2	0.1	0.2	0.3	0.3	0.3	0.2	0.1
22	Norway	0.1	0.0	0.0	0.1	0.1	0.1	0.1	0.1	0.2
23	Poland	—	0.3[d]	0.3	0.3	0.3	0.4	0.5	0.5	0.5[g]
24	Portugal	0.4[a]	0.4	0.4	0.5	0.5	0.4	0.3	0.3	0.3
25	Singapore	—	—	0.3	0.4	0.4	0.4	0.5	0.5	0.3
26	Spain	0.4	0.4	0.4	0.4	0.3	0.2	0.2	0.1	0.1
27	Sweden	0.1	0.1	0.1	0.1	0.1	0.1	0.1	0.1	0.1
28	Switzerland	0.2	0.1	0.2	0.1	0.2	0.2	0.2	0.2	0.2
29	U.K.	0.5	0.4	0.4	0.3	0.3	0.4	0.3	0.3	0.3
30	U.S.	0.2	0.2	0.2	0.3	0.3	0.4	0.4	0.4	0.4

[a] 1955–57, [b] 1954–57, [c] 1960–62, [d] 1959–62, [e] 1964–67, [f] 1990–92, [g] 1993–96, [h] 1993, 94, [i] 1993–95.

TABLE I-11. Age-adjusted Death Rates of Cancer

11. Trachea, bronchus and lung (male)

	Country	1953–1957	1958–1962	1963–1967	1968–1972	1973–1977	1978–1982	1983–1987	1988–1992	1993–1997
1	Australia	20.9	27.8	36.2	43.0	46.9	48.2	46.5	42.4	37.8
2	Austria	45.2[a]	48.8	51.3	51.6	51.2	49.1	47.8	45.2	41.5
3	Belgium	28.8[b]	37.7	49.2	60.0	69.9	77.8	78.7	72.8	69.1[g]
4	Bulgaria	—	—	36.8[e]	35.5	35.9	36.0	39.7	40.8	42.2
5	Canada	20.5	25.9	33.0	40.6	47.4	53.0	55.8	56.1	49.8
6	Chile	12.3[a]	12.9	15.0	18.2	19.4	20.7	21.8	21.7	21.0[h]
7	Costa Rica	—	—	6.8	8.6	10.6	14.4	15.7	15.4	13.5[i]
8	Denmark	21.4	29.2	37.2	43.4	46.8	53.4	54.8	51.3	49.1
9	Finland	47.7	58.2	62.0	67.8	65.4	64.4	56.8	47.7	40.7
10	France	16.7	21.9	27.7	31.1	36.8	42.1	44.9	47.0	46.5
11	Germany	—	—	—	—	—	—	—	48.2[f]	45.9
12	Greece	—	—	30.6	33.1	40.8	44.8	47.9	49.2	49.8
13	Hong Kong	—	21.6[c]	29.9	39.0	47.6	55.4	55.8	55.3	52.0
14	Hungary	22.4[a]	28.0	35.7	41.4	47.7	58.8	69.2	77.8	84.8
15	Iceland	8.3	10.8	13.4	15.0	17.5	25.1	26.2	30.1	30.5
16	Ireland	19.6	25.8	31.2	39.3	45.4	46.8	50.3	46.9	42.7
17	Italy	15.1	21.5	29.6	38.2	44.9	52.9	57.9	57.6	52.6
18	Japan	5.8	9.8	13.2	16.3	19.8	24.2	27.7	30.2	31.5
19	Mexico	—	5.8	6.6	7.7	9.6	12.4	15.0	16.3	16.4[i]
20	Netherlands	31.9	42.4	54.5	65.1	72.7	77.6	76.3	69.4	61.1
21	New Zealand	25.7	30.6	37.3	45.0	49.0	48.8	48.9	42.6	37.4
22	Norway	8.5	12.0	14.7	19.0	22.1	26.4	29.5	30.7	31.6
23	Poland	—	18.1[d]	28.1	36.7	45.6	54.6	64.7	70.4	71.4[g]
24	Portugal	7.6[a]	8.7	10.9	13.5	15.5	20.1	23.9	25.7	29.4
25	Singapore	—	—	31.0	37.2	47.4	54.9	55.3	49.3	44.0
26	Spain	11.8	16.1	19.2	22.6	28.6	34.4	40.0	46.2	48.0
27	Sweden	10.8	14.6	16.9	20.4	24.1	24.6	24.2	23.6	22.3
28	Switzerland	27.2	31.4	37.0	41.8	47.4	48.8	48.3	44.6	37.9
29	U.K.	52.5	62.9	70.1	74.1	74.1	70.7	65.2	57.4	47.6
30	U.S.	25.2	31.7	38.9	47.0	52.1	55.9	56.9	56.8	53.0

[a] 1955–57, [b] 1954–57, [c] 1960–62, [d] 1959–62, [e] 1964–67, [f] 1990–92, [g] 1993–96, [h] 1993, 94, [i] 1993–95.

by Site and Year (1953–57 to 1993–97)
11. Trachea, bronchus and lung (female)

	Country	1953–1957	1958–1962	1963–1967	1968–1972	1973–1977	1978–1982	1983–1987	1988–1992	1993–1997
1	Australia	3.3	3.5	4.4	6.0	7.6	9.7	11.4	12.9	13.6
2	Austria	5.8[a]	5.9	6.0	6.3	6.7	7.4	8.4	9.1	10.1
3	Belgium	3.6[b]	4.0	4.4	4.6	5.7	6.2	7.0	8.3	9.5[g]
4	Bulgaria	—	—	7.0[e]	6.2	6.1	5.7	6.6	6.3	6.7
5	Canada	3.6	3.8	5.0	6.6	9.5	13.4	17.7	21.2	23.4
6	Chile	4.4[a]	4.6	5.3	5.3	5.0	5.4	5.9	6.1	6.7[h]
7	Costa Rica	—	—	3.9	5.0	5.0	6.5	5.9	5.5	5.1[i]
8	Denmark	4.4	5.3	6.9	8.8	11.0	14.9	20.7	24.0	27.7
9	Finland	4.0	3.6	4.0	4.2	4.5	5.6	6.2	6.8	6.9
10	France	3.4	3.4	3.8	3.4	3.5	3.8	4.4	5.2	6.1
11	Germany	—	—	—	—	—	—	—	8.2[f]	9.3
12	Greece	—	—	5.9	5.8	6.4	6.4	6.4	7.0	7.0
13	Hong Kong	—	11.2[c]	15.6	19.3	22.5	23.6	23.9	23.5	20.5
14	Hungary	5.5[a]	6.5	7.3	7.6	8.6	10.0	12.0	15.2	19.0
15	Iceland	3.9	5.3	7.5	9.3	10.9	19.6	19.2	25.2	25.1
16	Ireland	5.6	6.1	7.4	10.5	13.4	15.6	17.6	18.5	17.5
17	Italy	3.2	3.8	4.5	4.7	5.4	6.0	6.9	7.4	7.8
18	Japan	2.1	3.7	4.6	5.3	6.0	7.0	7.7	8.1	8.4
19	Mexico	—	3.4	3.5	4.0	4.3	4.9	5.8	5.9	6.0[i]
20	Netherlands	3.1	3.3	3.5	3.8	4.5	6.1	8.2	10.6	13.7
21	New Zealand	3.3	4.4	5.3	8.1	11.1	13.4	14.8	17.4	18.2
22	Norway	2.4	2.6	2.8	3.7	4.5	5.7	8.1	10.5	13.7
23	Poland	—	3.6[d]	4.3	5.1	5.6	6.8	8.2	9.7	11.0[g]
24	Portugal	2.4[a]	2.3	2.5	2.9	3.3	3.6	3.9	4.4	4.6
25	Singapore	—	—	11.4	12.1	14.8	17.4	18.8	16.5	16.3
26	Spain	2.9	3.5	3.7	4.0	4.0	3.8	3.6	3.5	3.9
27	Sweden	3.7	3.9	4.1	4.8	6.0	7.3	8.6	10.3	11.8
28	Switzerland	3.2	3.0	3.4	3.5	4.4	5.2	6.5	7.5	9.1
29	U.K.	6.8	8.1	10.2	12.6	15.1	17.7	19.9	21.1	20.6
30	U.S.	4.1	4.7	6.3	9.4	12.8	17.1	21.3	24.9	26.5

[a] 1955–57, [b] 1954–57, [c] 1960–62, [d] 1959–62, [e] 1964–67, [f] 1990–92, [g] 1993–96, [h] 1993, 94, [i] 1993–95.

TABLE I-12. Age-adjusted Death Rates of Cancer

12. Skin (male)

	Country	1953–1957	1958–1962	1963–1967	1968–1972	1973–1977	1978–1982	1983–1987	1988–1992	1993–1997
1	Australia	3.8	4.2	4.5	4.7	5.2	5.9	6.3	6.9	6.9
2	Austria	1.9[a]	1.7	2.0	2.1	2.2	2.4	3.1	3.7	3.1
3	Belgium	1.6[b]	1.6	1.6	1.5	1.4	1.6	1.6	2.0	1.8[g]
4	Bulgaria	—	—	1.6[e]	1.7	1.4	1.4	1.6	1.5	1.7
5	Canada	1.8	1.8	1.9	1.8	1.8	1.9	2.2	2.5	2.5
6	Chile	0.9[a]	0.8	1.1	1.4	1.1	0.8	0.7	0.8	—
7	Costa Rica	—	—	1.6	1.8	0.9	0.7	0.7	0.8	—
8	Denmark	2.0	2.0	2.0	2.6	2.6	2.7	3.2	3.6	3.1
9	Finland	1.7	1.9	2.1	2.6	2.8	2.6	2.5	2.5	2.7
10	France	2.0	2.0	1.9	1.7	1.7	1.7	1.7	1.7	1.8
11	Germany	—	—	—	—	—	—	—	2.2[f]	2.1
12	Greece	—	—	1.0	0.9	1.0	1.0	1.1	1.0	1.2
13	Hong Kong	—	0.5[c]	0.6	0.6	0.8	0.4	0.5	0.5	0.6
14	Hungary	2.4[a]	2.5	2.3	2.6	2.9	2.8	2.9	3.4	3.6
15	Iceland	0.0	1.5	0.3	1.1	1.0	2.4	1.0	1.5	1.7
16	Ireland	2.7	3.0	2.5	2.5	2.2	2.2	2.8	3.0	2.2
17	Italy	1.9	1.7	1.7	1.7	1.4	1.9	2.0	2.1	2.1
18	Japan	1.0	1.0	0.9	0.8	0.8	0.6	0.5	0.4	0.4
19	Mexico	—	0.7	0.5	0.7	0.8	0.4	0.4	0.4	—
20	Netherlands	1.6	1.7	1.6	1.8	1.9	2.1	2.4	2.3	2.5
21	New Zealand	3.3	2.7	3.2	4.1	4.8	5.9	6.2	6.5	6.5
22	Norway	1.7	1.8	2.2	2.7	3.6	3.3	3.8	3.8	4.1
23	Poland	—	0.9[d]	1.7	1.9	2.0	2.1	2.5	2.6	2.9[g]
24	Portugal	1.2[a]	1.4	1.7	1.8	1.9	1.3	1.1	1.7	1.7
25	Singapore	—	—	1.2	1.2	1.4	0.7	1.0	0.7	0.7
26	Spain	1.6	1.6	1.6	1.2	1.4	1.4	2.0	1.9	2.0
27	Sweden	1.4	1.8	1.9	2.2	2.4	2.8	3.0	3.1	3.0
28	Switzerland	2.2	2.4	2.5	2.6	3.2	3.2	3.8	3.9	—
29	U.K.	1.8	1.6	1.5	1.6	1.7	1.8	2.0	2.1	2.3
30	U.S.	2.4	2.4	2.6	2.4	2.7	2.9	3.4	3.5	3.4

[a] 1955–57, [b] 1954–57, [c] 1960–62, [d] 1959–62, [e] 1964–67, [f] 1990–92, [g] 1993–96.

by Site and Year (1953–57 to 1993–97)
12. Skin (female)

	Country	1953–1957	1958–1962	1963–1967	1968–1972	1973–1977	1978–1982	1983–1987	1988–1992	1993–1997
1	Australia	2.3	2.3	2.6	2.6	2.7	2.7	3.0	2.9	2.8
2	Austria	1.5[a]	1.6	1.6	1.7	1.5	1.7	1.8	1.9	2.0
3	Belgium	1.3[b]	1.1	1.1	1.0	1.0	1.0	1.0	1.3	1.4[g]
4	Bulgaria	—	—	1.1[e]	1.3	0.9	1.1	1.1	1.0	1.1
5	Canada	1.2	1.2	1.3	1.3	1.2	1.2	1.3	1.2	1.3
6	Chile	0.6[a]	0.6	0.9	1.0	1.0	0.5	0.6	0.7	—
7	Costa Rica	—	—	1.3	0.7	0.9	0.3	0.3	0.5	—
8	Denmark	1.6	1.8	1.9	2.0	2.2	2.1	2.2	2.6	2.1
9	Finland	1.4	1.4	1.4	1.7	1.6	1.4	1.4	1.5	1.4
10	France	1.7	1.6	1.4	1.3	1.3	1.2	1.2	1.1	1.3
11	Germany	—	—	—	—	—	—	—	1.4[f]	1.3
12	Greece	—	—	0.9	0.8	0.9	0.8	0.8	0.8	0.8
13	Hong Kong	—	0.3[c]	0.4	0.4	0.5	0.3	0.3	0.3	0.3
14	Hungary	1.7[a]	2.0	1.9	2.0	2.2	2.0	2.0	2.1	2.2
15	Iceland	0.5	0.5	1.1	1.6	1.2	1.2	1.1	0.5	1.3
16	Ireland	2.1	1.8	2.1	2.1	1.8	2.2	2.2	2.2	1.4
17	Italy	1.3	1.2	1.2	1.1	1.0	1.2	1.3	1.3	1.3
18	Japan	0.7	0.7	0.6	0.6	0.5	0.4	0.3	0.3	0.3
19	Mexico	—	0.7	0.4	0.8	0.6	0.3	0.3	0.3	—
20	Netherlands	1.4	1.2	1.3	1.3	1.3	1.4	1.5	1.7	1.8
21	New Zealand	1.8	2.2	2.4	2.5	3.2	3.2	3.6	3.4	3.4
22	Norway	1.5	1.3	1.6	1.8	2.0	1.9	2.3	2.1	2.4
23	Poland	—	0.7[d]	1.5	1.6	1.6	1.6	1.8	1.9	2.0[g]
24	Portugal	1.2[a]	1.1	1.3	1.4	1.3	0.9	0.7	1.0	1.1
25	Singapore	—	—	1.2	0.8	0.7	0.7	0.6	0.5	0.6
26	Spain	1.2	1.2	1.1	0.8	0.9	0.8	1.0	1.1	1.2
27	Sweden	1.0	1.2	1.3	1.5	1.5	1.9	1.8	1.8	1.7
28	Switzerland	1.8	1.9	1.8	1.7	1.9	2.0	2.3	2.4	—
29	U.K.	1.3	1.2	1.2	1.3	1.5	1.5	1.5	1.6	1.7
30	U.S.	1.5	1.5	1.5	1.4	1.5	1.5	1.5	1.5	1.5

[a] 1955–57, [b] 1954–57, [c] 1960–62, [d] 1959–62, [e] 1964–67, [f] 1990–92, [g] 1993–96.

TABLE I-13. Age-adjusted Death Rates of Cancer by Site and Year (1953–57 to 1993–97)

13. Breast (female)

	Country	1953–1957	1958–1962	1963–1967	1968–1972	1973–1977	1978–1982	1983–1987	1988–1992	1993–1997
1	Australia	20.1	19.1	19.5	20.0	20.1	19.4	20.7	20.5	19.5
2	Austria	15.0[a]	15.7	17.4	18.4	19.7	19.7	21.9	22.1	21.0
3	Belgium	20.1[b]	20.6	21.4	23.0	23.5	25.8	26.2	26.0	25.4[g]
4	Bulgaria	—	—	8.9[e]	10.4	12.1	13.3	14.8	15.7	16.0
5	Canada	22.9	23.3	24.0	23.9	23.7	23.1	23.9	23.3	21.1
6	Chile	8.4[a]	9.4	9.9	12.2	11.8	12.0	12.7	12.6	12.0[h]
7	Costa Rica	—	—	8.1	8.6	8.7	9.9	12.3	11.8	12.7[i]
8	Denmark	24.4	24.3	24.7	25.9	26.3	25.4	27.4	27.8	27.4
9	Finland	12.4	13.5	14.1	14.7	15.5	15.2	16.4	16.9	16.6
10	France	14.8	15.7	17.0	17.4	18.4	18.7	19.3	19.7	19.6
11	Germany	—	—	—	—	—	—	—	22.2[f]	21.8
12	Greece	—	—	8.0	10.4	12.1	14.6	15.2	15.3	15.9
13	Hong Kong	—	8.8[c]	8.9	9.0	9.4	8.6	8.7	9.1	8.9
14	Hungary	12.1[a]	12.6	14.2	16.6	18.9	20.6	21.4	22.8	23.9
15	Iceland	12.4	21.5	20.4	22.0	18.1	18.5	21.2	23.4	25.3
16	Ireland	19.7	20.0	21.7	23.8	26.0	26.6	26.1	27.7	25.5
17	Italy	13.9	14.6	16.2	17.7	18.6	19.2	20.4	20.6	19.8
18	Japan	3.8	3.8	3.9	4.3	4.9	5.4	5.8	6.4	7.4
19	Mexico	—	3.9	4.1	4.8	5.6	6.2	7.1	8.3	9.2[i]
20	Netherlands	23.2	24.3	26.1	27.0	26.6	26.2	26.4	26.9	25.9
21	New Zealand	21.9	22.2	23.5	24.2	24.9	25.5	26.2	25.9	23.7
22	Norway	17.4	17.1	17.2	18.2	18.0	18.3	18.1	18.9	19.1
23	Poland	—	6.4[d]	10.5	11.7	13.2	14.6	15.1	15.8	16.0[g]
24	Portugal	10.6[a]	11.5	12.5	13.5	14.0	15.1	16.6	18.0	17.6
25	Singapore	—	—	10.2	10.0	10.1	13.4	13.1	13.1	13.9
26	Spain	6.0	7.9	9.4	10.5	12.6	13.7	15.4	17.2	16.9
27	Sweden	19.0	19.3	18.7	19.2	19.6	18.5	18.0	17.9	16.7
28	Switzerland	22.2	21.8	22.6	23.8	24.0	24.1	25.2	24.2	21.7
29	U.K.	23.4	23.7	24.6	26.3	27.4	28.1	29.0	28.2	24.8
30	U.S.	21.7	21.5	22.1	22.4	22.3	22.0	22.4	22.2	20.2

[a] 1955–57, [b] 1954–57, [c] 1960–62, [d] 1959–62, [e] 1964–67, [f] 1990–92, [g] 1993–96, [h] 1993, 94, [i] 1993–95.

TABLE I-14. Age-adjusted Death Rates of Cancer by Site and Year (1953–57 to 1993–97)

14. Uterus

	Country	1953–1957	1958–1962	1963–1967	1968–1972	1973–1977	1978–1982	1983–1987	1988–1992	1993–1997
1	Australia	11.1	9.9	8.7	8.0	6.9	5.8	5.5	4.6	4.1
2	Austria	21.4[a]	19.6	18.1	17.0	13.9	11.3	9.7	8.1	6.7
3	Belgium	14.9[b]	14.3	12.4	10.7	8.3	7.8	6.7	5.6	5.3[g]
4	Bulgaria	—	—	7.2[e]	7.5	7.4	7.7	8.9	10.3	10.3
5	Canada	13.7	12.1	10.8	9.2	7.2	6.1	5.3	4.6	4.2
6	Chile	20.3[a]	20.2	20.9	22.2	20.3	17.6	15.7	14.6	13.9[h]
7	Costa Rica	—	—	26.7	19.8	16.6	15.0	15.5	13.4	14.5[i]
8	Denmark	18.4	18.6	17.7	14.7	12.8	11.6	9.8	8.8	7.3
9	Finland	12.0	11.2	10.3	8.5	6.5	5.4	4.5	4.2	3.7
10	France	12.9	12.3	11.3	10.2	9.3	7.8	6.6	5.7	5.0
11	Germany	—	—	—	—	—	—	—	6.6[f]	5.8
12	Greece	—	—	6.4	5.9	6.0	5.3	4.6	4.2	3.4
13	Hong Kong	—	14.7[c]	12.4	10.7	9.1	6.8	6.4	5.4	5.1
14	Hungary	22.8[a]	21.2	19.0	16.6	16.4	14.5	12.8	11.8	11.2
15	Iceland	12.2	14.8	15.8	12.3	8.3	5.5	6.0	4.9	5.0
16	Ireland	9.2	7.9	8.0	8.1	7.2	6.3	6.0	5.7	5.5
17	Italy	13.7	13.7	13.2	12.1	10.4	8.7	7.0	5.6	4.7
18	Japan	19.1	16.0	13.6	11.3	8.9	6.9	5.2	4.2	3.9
19	Mexico	—	19.9	19.3	19.4	18.6	17.8	18.5	17.9	16.3[i]
20	Netherlands	10.9	10.6	10.3	9.5	7.9	6.4	5.5	4.8	4.0
21	New Zealand	11.0	10.7	9.8	8.8	8.4	8.1	7.7	7.1	5.6
22	Norway	10.6	9.7	9.0	9.0	8.1	8.1	7.0	6.9	5.9
23	Poland	—	12.5[d]	16.0	15.3	13.4	12.6	12.5	11.9	11.1[g]
24	Portugal	14.2[a]	14.1	13.2	13.3	10.9	9.0	8.0	7.2	6.8
25	Singapore	—	—	14.6	12.3	11.0	10.2	10.0	8.0	7.7
26	Spain	8.9	9.7	9.9	8.9	8.4	6.9	5.8	5.3	4.7
27	Sweden	10.7	11.1	9.8	9.7	8.2	6.8	5.6	4.9	4.5
28	Switzerland	13.4	13.1	12.3	11.5	9.4	8.3	7.0	5.8	4.6
29	U.K.	11.2	10.9	10.1	9.5	8.6	8.1	7.6	6.7	5.2
30	U.S.	15.4	13.2	11.4	9.2	7.5	6.3	5.6	5.2	4.9

[a] 1955–57, [b] 1954–57, [c] 1960–62, [d] 1959–62, [e] 1964–67, [f] 1990–92, [g] 1993–96, [h] 1993, 94, [i] 1993–95.

TABLE I-15. Age-adjusted Death Rates of Cancer by Site and Year (1953-57 to 1993-97)

15. Ovary and other uterine adnexa

	Country	1953–1957	1958–1962	1963–1967	1968–1972	1973–1977	1978–1982	1983–1987	1988–1992	1993–1997
1	Australia	6.3[a]	6.0	6.5	6.3	6.4	6.0	5.9	5.6	5.3
2	Austria	—	—	—	9.2[b]	8.9	8.7	8.2	8.1	6.9
3	Belgium	5.2[a]	5.6	5.8	7.1	7.1	7.0	7.1	7.2	6.9[g]
4	Bulgaria	—	—	—	3.8	4.0	4.8	4.9	4.0	4.9
5	Canada	7.3[a]	7.2	7.5	7.6	7.2	6.8	6.3	6.0	5.8
6	Chile	1.7[a]	1.8	2.5	—	—	—	—	—	—
7	Costa Rica	—	—	—	—	—	—	—	—	—
8	Denmark	10.3[a]	10.8	11.3	12.1	10.7	10.8	9.8	9.9	9.6
9	Finland	5.1[a]	5.6	6.1	6.6	6.9	6.4	6.3	6.7	6.3
10	France	3.0[a]	3.5	3.9	4.3	4.9	5.5	5.8	5.8	5.6
11	Germany	—	—	—	—	—	—	—	7.5[f]	7.0
12	Greece	—	—	—	1.3	1.8	2.6	3.0	3.2	3.8
13	Hong Kong	—	—	—	3.5	3.4	3.0	3.1	3.0	3.0
14	Hungary	—	—	—	6.3[c]	7.0	7.2	7.2	7.1	6.5
15	Iceland	—	—	—	—	7.4	8.1	8.4	8.6	7.6
16	Ireland	4.3[a]	4.8	5.4	6.0	7.4	6.9	8.1	8.9	8.5
17	Italy	2.6[a]	3.0	3.2	3.6	3.8	4.2	4.8	5.0	4.8
18	Japan	1.3[a]	1.5	1.8	2.1	2.5	3.0	3.2	3.4	3.5
19	Mexico	—	—	—	—	—	—	—	—	—
20	Netherlands	7.7[a]	7.8	8.2	9.3	9.3	8.2	8.0	8.0	7.3
21	New Zealand	7.0[a]	7.7	7.9	8.3	7.7	7.8	7.0	6.7	6.5
22	Norway	7.9[a]	8.0	8.3	8.8	8.4	8.2	8.9	8.0	8.0
23	Poland	—	—	3.8	—	—	6.1[d]	6.4	6.9	6.8[g]
24	Portugal	—	—	—	—	—	2.4[d]	3.0	3.2	3.5
25	Singapore	—	—	—	2.5	2.8	4.0	3.8	3.6	4.3
26	Spain	0.5[a]	0.7	0.9	1.1	1.8	2.4	3.1	3.7	4.2
27	Sweden	8.3[a]	8.9	9.3	9.6	9.5	9.0	8.1	7.6	7.3
28	Switzerland	7.8[a]	7.9	8.3	8.3	8.3	8.1	7.0	6.9	—
29	U.K.	—	8.0	—	8.9	8.7	8.6	8.6	8.4	8.1
30	U.S.	7.4[a]	7.4	7.4	7.4	7.1	6.5[e]	6.3	6.3	6.0

[a] 1955–57, [b] 1969–72, [c] 1970–72, [d] 1980–82, [e] 1979–82, [f] 1990–92, [g] 1993–96.

TABLE I-16. Age-adjusted Death Rates of Cancer by Site and Year (1953–57 to 1993–97)

16. Prostate

	Country	1953–1957	1958–1962	1963–1967	1968–1972	1973–1977	1978–1982	1983–1987	1988–1992	1993–1997
1	Australia	15.1	14.7	14.5	15.4	15.6	15.2	16.1	18.0	18.5
2	Austria	12.7[a]	13.0	13.6	14.0	14.8	15.4	15.8	17.2	17.1
3	Belgium	12.9[b]	14.3	15.7	15.2	16.1	17.5	17.3	18.3	19.2[g]
4	Bulgaria	—	—	6.0[e]	6.5	6.1	6.3	7.4	8.0	8.8
5	Canada	12.9	13.4	13.0	13.9	14.3	14.5	15.7	17.0	16.1
6	Chile	6.7[a]	8.7	9.1	10.6	11.8	11.0	12.4	13.8	15.3[h]
7	Costa Rica	—	—	9.3	9.3	9.4	10.6	14.4	17.1	19.2[i]
8	Denmark	13.5	14.2	14.3	12.9	13.5	15.9	17.8	18.6	19.9
9	Finland	9.9	11.9	11.3	13.4	15.3	16.3	16.9	17.7	18.3
10	France	11.9	14.7	15.6	14.9	15.0	15.3	16.5	17.0	15.7
11	Germany	—	—	—	—	—	—	—	16.3[f]	16.7
12	Greece	—	—	5.2	5.8	6.6	7.2	7.9	8.4	9.3
13	Hong Kong	—	1.5[c]	2.1	2.4	2.1	2.4	2.7	2.8	3.6
14	Hungary	8.0[a]	10.5	12.7	14.5	15.9	15.8	15.6	15.8	17.5
15	Iceland	8.2	7.1	10.2	12.2	12.7	12.4	18.5	20.7	19.8
16	Ireland	8.0	9.7	11.2	12.7	13.6	14.0	15.4	17.9	18.9
17	Italy	6.8	8.2	9.4	10.4	10.5	10.8	11.6	11.5	11.2
18	Japan	0.9	1.5	1.8	2.0	2.4	2.8	3.3	3.8	4.8
19	Mexico	—	3.5	3.5	5.1	5.9	6.8	9.0	10.7	12.4[i]
20	Netherlands	12.6	13.3	14.3	15.0	15.4	16.0	17.0	18.3	19.2
21	New Zealand	14.3	13.6	14.0	14.9	16.9	16.0	17.2	18.7	19.4
22	Norway	14.4	14.9	16.5	17.0	18.2	19.9	20.8	22.0	23.9
23	Poland	—	3.7[d]	7.4	8.3	8.0	8.4	9.2	9.7	10.9[g]
24	Portugal	8.5[a]	9.7	11.6	13.2	13.4	13.8	13.0	14.6	17.3
25	Singapore	—	—	2.3	2.3	1.9	2.9	4.2	3.9	5.4
26	Spain	6.8	9.3	11.0	11.8	12.3	12.6	12.7	13.1	13.9
27	Sweden	13.1	16.9	17.7	19.0	21.6	19.6	18.9	20.9	21.7
28	Switzerland	14.5	15.7	16.3	18.3	19.4	19.8	21.7	22.4	20.1
29	U.K.	11.4	11.9	12.2	11.8	12.1	12.4	14.6	16.7	16.7
30	U.S.	14.3	13.7	13.6	13.8	14.4	14.9	15.5	17.0	16.2

[a] 1955-57, [b] 1954-57, [c] 1960-62, [d] 1959-62, [e] 1964-67, [f] 1990-92, [g] 1993-96, [h] 1993, 94, [i] 1993-95.

TABLE I-17. Age-adjusted Death Rates of Cancer

17. Bladder (male)

	Country	1953–1957	1958–1962	1963–1967	1968–1972	1973–1977	1978–1982	1983–1987	1988–1992	1993–1997
1	Australia	4.7[a]	4.9	4.9	5.3	5.0	5.1	4.8	4.4	4.1
2	Austria	—	—	—	7.3[b]	6.9	6.7	6.4	5.8	5.0
3	Belgium	4.5[a]	5.5	6.3	7.1	8.1	8.6	8.2	7.6	7.7[g]
4	Bulgaria	—	—	—	3.9	4.0	4.0	4.4	4.5	4.9
5	Canada	5.4[a]	5.5	5.4	5.6	5.3	5.0	4.7	4.5	4.2
6	Chile	1.8[a]	1.8	2.2	—	—	2.7[d]	2.7	2.7	2.8[h]
7	Costa Rica	—	—	—	—	—	2.2[d]	2.6	2.1	1.6[i]
8	Denmark	6.1[a]	6.5	7.5	7.9	8.3	9.1	9.7	9.2	9.0
9	Finland	4.0[a]	4.5	4.5	5.2	5.0	4.8	4.4	4.3	3.9
10	France	3.4[a]	4.3	5.2	5.6	6.1	6.7	6.8	6.7	6.5
11	Germany	—	—	—	—	—	—	—	6.9[f]	6.4
12	Greece	—	—	—	5.1	5.3	6.2	6.7	6.8	6.6
13	Hong Kong	—	—	—	4.0	5.3	4.5	4.2	4.1	3.4
14	Hungary	—	—	—	5.8[c]	6.3	6.9	7.1	7.6	8.1
15	Iceland	—	—	—	—	3.0	4.6	4.0	4.2	4.8
16	Ireland	3.3[a]	3.3	3.5	3.8	4.3	4.4	4.5	4.7	4.3
17	Italy	4.1[a]	4.9	5.6	6.5	7.4	8.2	9.1	8.9	7.6
18	Japan	1.7[a]	2.1	2.3	2.3	2.4	2.5	2.3	2.3	2.4
19	Mexico	—	—	—	—	—	1.3[e]	1.3	1.4	1.5[i]
20	Netherlands	4.6[a]	5.0	6.2	6.8	7.0	7.4	7.4	7.2	6.3
21	New Zealand	4.3[a]	5.3	5.0	5.1	5.6	5.5	4.6	4.5	4.3
22	Norway	3.6[a]	3.7	4.5	5.0	5.5	5.7	5.8	5.7	5.6
23	Poland	—	—	4.9	—	—	6.7[d]	7.1	7.7	8.1[g]
24	Portugal	—	—	—	—	—	4.7[d]	4.9	5.0	5.2
25	Singapore	—	—	—	2.9	4.6	2.9	3.1	2.6	2.5
26	Spain	3.9[a]	4.3	4.6	5.3	7.0	7.3	7.8	8.5	8.5
27	Sweden	2.6[a]	3.2	3.9	4.4	4.8	4.4	4.2	4.3	4.2
28	Switzerland	4.7[a]	4.6	5.0	5.7	6.0	6.6	6.6	6.7	5.3
29	U.K.	—	7.0	—	7.9	7.9	7.6	7.5	7.4	6.6
30	U.S.	5.2[a]	5.2	5.1	5.1	5.0	4.5[e]	4.0	3.9	3.8

[a] 1955–57, [b] 1969–72, [c] 1970–72, [d] 1980–82, [e] 1979–82, [f] 1990–92, [g] 1993–96, [h] 1994, 95, [i] 1993–95.

by Site and Year (1953–57 to 1993–97)
17. Bladder (female)

	Country	1953–1957	1958–1962	1963–1967	1968–1972	1973–1977	1978–1982	1983–1987	1988–1992	1993–1997
1	Australia	1.6[a]	1.5	1.6	1.6	1.6	1.5	1.4	1.4	1.2
2	Austria	—	—	—	1.6[b]	1.7	1.8	1.7	1.6	1.4
3	Belgium	1.5[a]	1.7	1.8	1.7	1.8	1.9	1.9	1.7	1.7[g]
4	Bulgaria	—	—	—	0.9	0.8	0.8	0.9	1.0	1.0
5	Canada	2.1[a]	1.9	1.9	1.6	1.6	1.4	1.3	1.3	1.2
6	Chile	0.8[a]	0.8	1.0	—	—	1.1[d]	1.0	0.9	1.1[h]
7	Costa Rica	—	—	—	—	—	0.6[d]	0.7	0.8	0.9[i]
8	Denmark	2.1[a]	2.3	2.4	2.2	2.7	2.4	2.5	2.4	2.6
9	Finland	0.9[a]	1.0	1.2	1.0	1.2	1.0	0.8	0.9	0.9
10	France	1.1[a]	1.2	1.3	1.3	1.3	1.3	1.3	1.2	1.2
11	Germany	—	—	—	—	—	—	—	1.7[f]	1.7
12	Greece	—	—	—	1.2	1.0	1.1	1.4	1.2	1.1
13	Hong Kong	—	—	—	1.8	1.9	1.7	1.3	1.2	1.0
14	Hungary	—	—	—	1.1[c]	1.1	1.3	1.4	1.6	1.6
15	Iceland	—	—	—	—	2.1	1.5	2.3	1.7	1.6
16	Ireland	1.3[a]	1.5	1.5	1.4	1.7	1.3	1.5	1.4	1.5
17	Italy	1.1[a]	1.2	1.2	1.2	1.3	1.4	1.4	1.3	1.2
18	Japan	0.9[a]	1.0	1.0	1.0	0.9	0.8	0.7	0.7	0.7
19	Mexico	—	—	—	—	—	0.5[e]	0.5	0.5	0.5[i]
20	Netherlands	1.8[a]	1.7	1.9	1.8	1.7	1.6	1.7	1.7	1.6
21	New Zealand	1.6[a]	1.5	1.4	1.7	1.7	1.4	1.4	1.5	1.4
22	Norway	1.7[a]	1.8	1.7	1.7	1.8	1.8	1.8	1.7	1.8
23	Poland	—	—	0.9	—	—	0.9[d]	1.0	1.0	1.1[g]
24	Portugal	—	—	—	—	—	1.1[d]	1.1	1.3	1.2
25	Singapore	—	—	—	0.9	1.1	1.0	1.3	0.8	0.7
26	Spain	0.8[a]	0.8	0.8	0.9	1.1	1.1	1.1	1.2	1.1
27	Sweden	1.2[a]	1.4	1.3	1.5	1.5	1.4	1.2	1.3	1.2
28	Switzerland	1.5[a]	1.6	1.5	1.6	1.7	1.6	1.8	1.5	1.5
29	U.K.	—	2.1	—	2.1	2.2	2.2	2.2	2.2	2.1
30	U.S.	2.1[a]	1.9	1.8	1.6	1.5	1.3[e]	1.2	1.2	1.2

[a] 1955–57, [b] 1969–72, [c] 1970–72, [d] 1980–82, [e] 1979–82, [f] 1990–92, [g] 1993–96, [h] 1994, 95, [i] 1993–95.

TABLE I-18. Age-adjusted Death Rates of Cancer

18. Thyroid gland (male)

	Country	1953–1957	1958–1962	1963–1967	1968–1972	1973–1977	1978–1982	1983–1987	1988–1992	1993–1997
1	Australia	0.3[a]	0.3	0.3	0.3	0.3	0.2	0.3	0.3	0.2
2	Austria	1.2[a]	1.2	1.1	1.1	1.0	0.9	0.7	0.6	0.7
3	Belgium	0.3[a]	0.4	0.4	0.5	0.3	0.3	0.5[g]	—	0.3[l]
4	Bulgaria	—	—	—	0.3	0.3	0.3	0.4[h]	0.3	0.3
5	Canada	0.4[a]	0.4	0.4	0.4	0.3	0.3	0.3	0.2	0.2
6	Chile	0.3[a]	0.4	0.4	—	—	—	—	—	—
7	Costa Rica	—	—	—	—	—	—	—	—	—
8	Denmark	0.4[a]	0.6	0.4	0.5	0.5	0.5	0.5	0.3	0.3
9	Finland	0.6[a]	0.5	0.6	0.6	0.6	0.6	0.5	0.4[i]	0.3
10	France	0.3[a]	0.3	0.3	0.4	0.4	0.4	0.4	0.4	0.3
11	Germany	—	—	—	—	—	—	—	0.5[j]	0.5
12	Greece	—	—	—	0.1	0.2	0.2	0.3	0.2	0.3
13	Hong Kong	—	—	—	0.6	0.4	0.4[d]	0.4	0.3[k]	0.2
14	Hungary	—	—	—	0.5[b]	0.6	0.6	0.7	0.6	0.6
15	Iceland	—	—	—	—	0.6	0.6	1.3	0.8	0.6
16	Ireland	0.3[a]	0.4	0.3	0.3	0.4	0.4	0.4	0.4	0.3
17	Italy	—	0.4	0.5	0.5[c]	0.6	0.5	0.5	0.5	0.4
18	Japan	0.1[a]	0.2	0.3	0.3	0.3	0.3	0.3	0.3	0.3
19	Mexico	—	—	—	—	—	—	—	—	—
20	Netherlands	0.3[a]	0.4	0.3	0.5	0.5	0.4	0.4	0.3	0.3
21	New Zealand	0.6[a]	0.4	0.4	0.5	0.4	0.4	0.3	0.2	0.3
22	Norway	0.6[a]	0.5	0.5	0.6	0.4	0.4	0.4	0.4	0.4
23	Poland	—	—	0.4	—	—	—	—	—	—
24	Portugal	—	—	—	—	—	—	0.3[h]	0.3	0.3
25	Singapore	—	—	—	0.4	0.5	0.9[e]	0.7	0.5	0.4
26	Spain	0.1[a]	0.1	0.2	0.2	0.2	0.2	0.2	0.3	0.2
27	Sweden	0.4[a]	0.5	0.5	0.6	0.6	0.5	0.4	0.3	0.3
28	Switzerland	1.6[a]	1.4	1.2	1.2	1.0	0.9	0.7	0.6	—
29	U.K.	—	0.3	—	0.3	0.3	0.3	0.3	0.3	0.2
30	U.S.	0.4[a]	0.3	0.3	0.3	0.3	0.3[f]	0.2	0.2	0.3

[a] 1955–57, [b] 1970–72, [c] 1969–72, [d] 1978–81, [e] 1978, 79, 81, 82, [f] 1979–82, [g] 1983, 84, 86, [h] 1984–87, [i] 1989–92, [j] 1990–92, [k] 1988, 89, 91, 92, [l] 1993–96.

by Site and Year (1953–57 to 1993–97)
18. Thyroid gland (female)

	Country	1953–1957	1958–1962	1963–1967	1968–1972	1973–1977	1978–1982	1983–1987	1988–1992	1993–1997
1	Australia	0.6[a]	0.6	0.5	0.5	0.5	0.4	0.4	0.3	0.3
2	Austria	1.7[a]	1.7	1.5	1.4	1.3	1.1	1.0	0.8	0.6
3	Belgium	0.6[a]	0.7	0.6	0.6	0.6	0.7	0.5[g]	—	0.4[l]
4	Bulgaria	—	—	—	0.6	0.6	0.6	0.5[h]	0.4	0.4
5	Canada	0.8[a]	0.7	0.6	0.6	0.5	0.4	0.3	0.3	0.3
6	Chile	0.7[a]	0.8	0.8	—	—	—	—	—	—
7	Costa Rica	—	—	—	—	—	—	—	—	—
8	Denmark	1.1[a]	0.9	0.9	0.8	0.8	0.6	0.6	0.5	0.4
9	Finland	1.0[a]	0.9	1.0	1.1	0.9	1.0	0.7	0.7[i]	0.5
10	France	0.6[a]	0.5	0.6	0.6	0.6	0.6	0.6	0.5	0.4
11	Germany	—	—	—	—	—	—	—	0.7[j]	0.6
12	Greece	—	—	—	0.2	0.3	0.4	0.4	0.3	0.3
13	Hong Kong	—	—	—	0.8	0.6	0.7[d]	0.7	0.7[k]	0.5
14	Hungary	—	—	—	0.9[b]	0.9	0.9	0.8	0.8	0.8
15	Iceland	—	—	—	—	1.6	1.3	1.3	0.8	0.7
16	Ireland	1.0[a]	1.0	0.9	1.2	0.7	0.7	0.7	0.5	0.6
17	Italy	—	0.7	0.7	0.8[c]	0.8	0.7	0.7	0.7	0.6
18	Japan	0.3[a]	0.4	0.5	0.6	0.6	0.6	0.5	0.5	0.5
19	Mexico	—	—	—	—	—	—	—	—	—
20	Netherlands	0.7[a]	0.7	0.7	0.7	0.7	0.6	0.5	0.5	0.4
21	New Zealand	0.6[a]	0.7	0.8	0.7	0.7	0.5	0.4	0.5	0.5
22	Norway	1.0[a]	0.9	0.7	0.7	0.7	0.7	0.6	0.5	0.5
23	Poland	—	—	0.6	—	—	—	—	—	—
24	Portugal	—	—	—	—	—	—	0.4[h]	0.5	0.5
25	Singapore	—	—	—	1.1	1.0	1.2[e]	0.9	0.9	0.8
26	Spain	0.3[a]	0.3	0.3	0.3	0.4	0.4	0.4	0.4	0.4
27	Sweden	0.8[a]	1.0	0.9	0.8	0.8	0.8	0.5	0.5	0.4
28	Switzerland	1.8[a]	1.6	1.4	1.4	1.2	1.0	0.8	0.7	—
29	U.K.	—	0.7	—	0.6	0.6	0.5	0.4	0.4	0.3
30	U.S.	0.6[a]	0.6	0.5	0.4	0.4	0.3[f]	0.3	0.3	0.3

[a] 1955–57, [b] 1970–72, [c] 1969–72, [d] 1978–81, [e] 1978, 79, 81, 82, [f] 1979–82, [g] 1983, 84, 86, [h] 1984–87, [i] 1989–92, [j] 1990–92, [k] 1988, 89, 91, 92, [l] 1993–96.

TABLE I-19. Age-adjusted Death Rates of Cancer

19. Leukemia (male)

	Country	1953–1957	1958–1962	1963–1967	1968–1972	1973–1977	1978–1982	1983–1987	1988–1992	1993–1997
1	Australia	5.3	6.2	6.4	6.6	6.4	6.3	6.4	6.0	5.9
2	Austria	5.9[a]	6.1	5.7	6.2	6.0	6.0	5.7	5.5	5.0
3	Belgium	4.8[b]	6.3	6.2	6.2	6.3	6.5	6.0	6.1	6.1[g]
4	Bulgaria	—	—	5.0[e]	4.5	4.7	4.5	4.8	4.4	5.0
5	Canada	6.0	6.6	6.9	7.0	7.1	6.8	6.6	6.1	5.6
6	Chile	3.2[a]	3.7	4.0	4.2	4.0	4.1	4.1	3.9	4.2[h]
7	Costa Rica	—	—	4.4	3.8	5.2	5.7	6.0	5.8	5.4[i]
8	Denmark	7.3	8.2	8.3	7.6	6.8	7.0	7.2	6.7	6.0
9	Finland	5.4	6.0	7.0	7.1	6.8	6.5	5.8	5.1	4.7
10	France	5.6	6.2	6.6	6.7	7.0	6.9	6.8	6.0	5.6
11	Germany	—	—	—	—	—	—	—	5.9[f]	5.6
12	Greece	—	—	7.3	7.1	7.0	6.5	6.1	5.6	5.9
13	Hong Kong	—	2.9[c]	3.3	3.2	3.6	4.1	3.8	3.7	3.3
14	Hungary	4.8[a]	5.5	6.2	6.1	6.4	6.6	7.4	7.2	7.2
15	Iceland	6.2	9.6	7.0	5.6	5.1	6.5	5.4	5.2	5.3
16	Ireland	4.1	5.0	5.5	6.1	5.5	5.7	5.5	6.0	5.2
17	Italy	4.9	5.9	6.5	7.0	6.8	6.8	6.7	6.6	6.1
18	Japan	2.7	3.3	3.8	3.9	4.3	4.4	4.5	4.3	4.1
19	Mexico	—	1.7	2.1	2.3	2.7	3.0	3.5	3.8	3.8[i]
20	Netherlands	5.9	6.7	7.1	6.8	6.5	6.3	5.8	5.6	5.4
21	New Zealand	6.6	6.6	6.7	6.8	7.0	6.4	6.1	6.6	6.2
22	Norway	6.7	7.0	7.0	6.9	6.1	6.1	5.6	4.6	4.5
23	Poland	—	4.3[d]	5.1	5.5	5.7	5.8	5.7	5.8	5.6[g]
24	Portugal	3.1[a]	4.2	5.1	5.4	5.5	5.4	5.3	5.0	5.0
25	Singapore	—	—	4.1	3.3	4.0	3.8	4.4	4.4	4.3
26	Spain	2.6	3.6	4.1	4.4	4.7	4.9	5.2	5.2	5.1
27	Sweden	6.6	7.3	7.1	6.9	6.7	6.4	5.0	4.9	4.6
28	Switzerland	5.9	6.4	6.3	6.8	6.2	5.9	6.2	5.7	5.2
29	U.K.	5.0	5.4	5.6	5.7	5.6	5.6	5.4	5.2	4.7
30	U.S.	7.1	7.5	7.5	7.3	6.9	6.8	6.4	6.4	6.3

[a] 1955–57, [b] 1954–57, [c] 1960–62, [d] 1959–62, [e] 1964–67, [f] 1990–92, [g] 1993–96, [h] 1993, 94, [i] 1993–95.

by Site and Year (1953–57 to 1993–97)
19. Leukemia (female)

	Country	1953–1957	1958–1962	1963–1967	1968–1972	1973–1977	1978–1982	1983–1987	1988–1992	1993–1997
1	Australia	4.1	4.5	4.3	4.4	4.2	4.0	3.9	3.7	3.6
2	Austria	4.1[a]	4.2	4.5	4.3	4.2	4.0	3.7	3.5	3.4
3	Belgium	4.1[b]	4.3	4.4	4.3	3.8	4.2	4.0	3.7	3.8[g]
4	Bulgaria	—	—	3.7[e]	3.6	3.6	3.6	3.5	2.9	3.2
5	Canada	4.3	4.6	4.6	4.6	4.3	4.2	4.1	3.8	3.4
6	Chile	2.4[a]	3.1	3.0	3.5	3.3	3.4	3.5	3.2	2.9[h]
7	Costa Rica	—	—	3.3	3.8	4.4	5.2	4.4	4.6	4.3[i]
8	Denmark	5.6	5.2	5.1	4.8	4.6	4.5	4.5	4.1	3.7
9	Finland	3.8	4.8	5.2	5.3	4.4	4.0	4.0	3.1	3.1
10	France	4.1	4.5	4.6	4.3	4.4	4.4	4.1	3.6	3.4
11	Germany	—	—	—	—	—	—	—	3.6[f]	3.5
12	Greece	—	—	5.0	4.7	4.4	4.1	3.9	3.5	3.6
13	Hong Kong	—	2.1[c]	3.0	2.6	2.8	3.2	2.8	2.7	2.6
14	Hungary	3.5[a]	3.9	4.2	4.2	4.4	4.5	4.5	4.5	4.6
15	Iceland	4.6	3.7	4.2	6.1	3.3	3.0	4.0	3.4	2.3
16	Ireland	3.2	3.4	3.7	3.6	3.4	3.6	3.7	3.4	3.1
17	Italy	3.7	4.3	4.7	4.8	4.6	4.4	4.3	4.0	3.8
18	Japan	1.9	2.6	2.9	3.0	3.1	3.0	2.9	2.7	2.6
19	Mexico	—	1.3	1.9	2.1	2.3	2.7	3.0	3.0	3.1[i]
20	Netherlands	4.5	5.0	5.0	4.9	4.2	4.1	3.7	3.5	3.1
21	New Zealand	5.2	5.4	5.1	4.8	4.3	3.9	4.6	3.8	3.8
22	Norway	5.0	4.8	4.8	4.7	4.1	3.9	3.5	3.1	2.8
23	Poland	—	3.1[d]	3.7	3.8	3.8	3.8	3.7	3.6	3.5[g]
24	Portugal	2.8[a]	3.2	4.0	4.4	3.9	4.1	3.5	3.7	3.4
25	Singapore	—	—	2.3	3.2	2.9	3.6	3.2	2.7	3.1
26	Spain	1.9	2.8	3.2	3.3	3.4	3.4	3.4	3.4	3.1
27	Sweden	4.7	5.2	5.1	4.9	4.7	4.3	3.6	3.3	3.1
28	Switzerland	4.1	4.5	4.5	4.6	4.0	4.0	3.6	3.6	2.9
29	U.K.	3.6	3.9	3.9	3.8	3.6	3.6	3.5	3.2	3.0
30	U.S.	4.9	4.9	4.9	4.6	4.2	4.1	4.0	3.8	3.7

[a] 1955–57, [b] 1954–57, [c] 1960–62, [d] 1959–62, [e] 1964–67, [f] 1990–92, [g] 1993–96, [h] 1993, 94, [i] 1993–95.

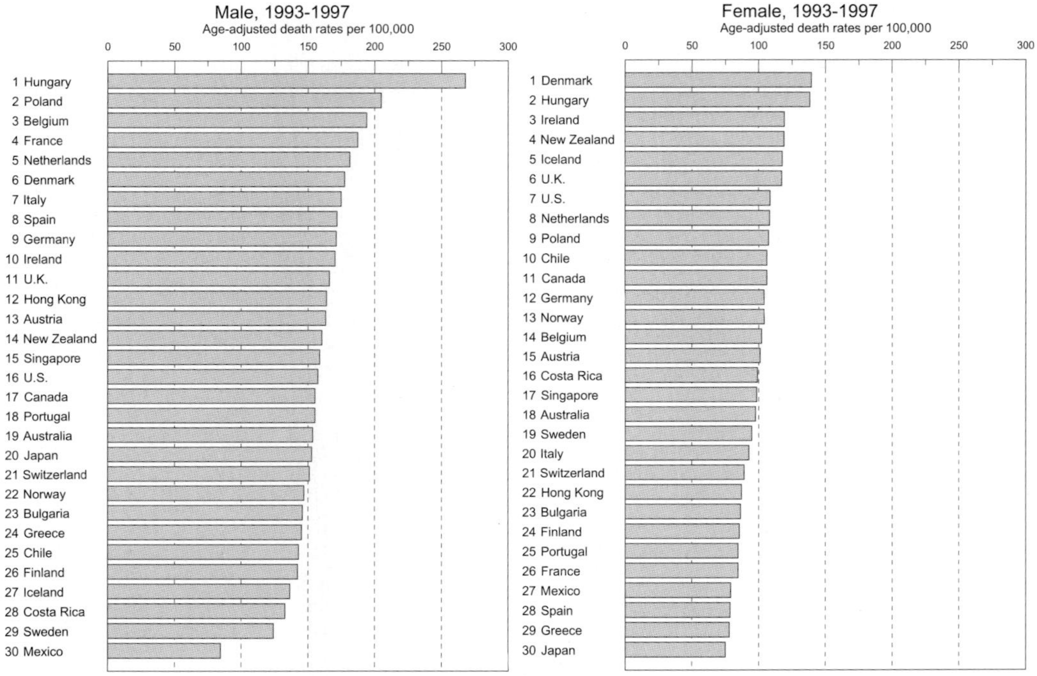

FIG. 1-1. Age-adjusted death rates for malignant neoplasm of all sites in 30 countries of the world (1993–1997)

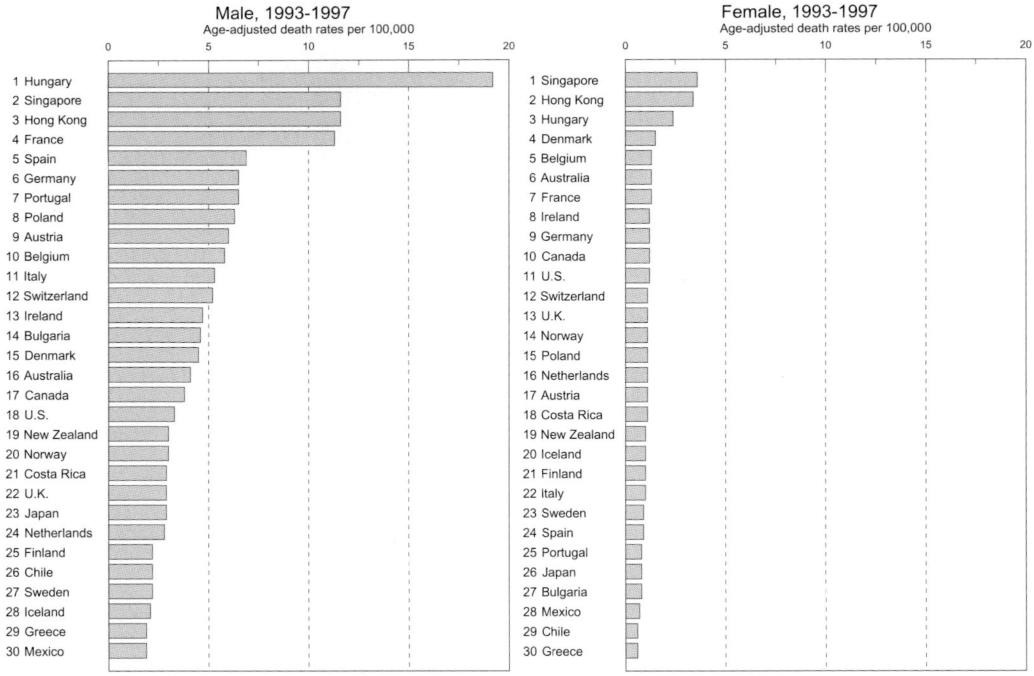

FIG. 1-2. Age-adjusted death rates of malignant neoplasm of lip, oral cavity and pharynx in 30 countries of the world (1993–1997)

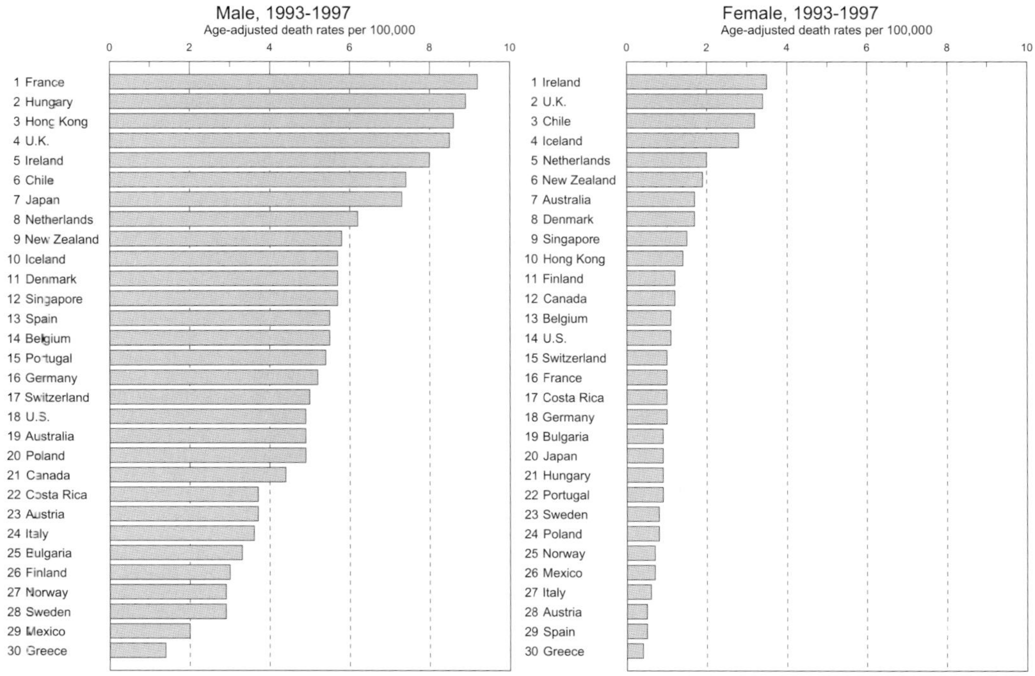

FIG. 1-3. Age-adjusted death rates of malignant neoplasm of esophagus in 30 countries of the world (1993–1997)

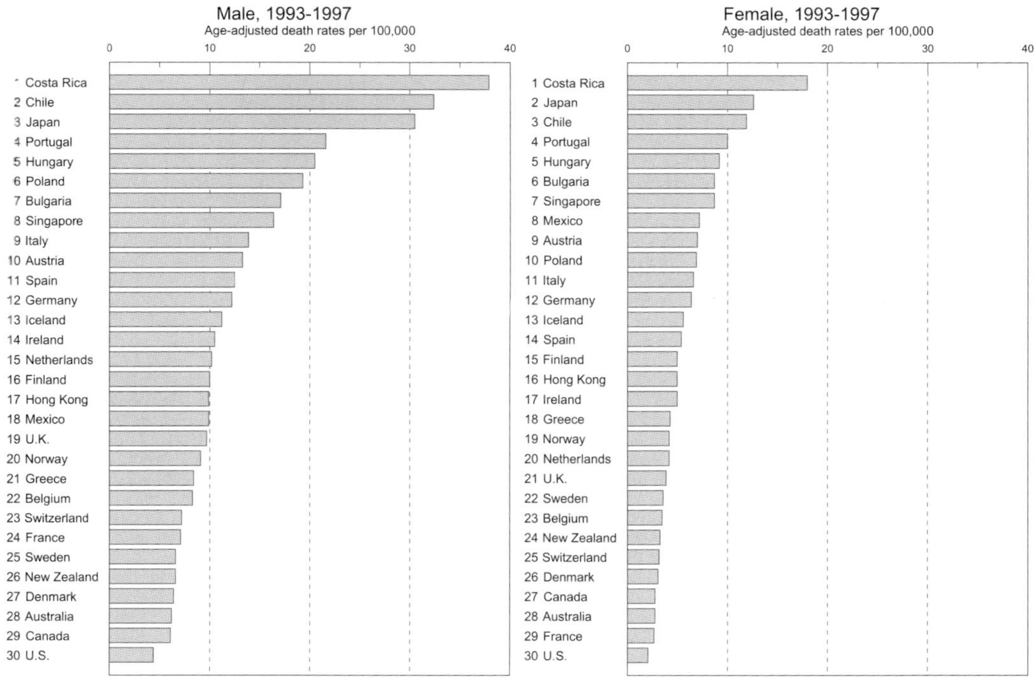

FIG. 1-4. Age-adjusted death rates of malignant neoplasm of stomach in 30 countries of the world (1993–1997)

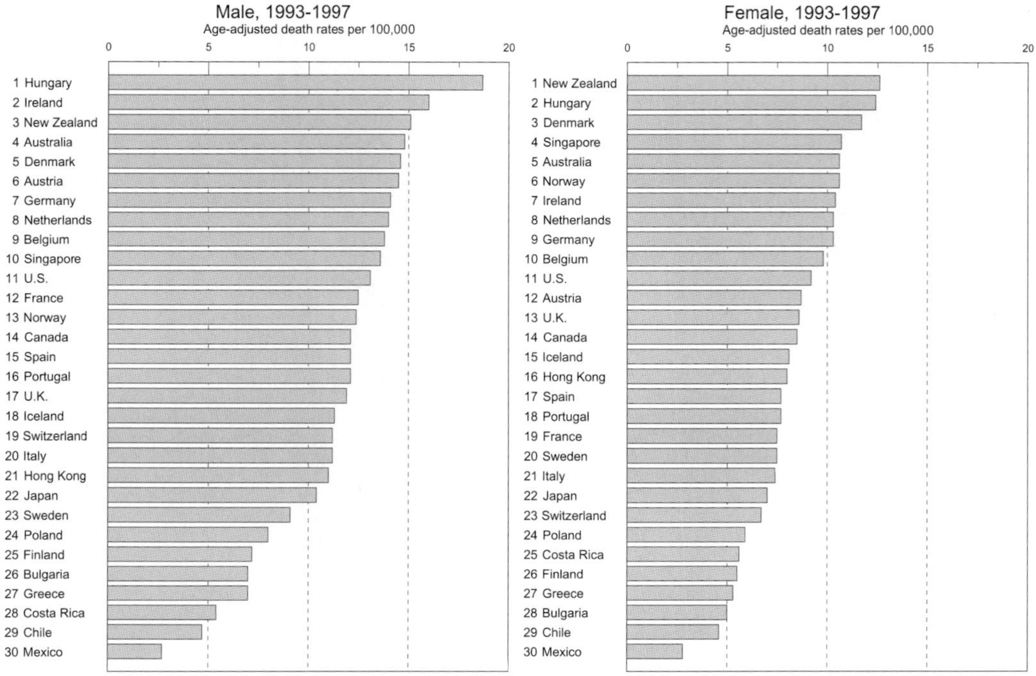

FIG. 1-5. Age-adjusted death rates of malignant neoplasm of intestine except rectum in 30 countries of the world (1993–1997)

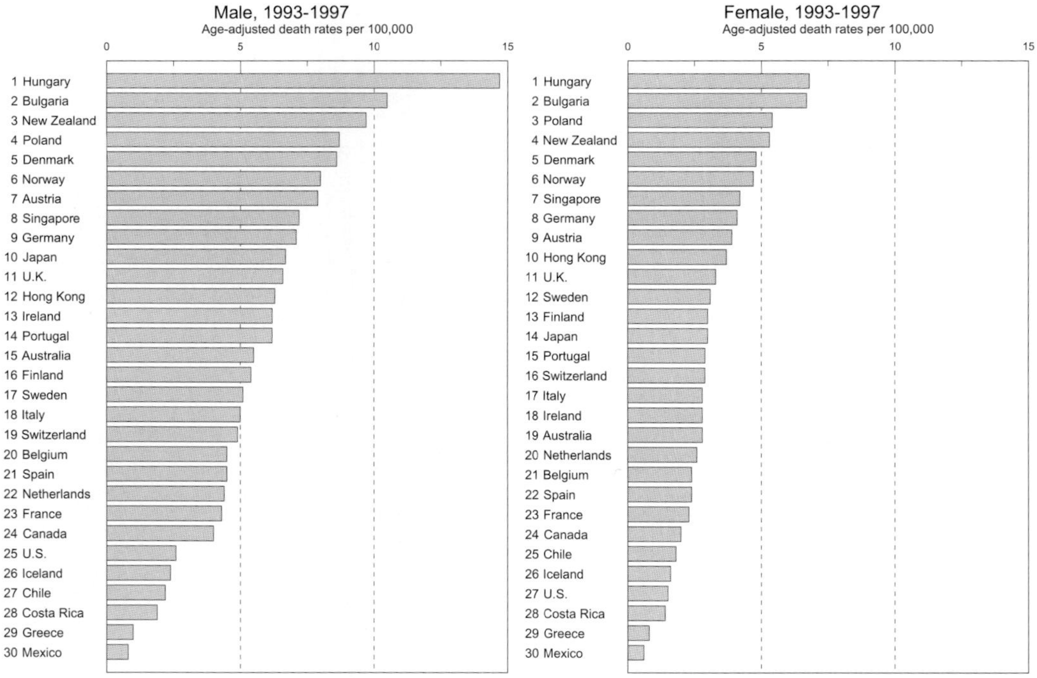

FIG. 1-6. Age-adjusted death rates of malignant neoplasm of rectum, rectosigmoid junction, and anus in 30 countries of the world (1993–1997)

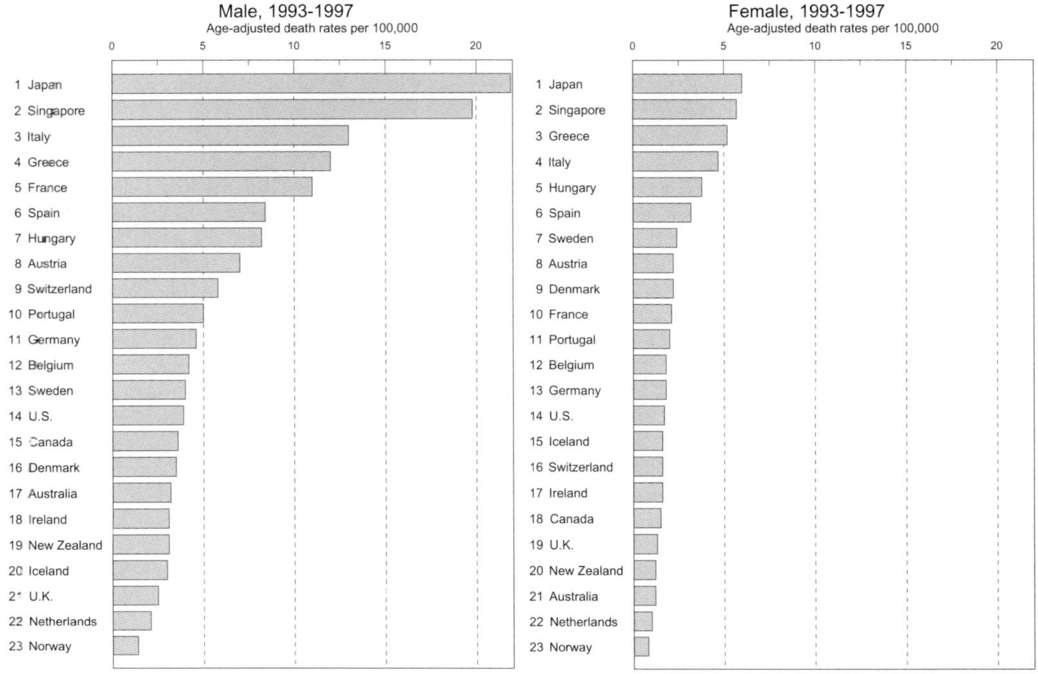

FIG. 1-7. Age-adjusted death rates of malignant neoplasm of liver and intrahepatic bile ducts in 30 countries of the world (1993–1997)

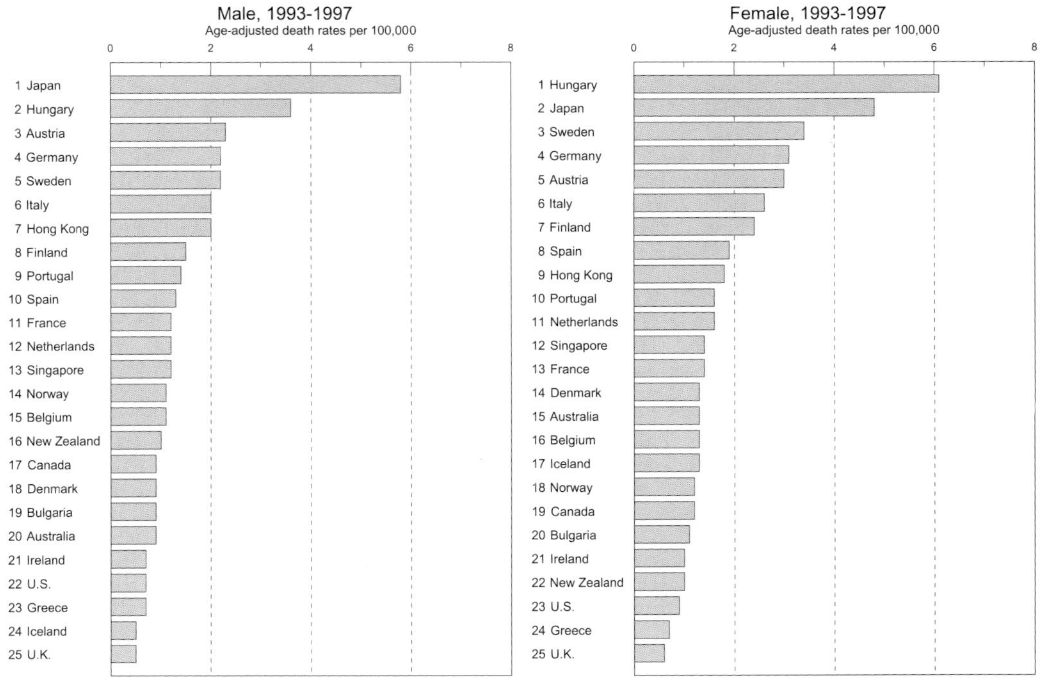

FIG. 1-8. Age-adjusted death rates of malignant neoplasm of gallbladder and extrahepatic bile ducts in 30 countries of the world (1993–1997)

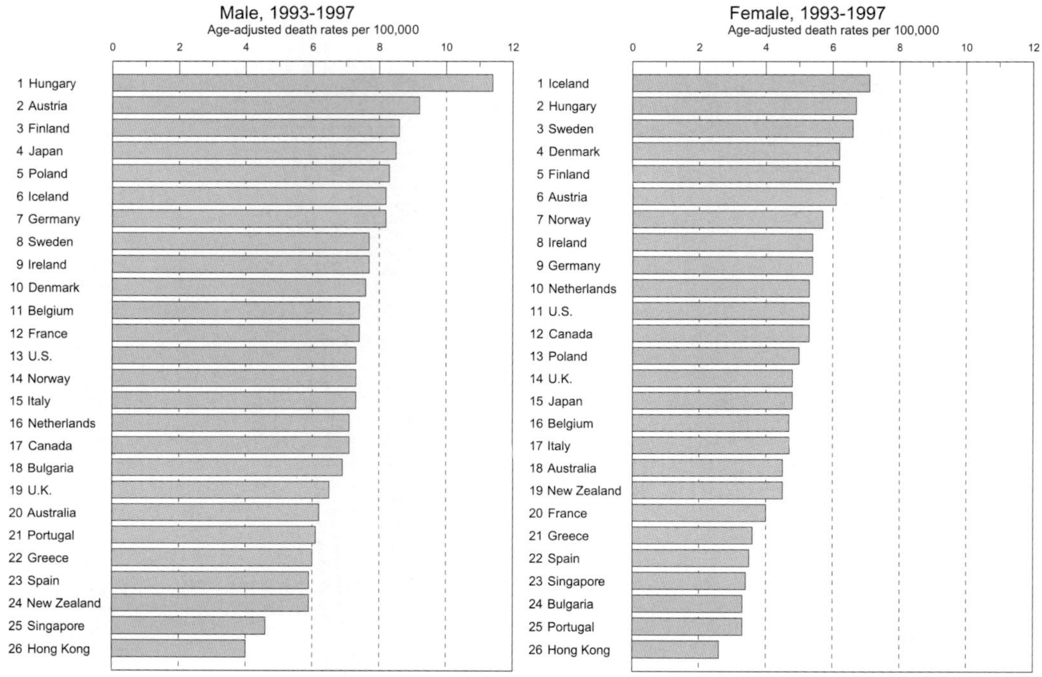

FIG. 1-9. Age-adjusted death rates of malignant neoplasm of pancreas in 30 countries of the world (1993–1997)

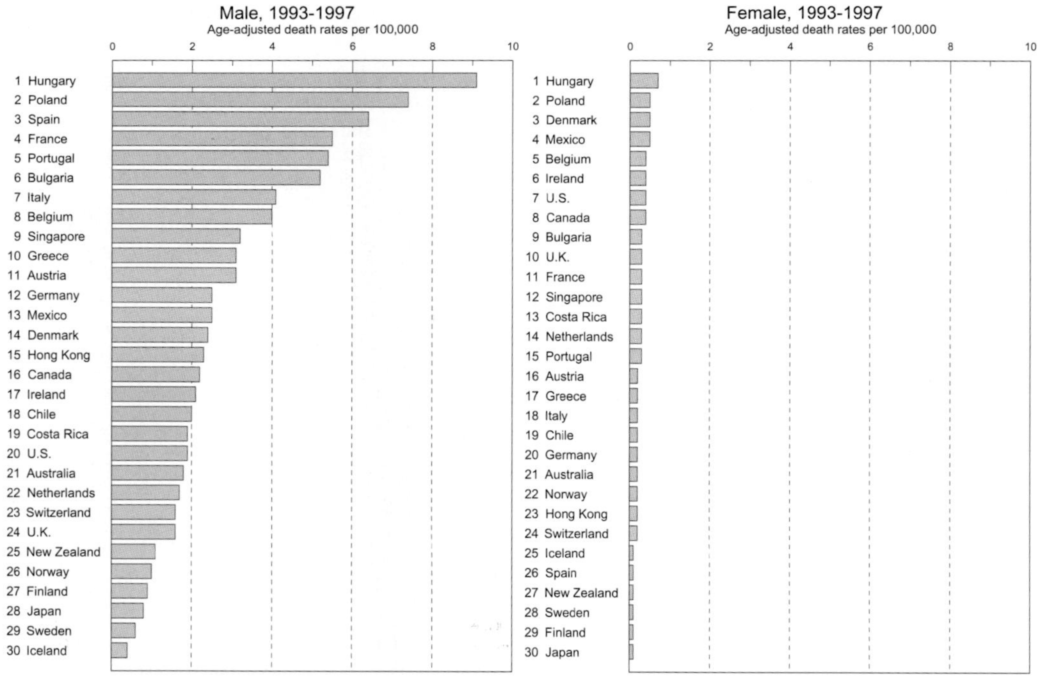

FIG. 1-10. Age-adjusted death rates of malignant neoplasm of larynx in 30 countries of the world (1993–1997)

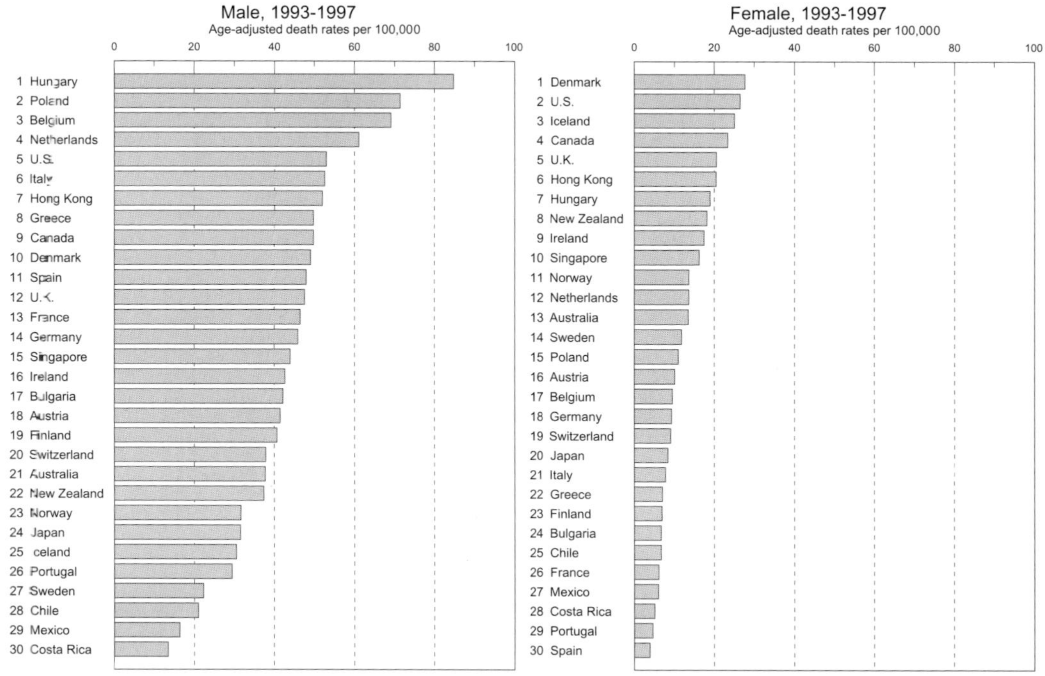

FIG. 1-11. Age-adjusted death rates of malignant neoplasm of trachea, bronchus and lung in 30 countries (1993–1997)

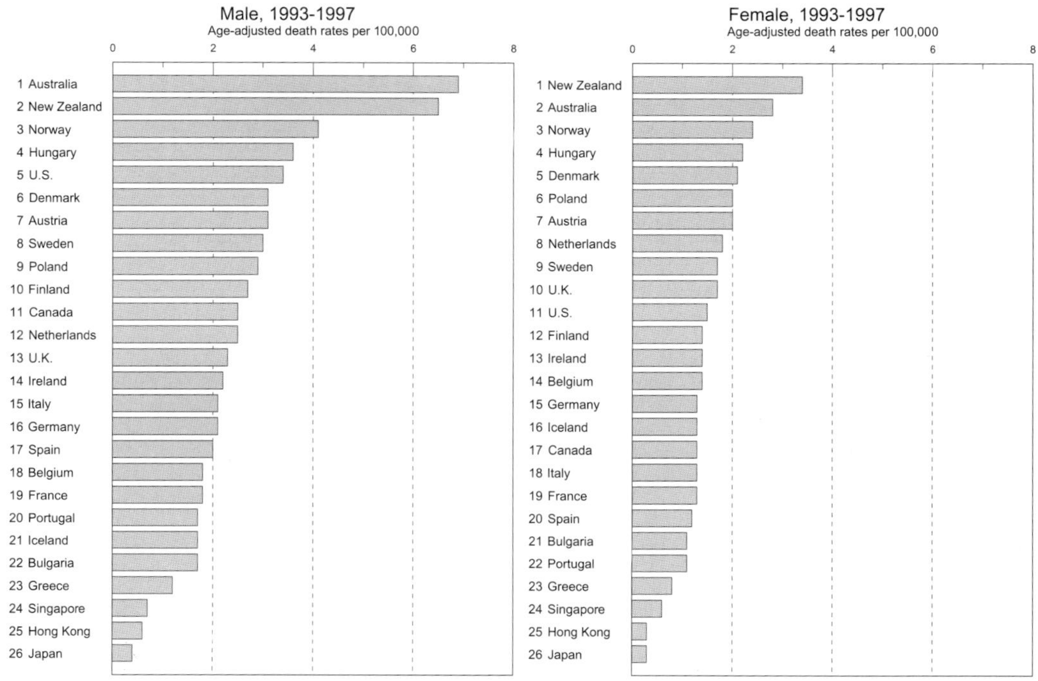

FIG. 1-12. Age-adjusted death rates of malignant neoplasm of skin in 30 countries of the world (1993–1997)

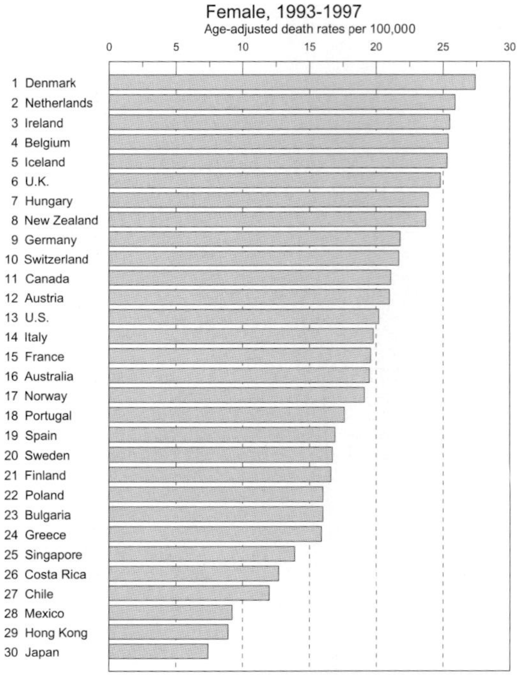

FIG. 1-13. Age-adjusted death rates of malignant neoplasm of breast (female) in 30 countries of the world (1993–1997)

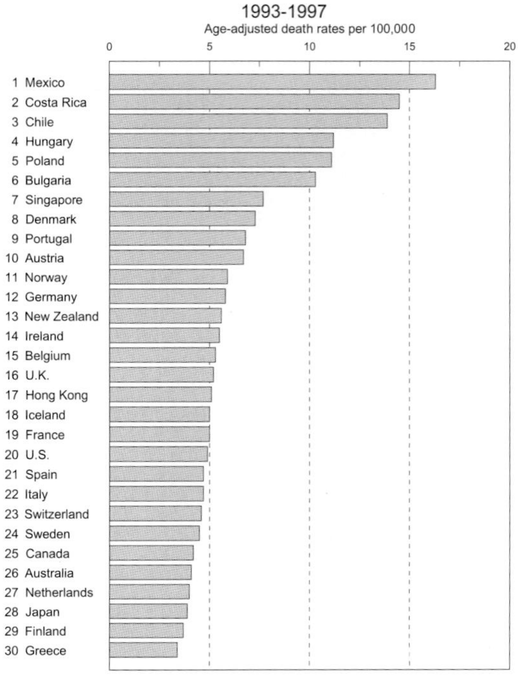

FIG. 1-14. Age-adjusted death rates of malignant neoplasm of uterus (all parts) in 30 Countries of the world (1993–1997)

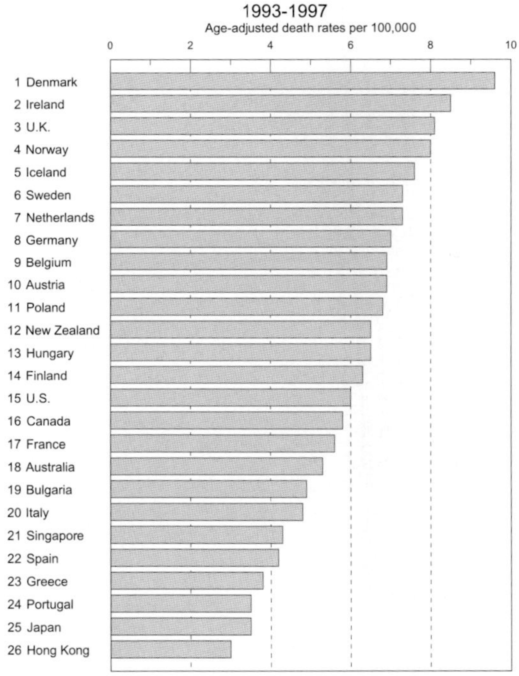

FIG. 1-15. Age-adjusted death rates of malignant neoplasm of ovary and other uterine adnexa in 30 countries of the world (1993–1997)

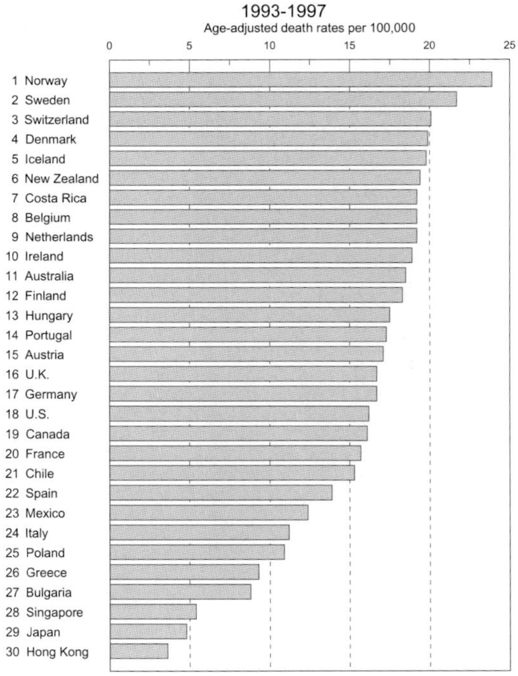

FIG. 1-16. Age-adjusted death rates of malignant neoplasm of prostate in 30 countries of the world (1993–1997)

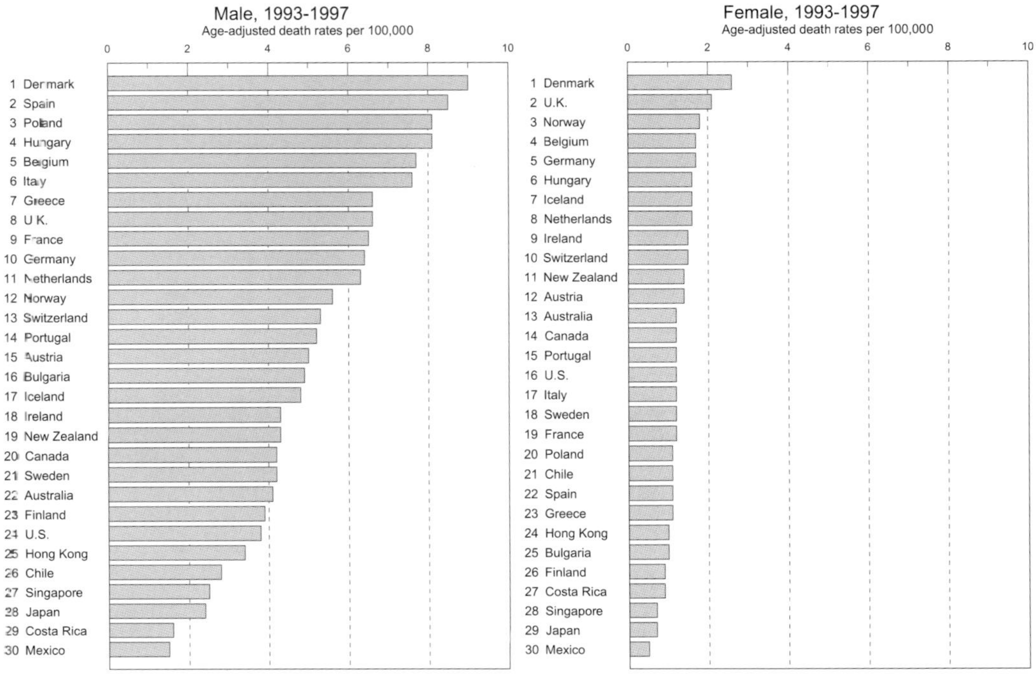

FIG. 1-17. Age-adjusted death rates of malignant neoplasm of bladder in 30 countries of the world (1993–1997)

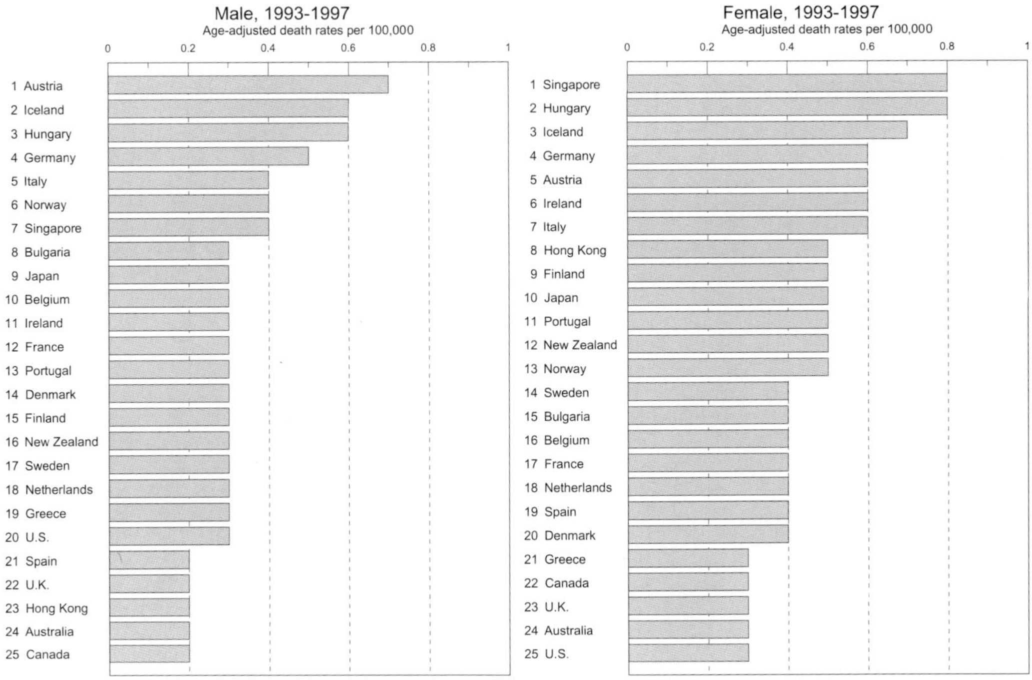

FIG. 1-18. Age-adjusted death rates of malignant neoplasm of thyroid gland in 30 countries of the world (1993–1997)

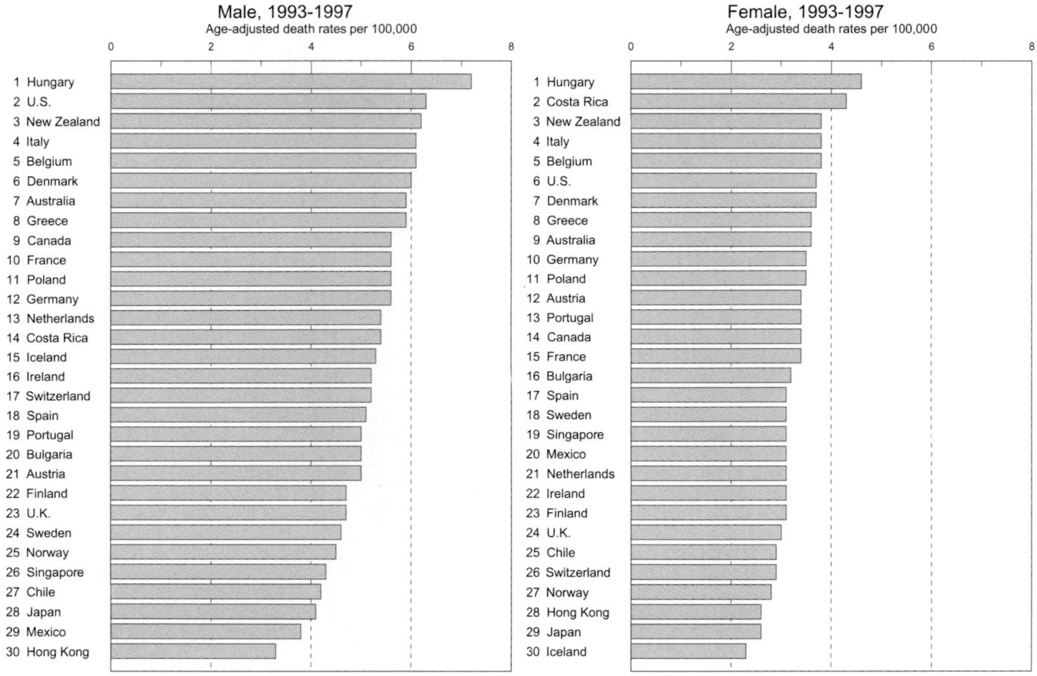

FIG. 1-19. Age-adjusted death rates of leukemia in 30 countries of the world (1993–1997)

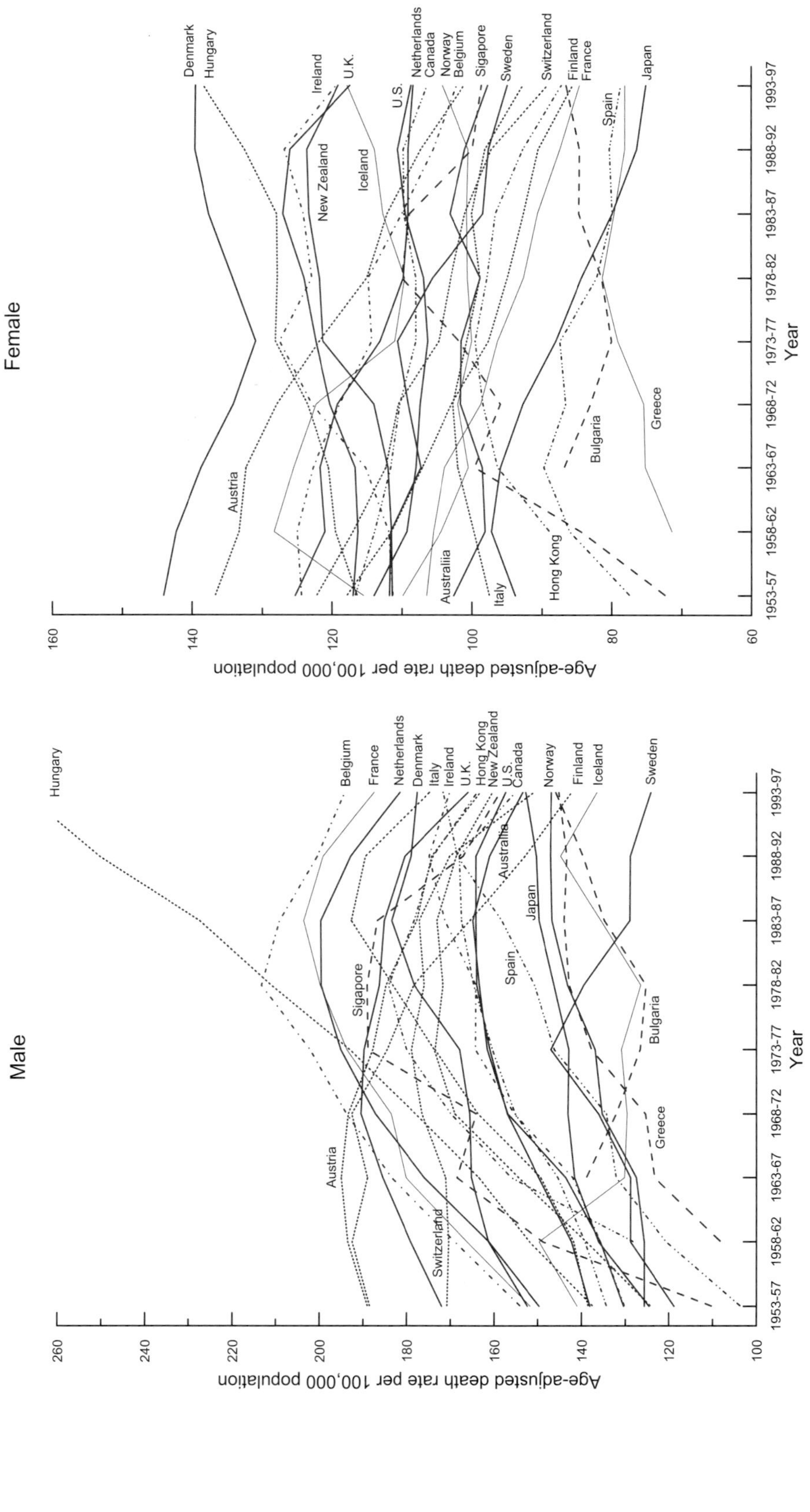

FIG. 2-1. Trends in age-adjusted death rates of malignant Neoplasm of all sites in 30 countries of the world (from 1953–57 to 1993–97)

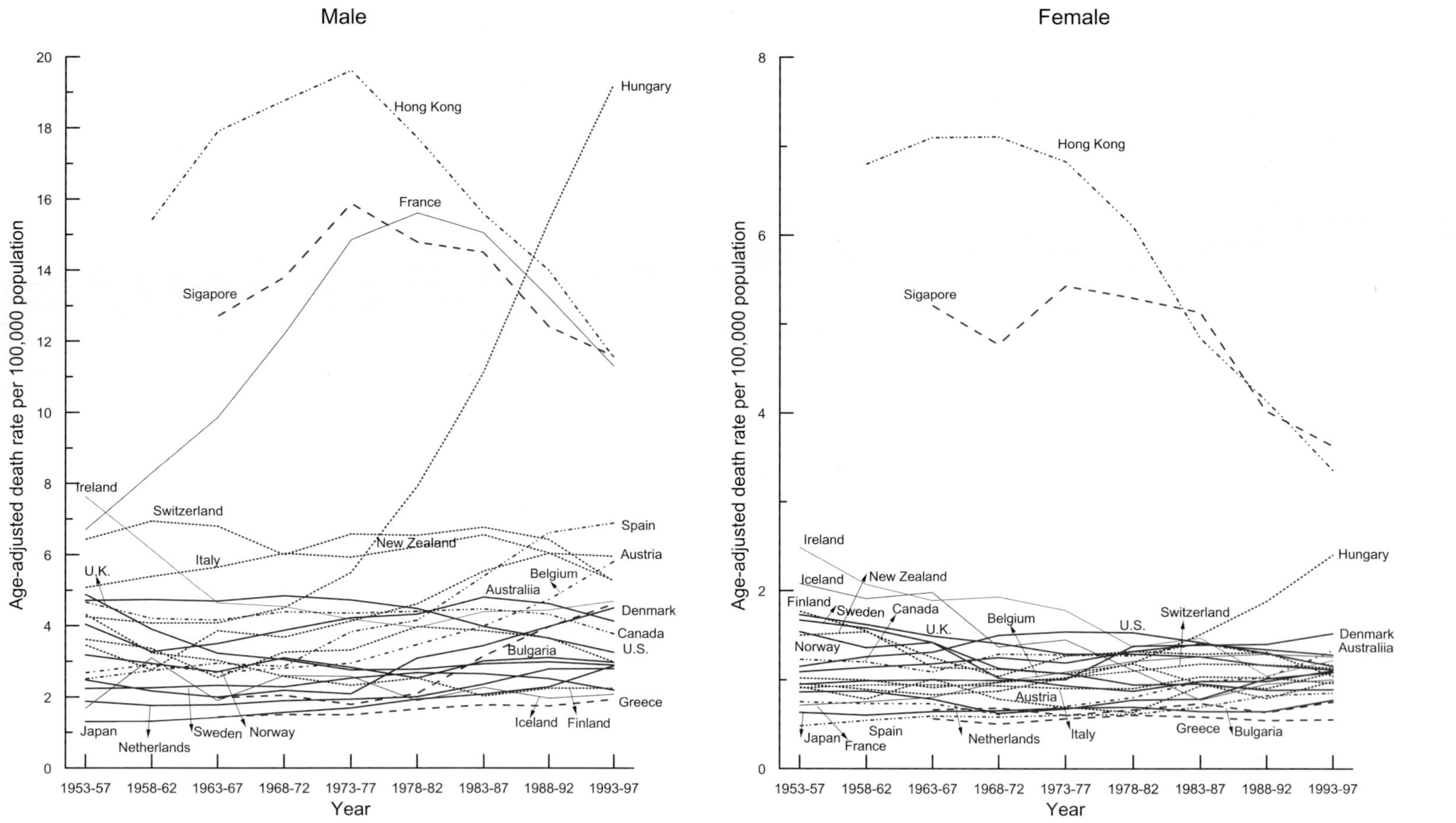

FIG. 2-2. Trends in age-adjusted death rates of malignant neoplasm of lip, oral cavity, and pharynx in 30 countries of the world (from 1953–57 to 1993–97)

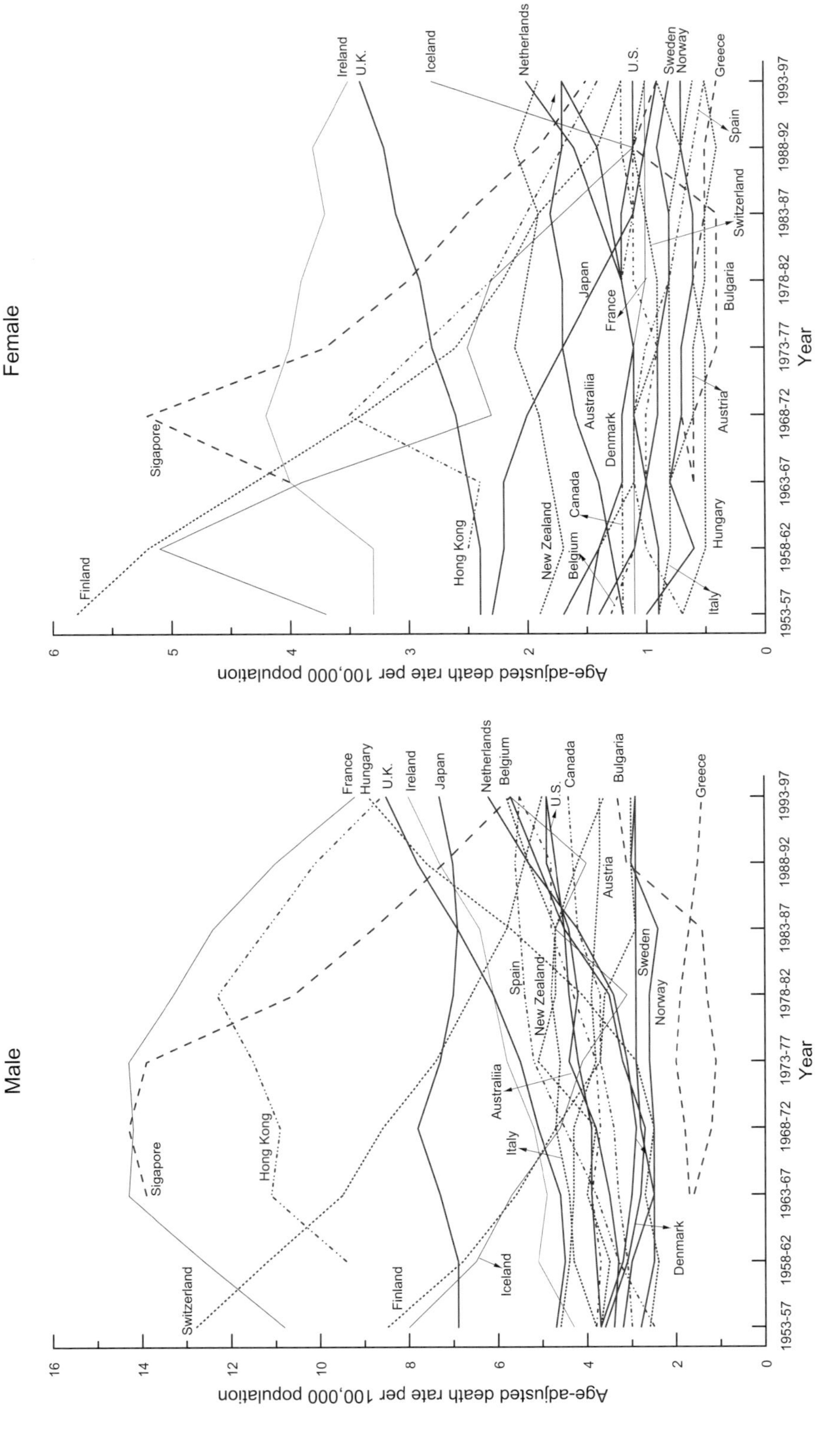

FIG. 2-3. Trends in age-adjusted death rates of malignant neoplasm of esophagus in 30 countries of the world (from 1953–57 to 1993–97)

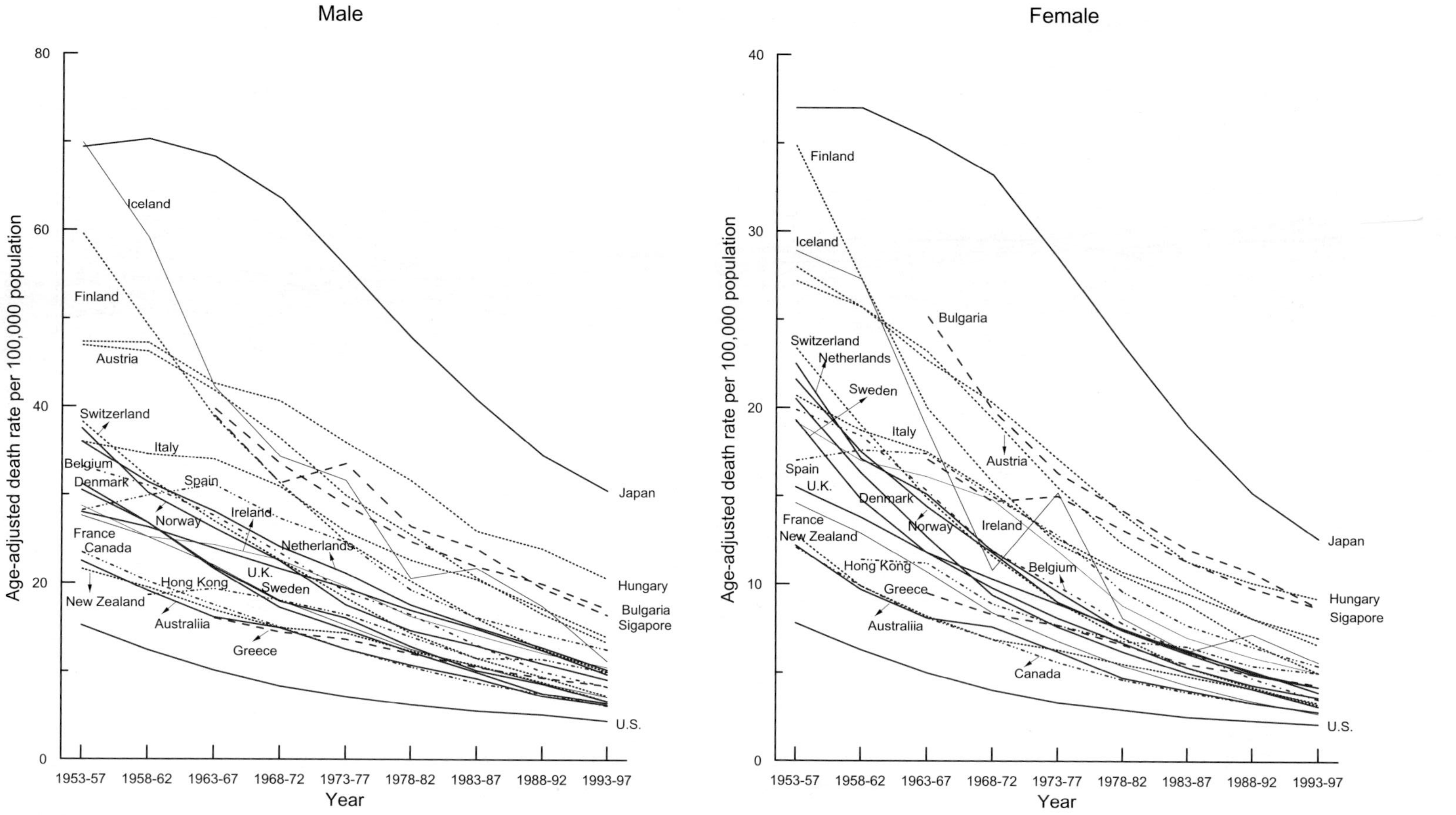

FIG. 2-4. Trends in age-adjusted death rates of malignant neoplasm of stomach in 30 countries of the world (from 1953–57 to 1993–97)

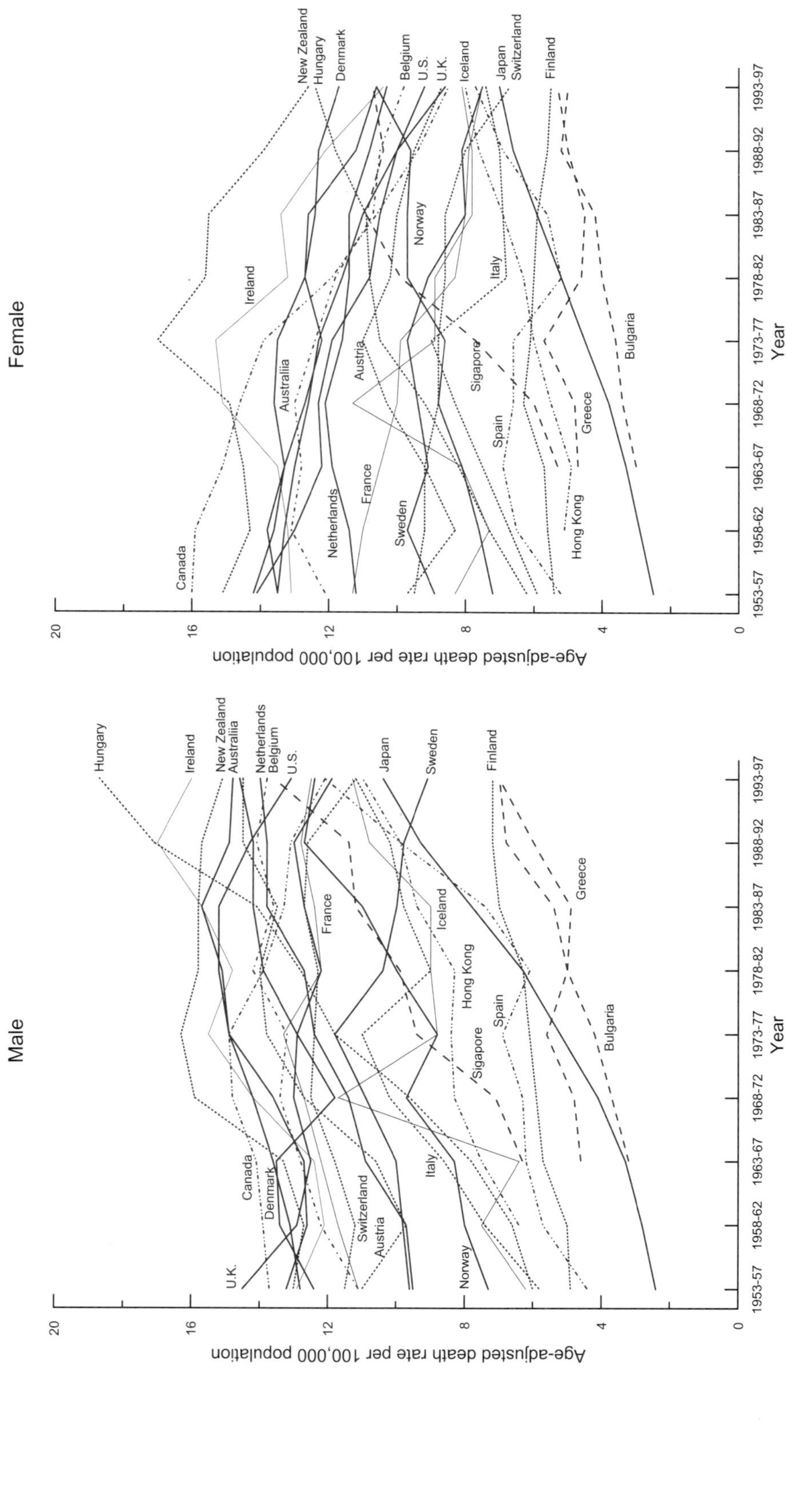

FIG. 2-5. Trends in age-adjusted death rates of malignant neoplasm of intestine except rectum in 30 countries of the world (from 1953–57 to 1993–97)

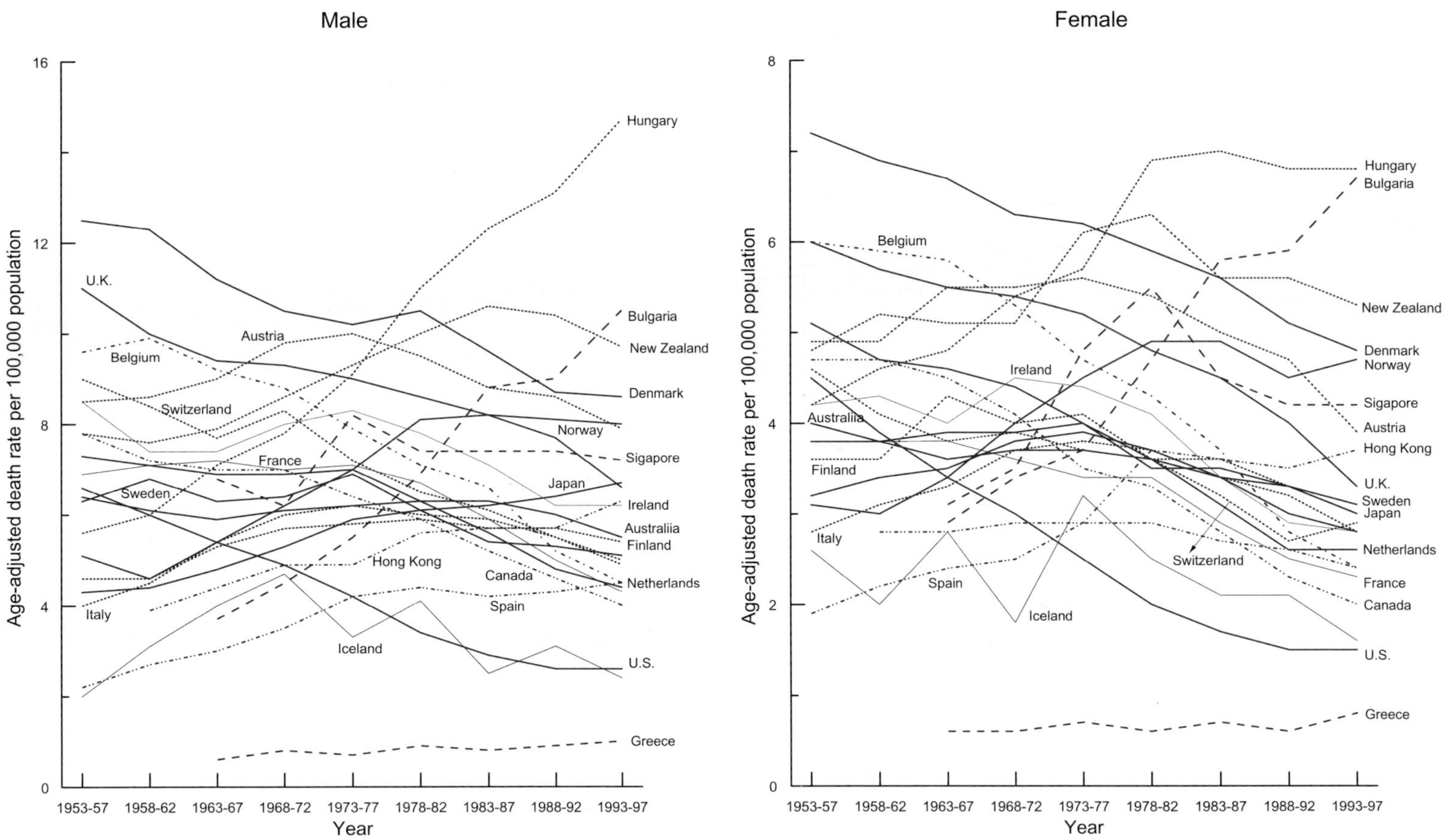

FIG. 2-6. Trends in age-adjusted death rates of malignant neoplasm of rectum, rectosigmoid junction, and anus in 30 countries of the world (from 1953–57 to 1993–97)

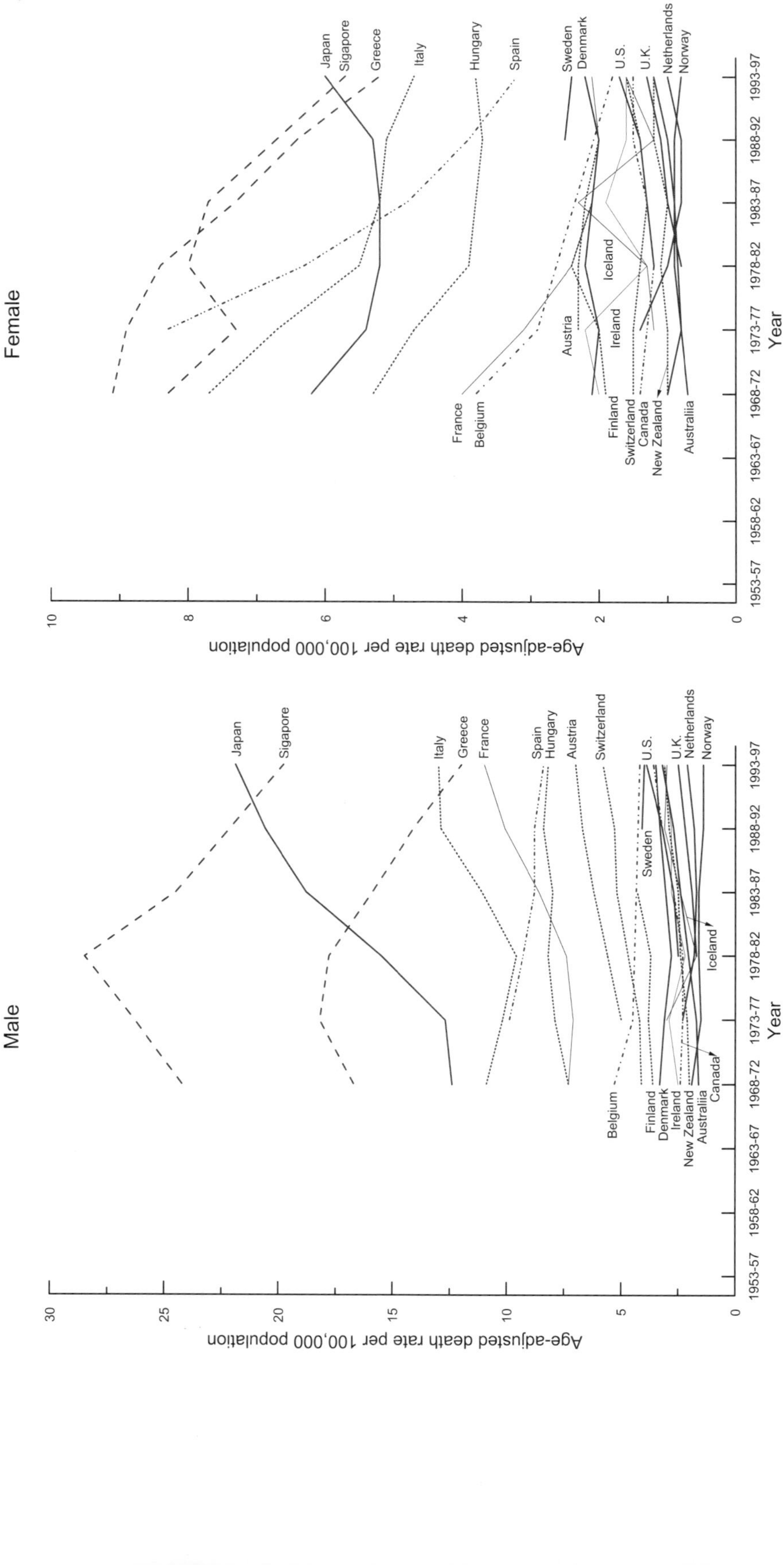

FIG. 2-7. Trends in age-adjusted death rates of malignant neoplasm of liver and intrahepatic bile ducts in 30 countries of the world (from 1953–57 to 1993–97)

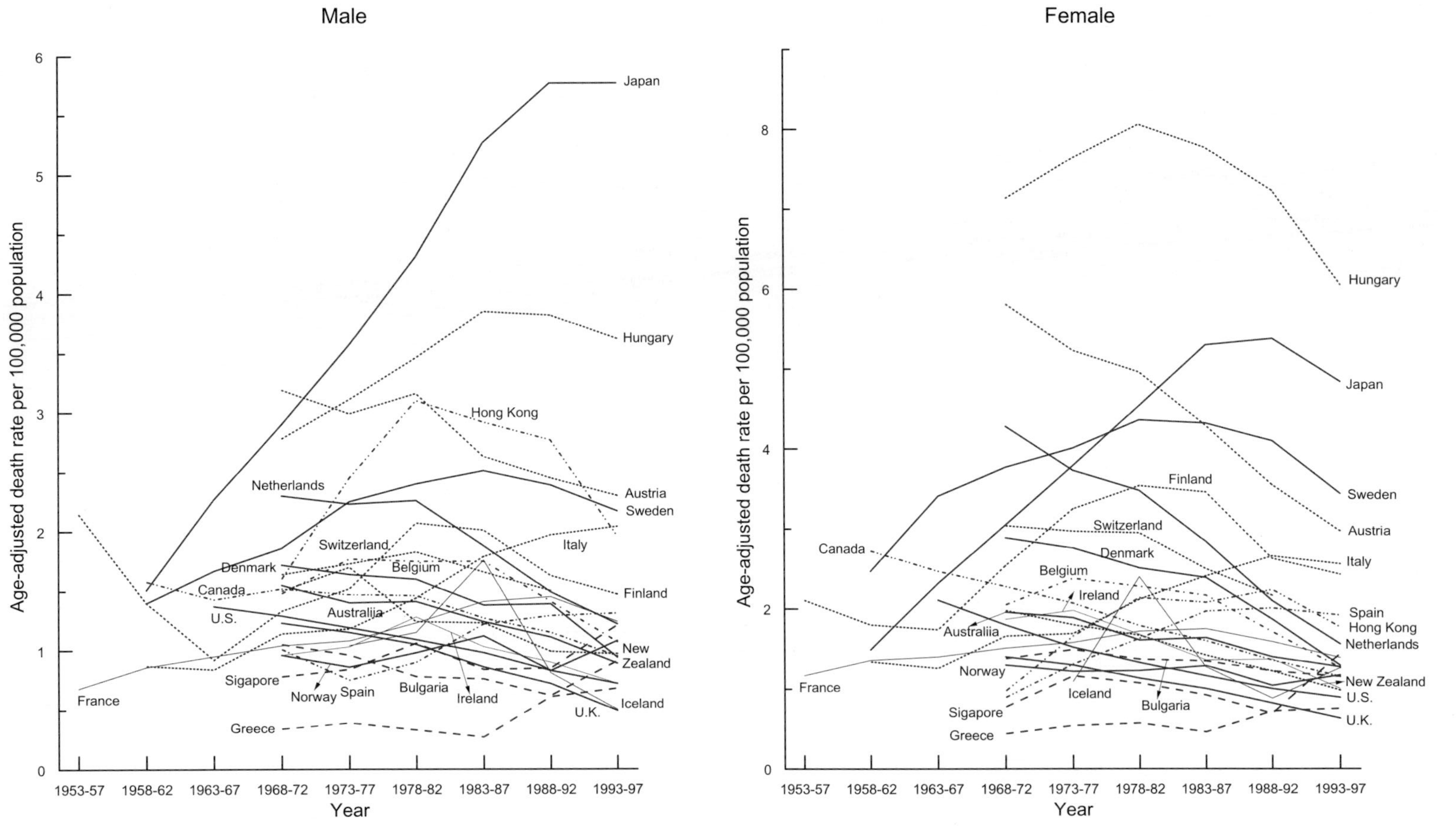

FIG. 2-8. Trends in age-adjusted death rates of malignant neoplasm of gallbladder and extrahepatic bile ducts in 30 countries of the world (from 1953–57 to 1993–97)

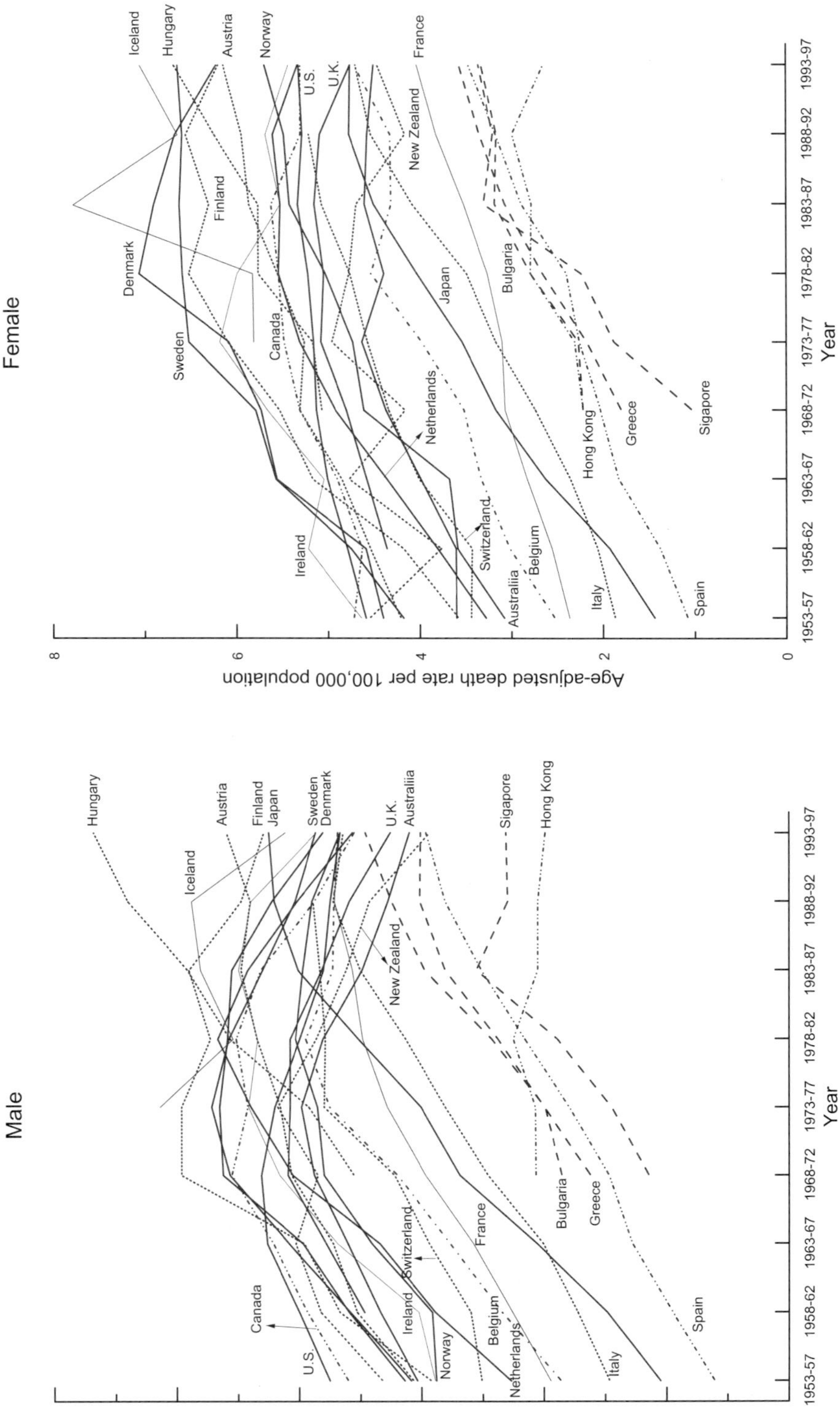

FIG. 2-9. Trends in age-adjusted death rates of malignant neoplasm of pancreas in 30 countries of the world (from 1953–57 to 1993–97)

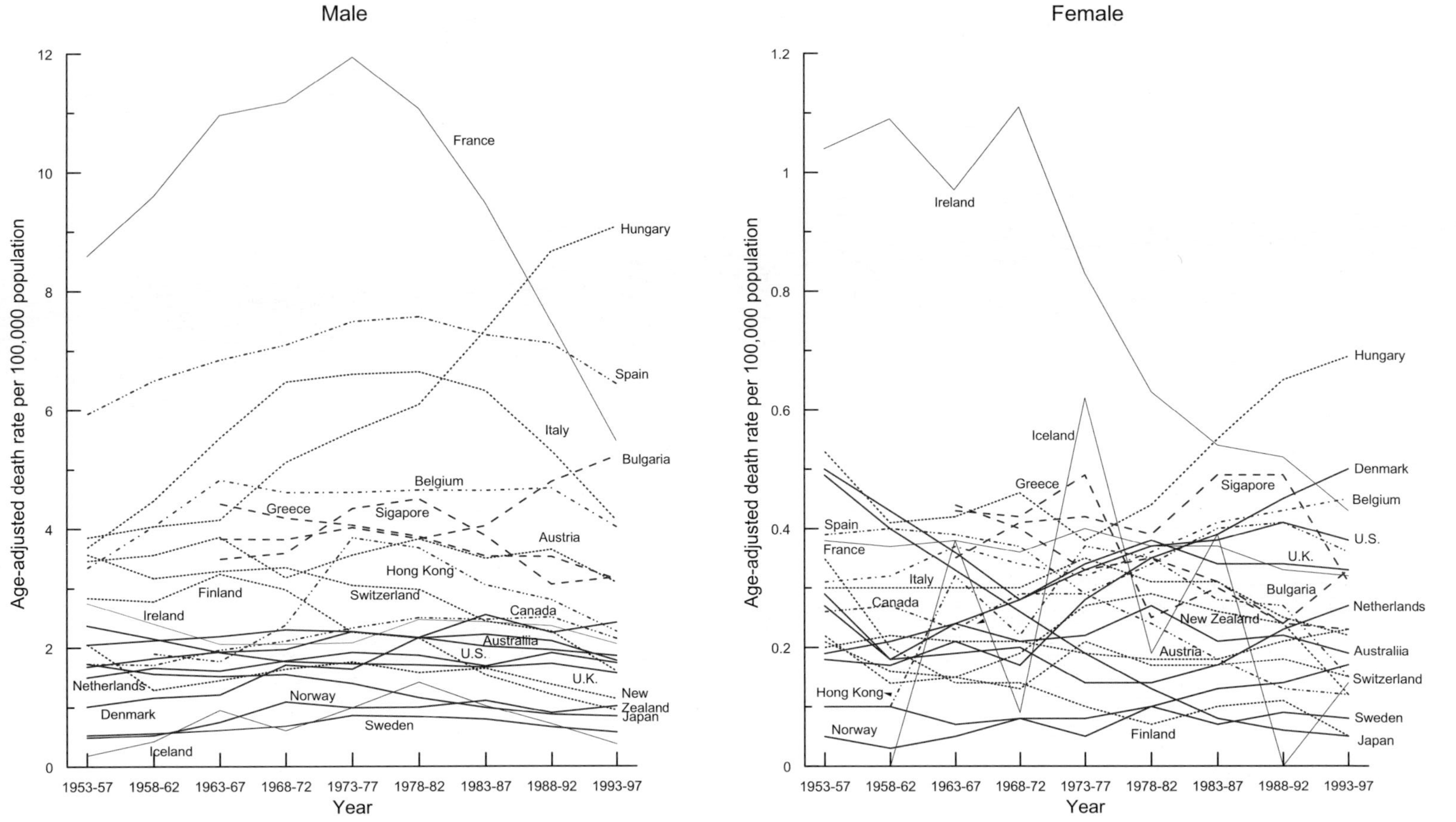

FIG. 2-10. Trends in age-adjusted death rates of malignant neoplasm of larynx in 30 countries of the world (from 1953–57 to 1993–97)

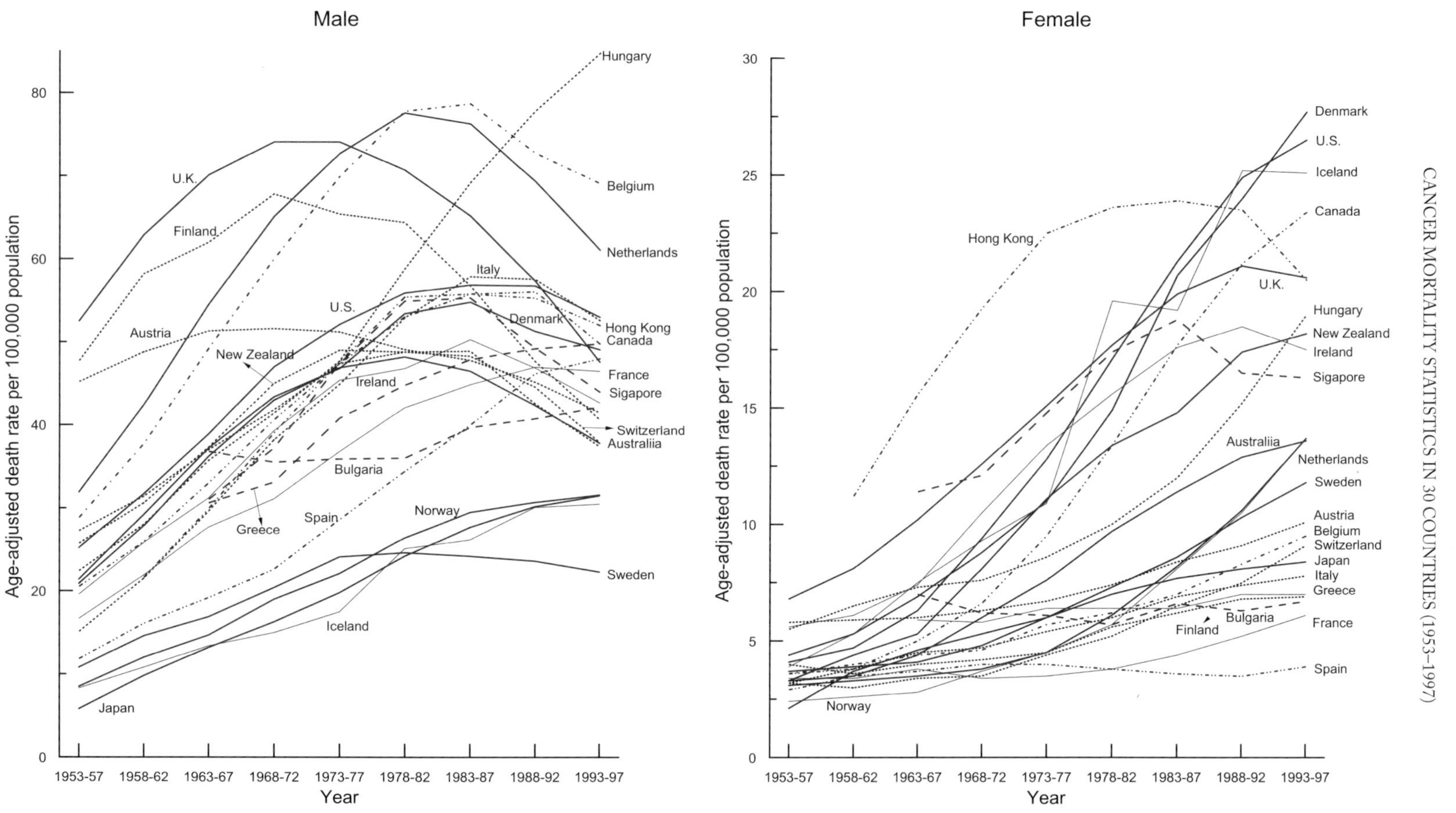

FIG. 2-11. Trends in age-adjusted death rates of malignant neoplasm of trachea, bronchus, and lung in 30 countries of the world (from 1953–57 to 1993–97)

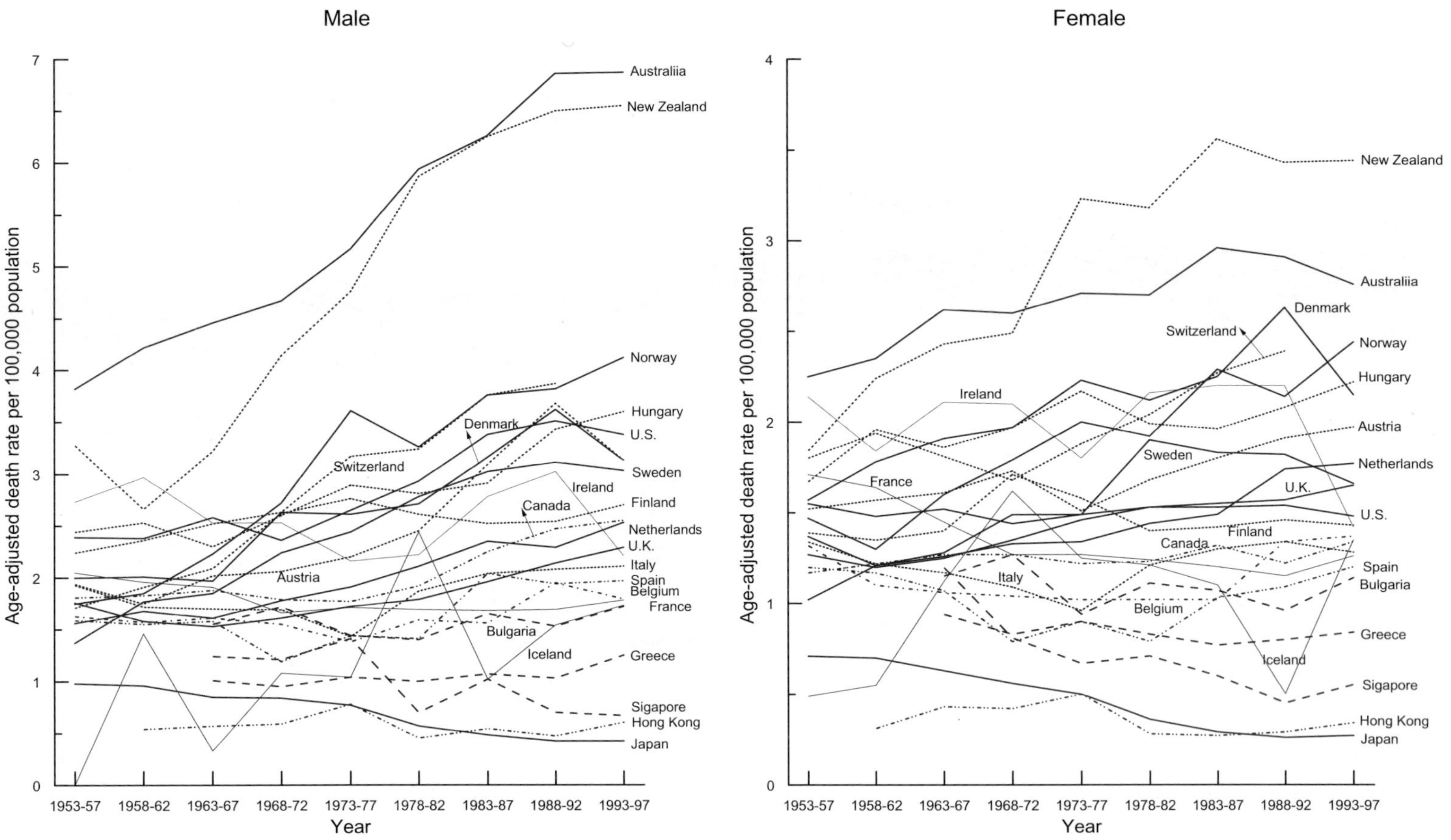

FIG. 2-12. Trends in age-adjusted death rates of malignant neoplasm of skin in 30 countries of the world (from 1953–57 to 1993–97)

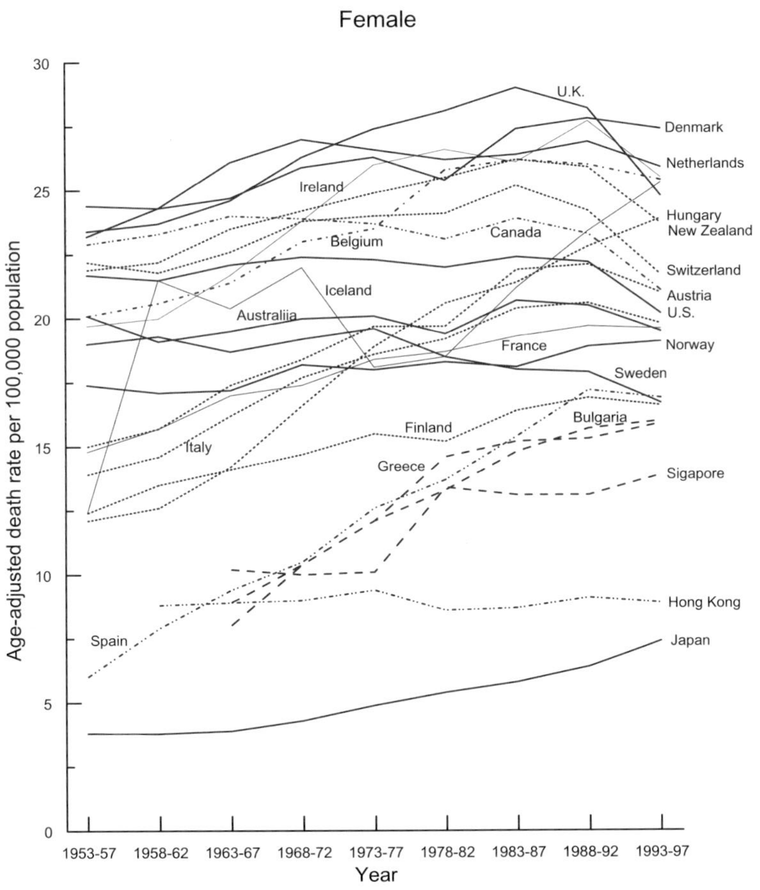

FIG. 2-13. Trends in age-adjusted death rates of malignant neoplasm of breast (female) in 30 countries of the world (from 1953–57 to 1993–97)

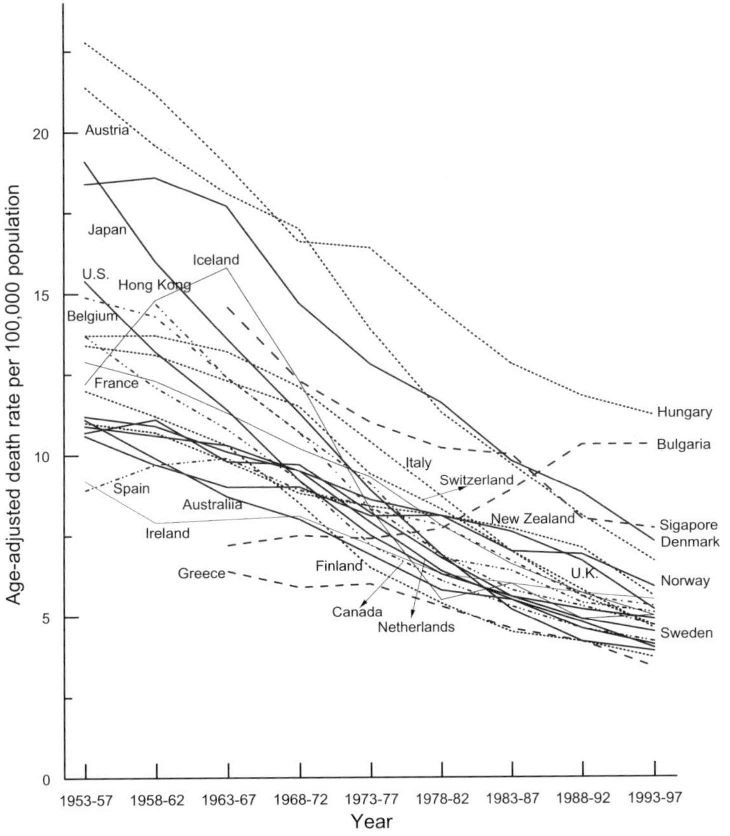

FIG. 2-14. Trends in age-adjusted death rates of malignant neoplasm of uterus (all parts) in 30 countries of the world (from 1953–57 to 1993–97)

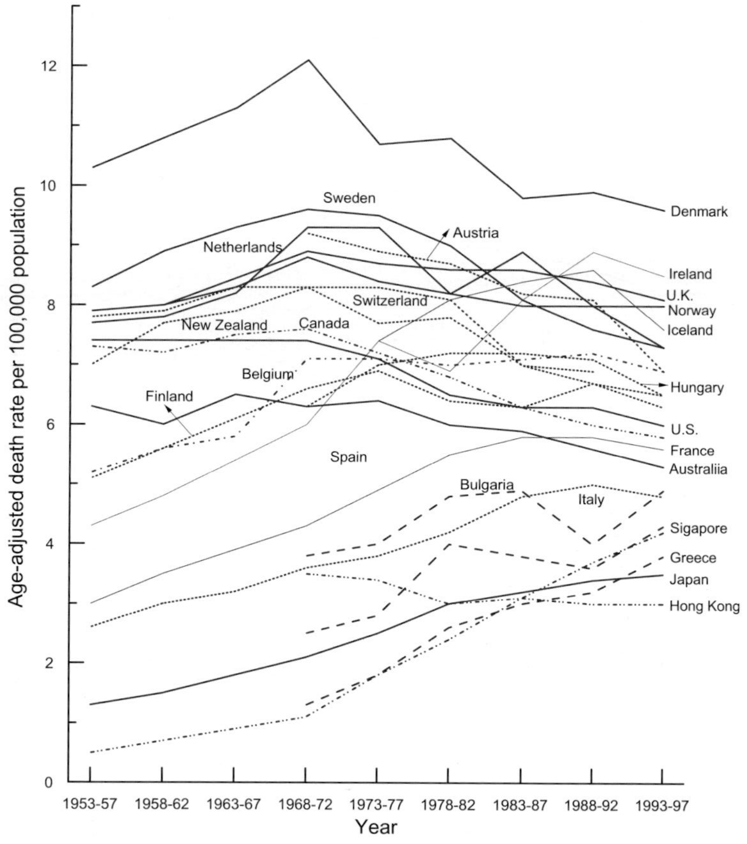

FIG. 2-15. Trends in age-adjusted death rates of malignant neoplasm of ovary and other uterine adnexa in 30 countries of the world (from 1953–57 to 1993–97)

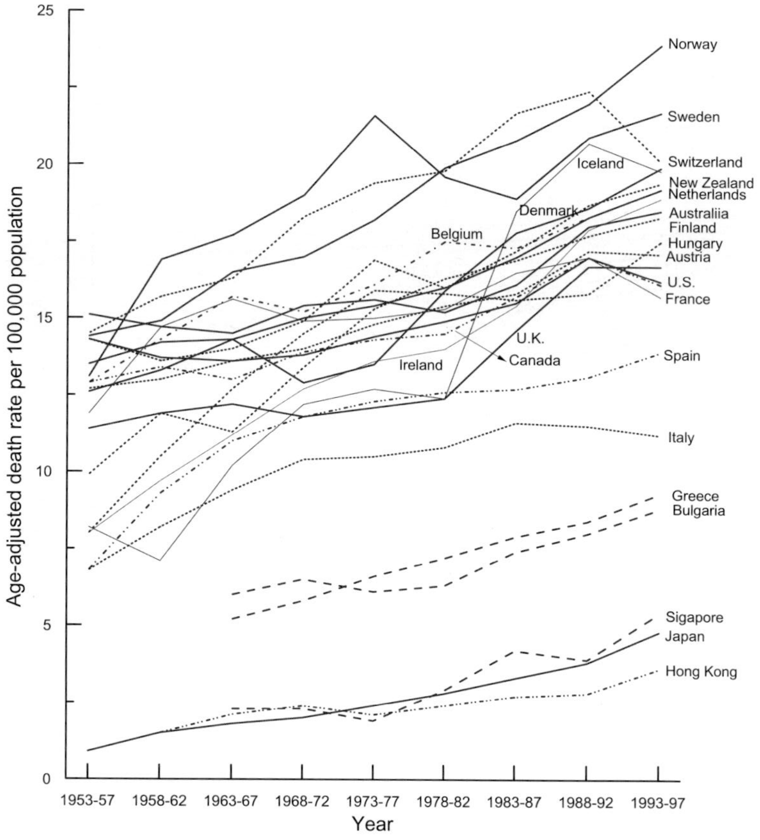

FIG. 2-16. Trends in age-adjusted death rates of malignant neoplasm of prostate in 30 countries of the world (from 1953–57 to 1993–97)

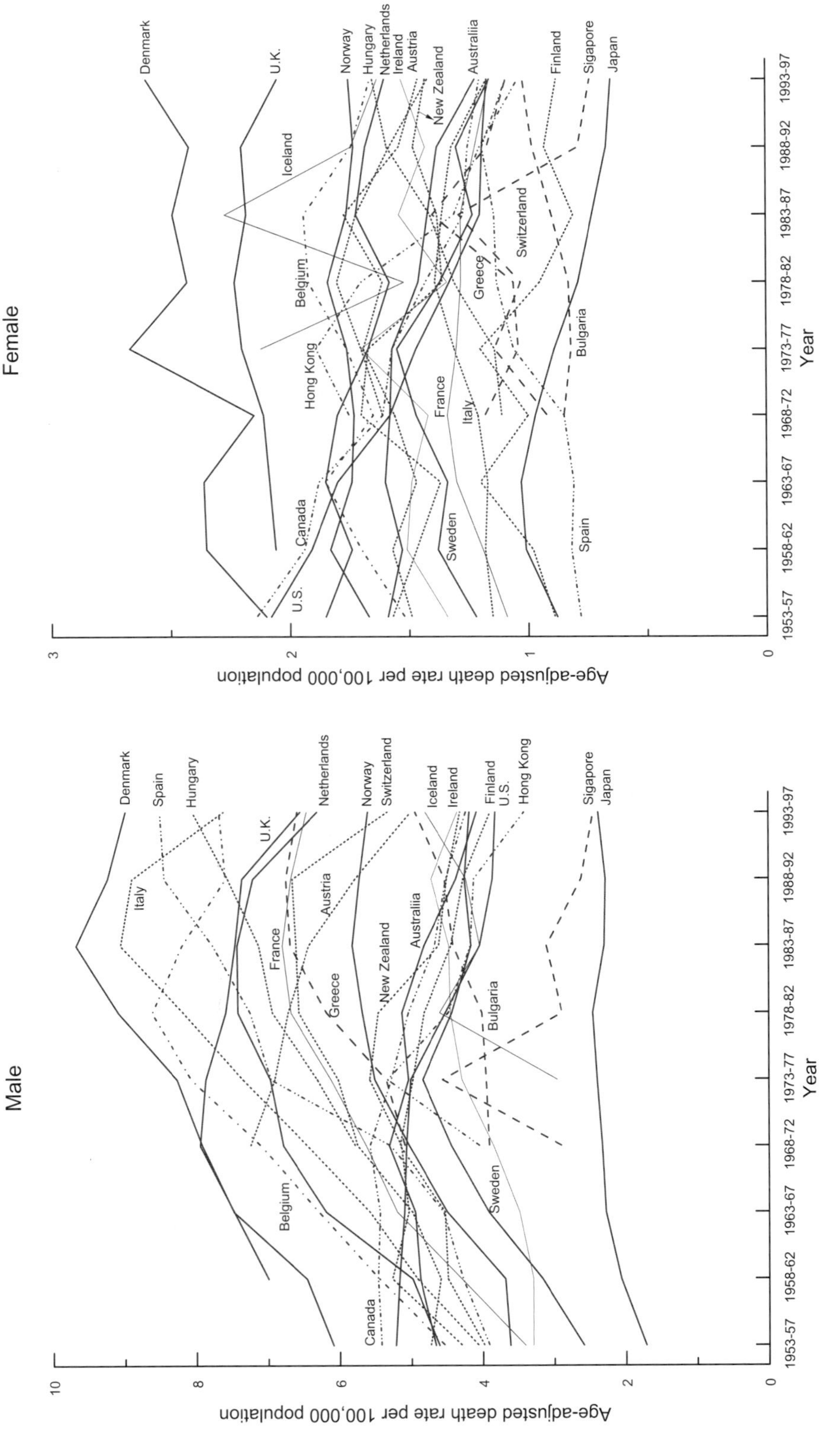

FIG. 2-17. Trends in age-adjusted death rates of malignant neoplasm of bladder in 30 countries of the world (from 1953–57 to 1993–97)

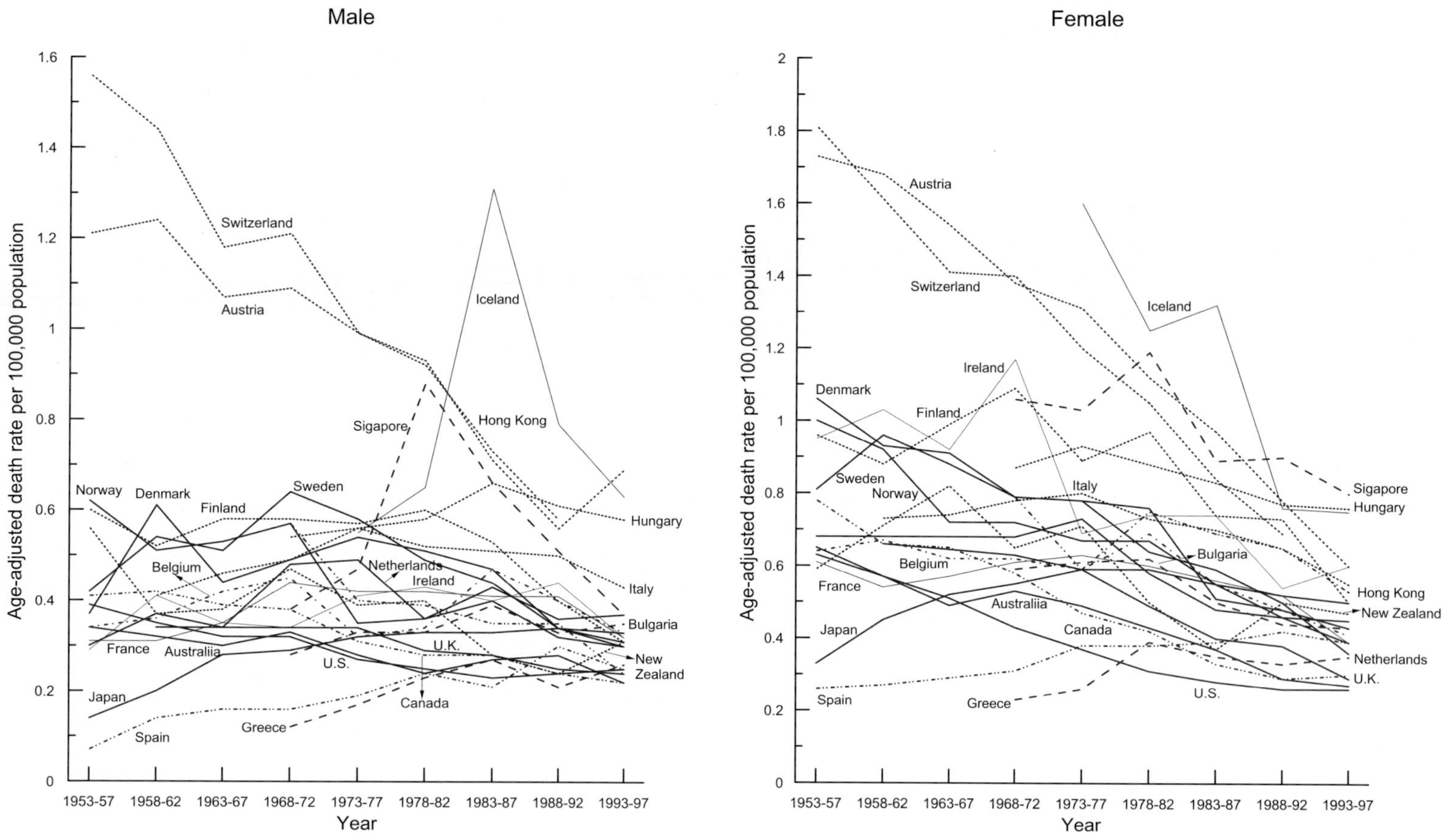

FIG. 2-18. Trends in age-adjusted death rates of malignant neoplasm of thyroid gland in 30 countries of the world (from 1953–57 to 1993–97)

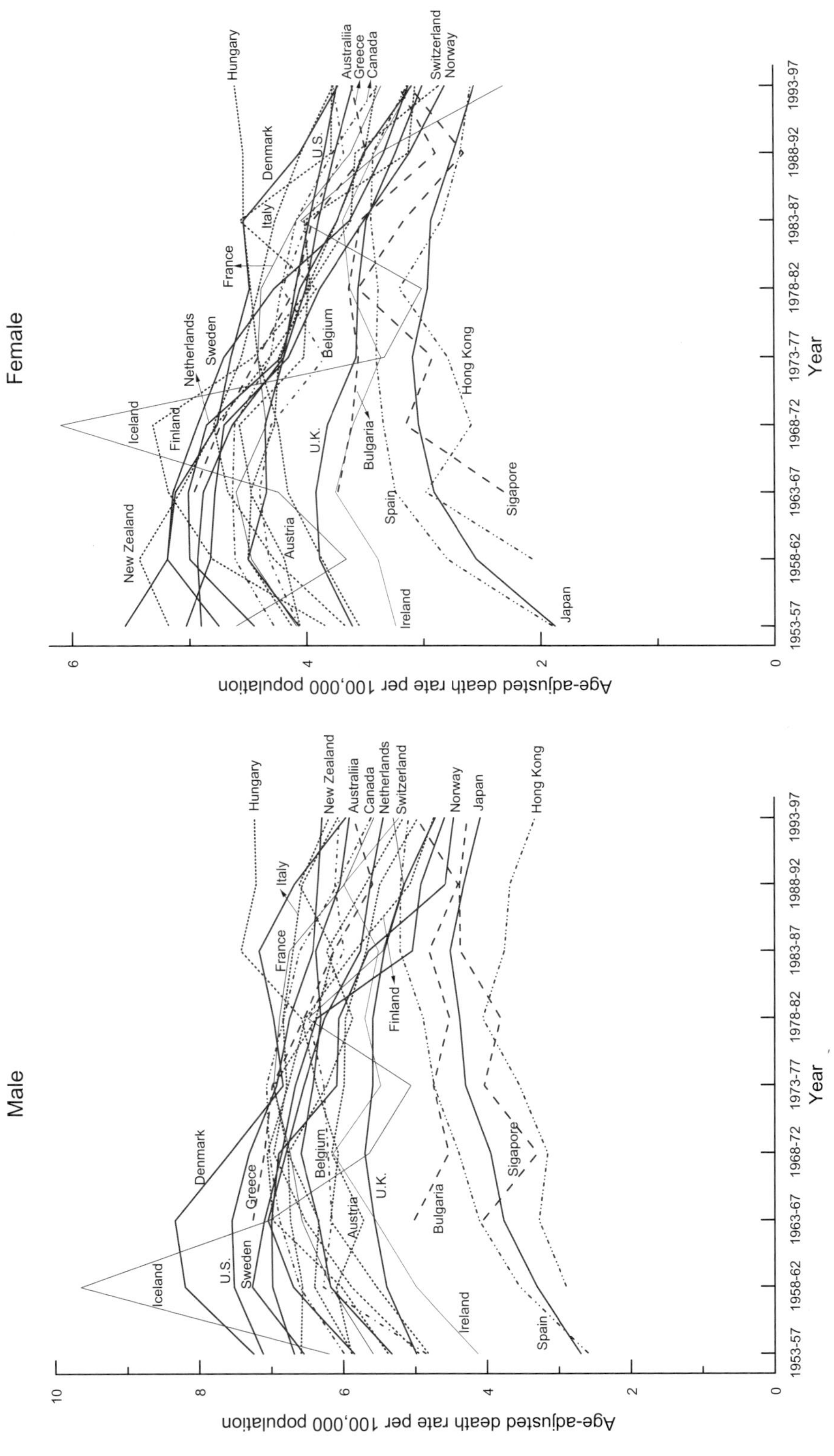

FIG. 2-19. Trends in age-adjusted death rates of leukemia in 30 countries of the world (from 1953–57 to 1993–97)